Neurological Disorders in Famous Artists – Part 2

Frontiers of Neurology and Neuroscience

Vol. 22

Series Editor

J. Bogousslavsky, Montreux

Neurological Disorders in Famous Artists – Part 2

Volume Editors

J. Bogousslavsky, Montreux
M.G. Hennerici, Mannheim

60 figures, 23 in color, and 6 tables, 2007

KARGER

Basel · Freiburg · Paris · London · New York ·
Bangalore · Bangkok · Singapore · Tokyo · Sydney

Julien Bogousslavsky, MD
Department of Neurology
Valmont Clinic
Genolier Swiss Medical
Network
CH–1823 Glion-sur-Montreux
(Switzerland)

Michael G. Hennerici, MD, PhD
Department of Neurology
University of Heidelberg
Universitätsklinikum Mannheim
Theodor Kutzer Ufer 1-3
DE–68135 Mannheim (Germany)

(As requested by the Library of Congress, CIP data for Part 1 (vol. 19) are printed).
Library of Congress Cataloging-in-Publication Data

Neurological disorders in famous artists / volume editors, J. Bogousslavsky,
F. Boller.
p. ; cm. – (Frontiers of neurology and neuroscience ; v. 19)
Includes bibliographical references and index.
ISBN 3-8055-7914-4 (hardcover : alk. paper)
1. Nervous system–Diseases. 2. Artists–Diseases
[DNLM: 1. Famous Persons–Case Reports. 2. Nervous System Diseases–Case
Reports.] I. Bogousslavsky, Julien. II. Boller, François. III. Series.
RC359.N46 2005
616.8–dc22
2005002444

Bibliographic Indices. This publication is listed in bibliographic services, including Current Contents® and Index Medicus.

www.karger.com
Printed in Switzerland on acid-free paper by Reinhardt Druck, Basel
ISSN 1660–4431
ISBN 978–3–8055–8265–0

Contents

VII **Preface**

1 **Painting after Right-Hemisphere Stroke – Case Studies of Professional Artists**
Bäzner, H.; Hennerici, M.G. (Mannheim)

14 **I and Me: Self-Portraiture in Brain Damage**
Blanke, O. (Lausanne/Geneva)

30 **Lovis Corinth: Integrating Hemineglect and Spatial Distortions**
Bäzner, H.; Hennerici, M.G. (Mannheim)

44 **Visconti and Fellini: From Left Social Neorealism to Right-Hemisphere Stroke**
Dieguez, S.; Assal, G. (Lausanne); Bogousslavsky, J. (Montreux)

75 **De novo Artistic Behaviour following Brain Injury**
Pollak, T.A.; Mulvenna, C.M.; Lythgoe, M.F. (London)

89 **Marcel Proust's Diseases and Doctors: The Neurological Story of a Life**
Bogousslavsky, J. (Montreux)

105 **Heinrich Heine and Syphilis**
auf der Horst, C. (Düsseldorf)

121 **Baudelaire's Aphasia: From Poetry to Cursing**
Dieguez, S. (Lausanne); Bogousslavsky, J. (Montreux)

150 **Memory and the Creation of Art: The Syndrome, as in de Kooning, of 'Creating in the Midst of Dementia'.**
An 'ArtScience' Study of Creation, Its 'Brain Methods' and Results
Espinel, C.H. (Washington, D.C.)

169 **Persisting Aphasia, Cerebral Dominance, and Painting in the Famous Artist Carl Fredrik Reuterswärd**
Colombo-Thuillard, F. (Fribourg); Assal, G. (Lausanne)

184 **Mozart in the Neurological Department – Who Has the Tic?**
Kammer, T. (Ulm)

193 **Hans von Bülow: Creativity and Neurological Disease in a Famous Pianist and Conductor**
Wöhrle, J.C. (Koblenz/Mannheim); Haas, F. (Karlsruhe)

206 **Synaesthesia, the Arts and Creativity: A Neurological Connection**
Mulvenna, C.M. (London)

223 **The Hallucinating Art of Heinrich Füssli**
Baumann, C.; Lentzsch, F.; Regard, M.; Bassetti, C. (Zürich)

236 **Author Index**

237 **Subject Index**

Preface

While artistic, literary, and musical creativity are perhaps the most fascinating of all human achievements, their basic brain counterparts remain poorly defined. It is likely that the brain participates as a whole in creativity, which can be defined as the ability to produce new and original works which stimulate interest or appeal esthetically. Creativity is a general feature of all humans, and everyone is indeed 'creative' on numerous occasions during his or her life. On the other hand, only a very limited number of individuals achieve what can be called 'extraordinary creativity', and which refers in particular to an ability to deconstruct established executive habits and tastes leading to truly novel productions, be it in science, art or other domains. When disease, especially brain disease, challenges the capabilities of one of these 'extraordinarily creative' individuals, the changes that consequently occur in their productions provide a unique opportunity to explore the mysteries of creativity, particularly in the artistic field.

Sometimes creativity is lost through disease and sometimes it is modified and occasionally, though more rarely, it may be enhanced or augmented. In the previous volume *Neurological Disorders in Famous Artists* edited by Dr. François Boller and one of the current editors, we presented a large series of famous painters, writers, poets, musicians, and philosophers who had developed some form of neurological dysfunction, and we focused on the influence of these pathologies on their work. We soon realized that several other artists whose style and output changed following a stroke, meningitis, or other cerebral disorder demanded a similar approach, since their personal lives and creative output were enormously modified by their disease.

Mozart, Baudelaire, de Kooning, Proust, Heine, von Bülow, Reuterswärd, Corinth, Füssli, Fellini, Visconti and others are all striking examples of how extraordinary creativity can be challenged and modified or destroyed or restored within the individual drama of disease. There are examples of de novo creativity following cerebral lesion, although we are not aware of any world-famous artist whose creativity first developed subsequent to brain damage. An alteration in the creativity of an artist can provide unique and fresh insights into the complex relationships between cerebral dysfunction and behavior. It may also be useful in better understanding the evolution of certain artists, particularly when the course of a disease corresponds with what is recognized as a new chapter in their work.

Julien Bogousslavsky
Michael G. Hennerici

Bogousslavsky J, Hennerici MG (eds): Neurological Disorders in Famous Artists – Part 2.
Front Neurol Neurosci. Basel, Karger, 2007, vol 22, pp 1–13

Painting after Right-Hemisphere Stroke – Case Studies of Professional Artists

H. Bäzner, M.G. Hennerici

Department of Neurology, University of Heidelberg, Universitätsklinikum Mannheim, Mannheim, Germany

Abstract

Changes in the style of professional artists as an immediate consequence of cerebrovascular disease are an intriguing phenomenon for the neuroscientist. While left-hemisphere damage is commonly provoking alterations in verbal production and comprehension, right-hemisphere stroke often leads to left-sided visuospatial neglect. We present a case series of 13 professional artists with right-hemisphere stroke and compare examples of their post-stroke artwork with their prestroke artwork.

Cerebrovascular disease and its related medical problems are very common. Brain lesions caused by stroke may result in devastating disability for the stroke victim. Through the continuously improving neurophysiological and neurosonological techniques and through the development of high-resolution neuroimaging technologies precise localization of lesions has become possible. Hence, pathophysiological mechanisms leading to stroke are better understood. Recent developments in neuropsychology have revealed certain regularities in the consequences of strokes depending on lesion extent and localization. Therefore, our knowledge is growing regarding the effects of stroke in the majority of patients. However, facing the specialized individual and highly developed skills of professional artists, and, moreover, lacking a reasonably large patient collective, only few authors have aimed at analyzing the consequences of stroke in professional visual artists systematically. On the other hand, some very interesting case reports have been produced, going back to the early 20th century. A seminal article including the cases of four German professional artists with right-hemisphere lesions has been published in 1974 by

Prof. Richard Jung, a clinical neurologist and researcher in neurophysiology, of Freiburg, Germany. In his paper he reported the cases of Anton Räderscheidt, Lovis Corinth, Otto Dix, and Johannes Thiel [Jung, 1974].

By reviewing the literature and by adding several additional cases, totaling a number of 13 professional visual artists, we will try to comment on common features of right-hemisphere damage with an emphasis on artistic production. We are well aware of the limitations of our effort, since the freedom of art rarely follows simplistic rules. Certainly artists and art historians will not always share the neurological point of view. Therefore we are obliged to interpret our observations with care.

(1) Anton Räderscheidt

Anton Räderscheidt (October 11, 1892 to March 8, 1970) started his artistic career in his birth town of Cologne. His portraits and figure paintings were shown in the famous 'Neue Sachlichkeit' exhibition in Mannheim in 1925. He was a protagonist of the 'Magischer Realismus' (magic realism), where persons and their surroundings were painted close to photographic art and the emotional content was reduced to a minimum as opposed to the contemporary expressionistic painters. His art being declared 'degenerate' by the Nazis, he emigrated from Germany in 1935, lived in Switzerland, England and France until 1949, when he returned to Cologne with his second wife, Gisèle. His artistic style changed after 1950, now inspired by abstract expressionism. On September 24, 1967, shortly before a large retrospective in Cologne, Räderscheidt suffered a stroke with severe visual disturbances and a mild left hemisyndrome. He had a homonymous hemianopsia to the left with a left-sided hemineglect, a disturbance of spatial orientation and an initially severe prosopagnosia. The problem of face recognition was so severe that he was unable to recognize even close relatives. This latter problem persisted over weeks [Jung, 1974; Herzog, 1991]. Beginning in December 1967 and continuing until June 1969, Räderscheidt painted an enormously large series of more than 60 self-portraits with the intention to compensate for the severe left-sided hemineglect. In Jung's 1974 paper, the improvement of his neglect was illustrated using five of these self-portraits. A set of four consecutive self-portraits [fig. 8b and 9a–c of Jung, 1974] were later repeatedly published [Gardner, 1977; Butter, 2004]. Räderscheidt is cited with the following remark concerning his stroke: 'Using all of my willpower, I intended to force my eyes to see correctly again.... A stroke has taken me away from the scene of life; offstage the play is going on with me. I am no longer the director of this play. I have to take care, not to miss my entrance in the play. My requisites obey to tricks only. Moreover, I am missing my loud colours.... The reproduction of my surroundings is a damned difficult thing. Nothing is staying in its place, nothing is keeping the shape. Perhaps I will be able to get hold of a

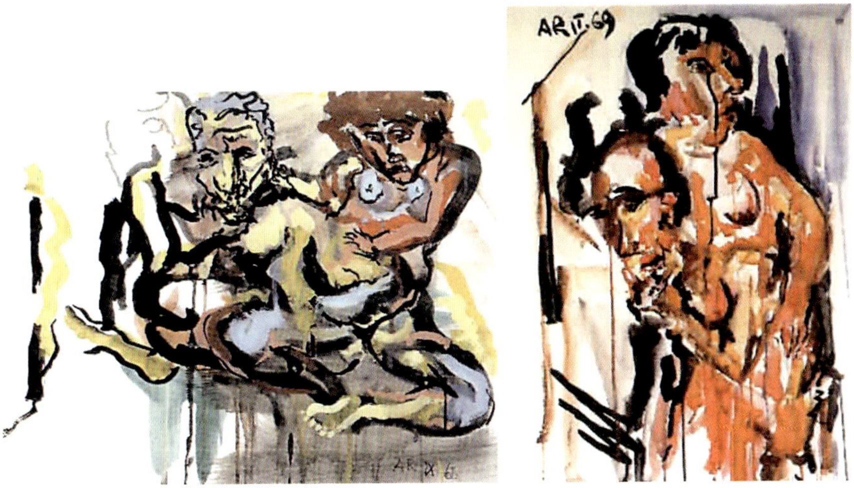

a *b*

***Fig. 1** **a**, **b**.* Anton Räderscheidt's poststroke paintings display ecstatic scenes, often depicting couples in close personal contact. Persons are grossly deformed, the artist using brighter colors and a larger variety of colors compared to his prestroke art. A moderate left-sided hemineglect can be noted (copyright VG Bild-Kunst, Bonn, 2007).

credible shape now if I can use this permanent motion.... In the past it felt like hunting [shape], now it feels more like catching a trout in moving water using bare hands.... Painting is like taming beasts of prey' [Richter, 1972; Herzog, 1991]. Neurological examination was not controlled until his death in March 1970; however, Jung assumes that his hemianopia was unchanged and that the painter learned to compensate for his neglect [Jung, 1974]. The change in artistic style in his late paintings displaying couples or nudes was discussed already by Jung who noticed a stronger affective relationship. Räderscheidt's son Pascal, who runs a remarkable web site (www.raederscheidt.com) presenting biographical data and a large collection of his father's artwork, says that his father referred to these paintings as 'Böse Bilder' (nasty paintings). These tempera paintings on cardboard, all in the same format, have been produced between June 1968 and August 1969. As to artistic expression, a total revolution occurred: compared to his earlier grouped figures and couples which lack any emotional content and avoid any personal contact, his poststroke paintings are overloaded with wild colorful brushstrokes, display ecstatic scenes, often depicting couples in close personal contact (fig. 1). Persons, who had previously been painted in a very realistic manner, are widely deformed, the artist uses brighter colors, and color variety is larger. His biographer Herzog [1991] describes the structure of the 'Böse Bilder' as 'acompository', and says, that the physiognomy of the figures is 'disfigured beyond recognition'. After June 1968, Räderscheidt's condition declined, although he still used to paint on every day. Again hospitalized between May and June 1969, his declining physical strength forced the painter to use smaller formats. Räderscheidt commented on his poststroke work in the last words of his diary as follows: 'After a 60 year long lasting fight with the material (form and colour), the material seems to have prevailed. My paintings become interesting to me, I start to enjoy them as a spectator' [Herzog, 1991].

(2) Otto Dix

Otto Dix (December 2, 1891 to July 25, 1969) was born in Untermdorf near Gera, studied in Düsseldorf and Dresden and became Professor of Arts of the Dresden Academy of Arts in 1927. He was well known in his early years for his naturalistic-veristic style, was painting large series of war scenes after being a soldier in the First World War. His portraits in the 1920s were often overcharacterized and displayed ugly human figures close to caricature. His paintings were classified as 'degenerate' and he was forced to leave the Academy of Arts in 1933. He moved to the Bodensee, where he stayed for more than 30 years until his death in 1969 [Schubert, 1980].

On November 13, 1967, Dix suffered a right-hemisphere stroke with left-sided hemiparesis, left hemineglect, partial hemianopia and mild spatioconstructive disturbances. Moreover, a reduced proprioception and apraxia of his left arm were noted by his treating neurologist, Prof. Baumgartner of Zürich. In the first 3 days following the stroke, Dix was unable to draw at all. On day 4 after the onset of symptoms, he was able to draw a simple and small sketch of a tree, with a unilateral shadowing giving the tree a plastic appearance. The left part of the paper was left free indicating his neglect. One week later, the neglect seemed widely compensated in a second sketch of a tree (both sketches are documented in Dix' patient chart in Zürich University Hospital and are reproduced by Jung [1974]). However, we cannot support Jung's view of an unchanged drawing style. His drawing was altered noticeably at least in his last self-portraits. The self-portrait with black collar (1968), small self-portrait (1968), self-portrait with a hand (1968) and self-portrait as a skull (1968) all share a missing resemblance with the painter. This is substantially different from the self-portraits Dix painted in 1957 (fig. 2b), 1964 (fig. 2c), and 1967 whose similitude is very close to the photographs showing Dix at the respective dates (fig. 2a). The self-portrait with black collar bears a certain resemblance to Dix, but spatial relations and facial structures are irritating, with his closed right eye seemingly protruded (fig. 2d). The painter's face appears to be supported on the left side of the portrait by a frame-like band seemingly preventing the painter's head from falling forward. The small self-portrait has much of a caricature (fig. 2e), and the self-portrait with a hand shows the painter's hand holding the

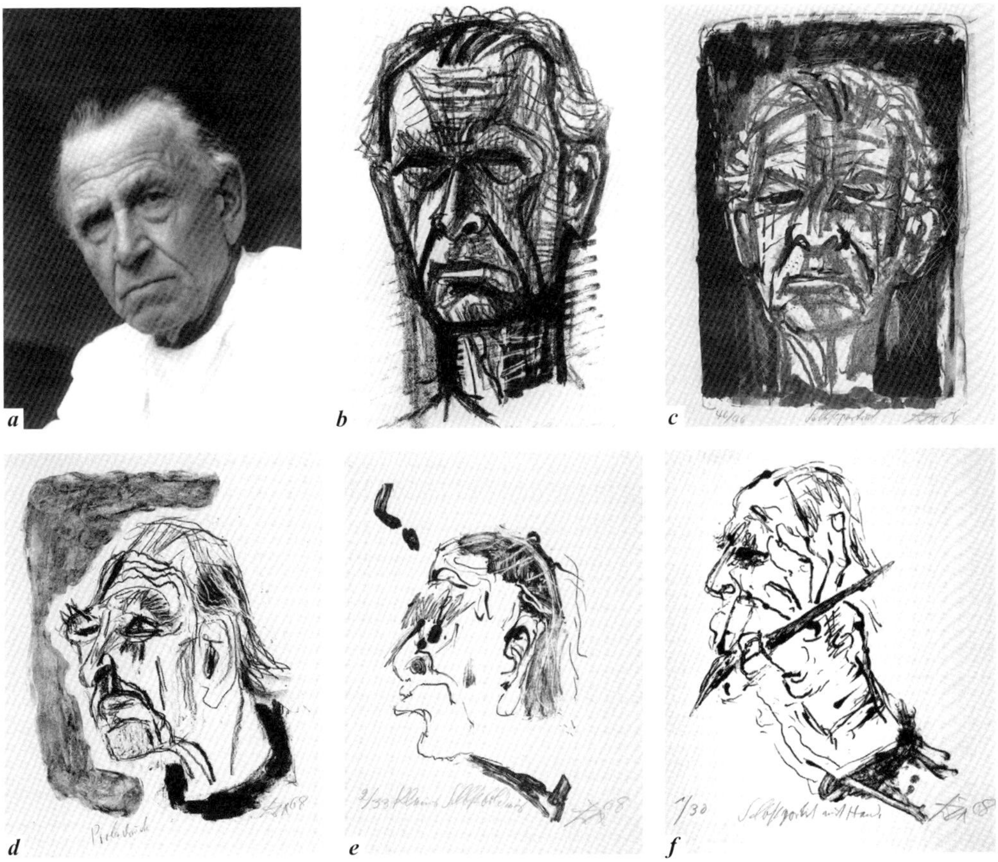

Fig. 2. 'Otto Dix' drawing style was altered noticeably in his last self-portraits. Self-portrait with black collar (1968, ***d***), small self-portrait (1968, ***e***), self-portrait with a hand (1968, ***f***) and self-portrait as a skull (1968, not shown) all share the absence of a resemblance to the painter. This is substantially different from the self-portraits Dix painted in 1957 (***b***), 1964 (***c***), and 1967 whose similitude is very close to the photographs showing Dix at the respective dates (***a***) (copyright VG Bild-Kunst, Bonn, 2007).

pencil in the forefront of the drawing covering most parts of the lower face (fig. 2f). On this right hand we count more than five fingers – the same observation can be made with certitude in his last large self-portrait with Marcella (1969), where Dix holds the little girl with both hands. On his right hand six fingers can be differentiated. Dix continued to paint until his death, working mostly on lithographs. He died of a second stroke on July 25, 1969 in Singen. Hans Kinkel, in his preface to Florian Karsch's catalogue of Dix' graphic art describes the painter's reaction to the stroke and the series of late self-portraits as an 'obsessingly urgent self-inquiry'. 'Lines became seismographic tracks; the structure was decomposed into flickering hieroglyphs. Outer appearance was replaced by inner similarity' [Kinkel, 1970].

(3) Johannes Thiel

Johannes Thiel (September 11, 1889 to July 31, 1962) travelled in Europe after studies at the Academies of Art in Munich and Stuttgart. He lived in Kirchzarten near Freiburg, producing landscape and figure paintings and book illustrations. His best artwork, according to Jung [1974], was his water color landscapes, where Thiel reached perfection in his 6th and 7th decade of life. He suffered two strokes with left-sided hemiparesis in 1959 (facial paresis on the left and mild weakness of the left hand with complete recovery) and 1960 (with a permanent left hand weakness) but recovered fairly well and was enormously productive until a third stroke in 1962 set an end to his life. Except for a portrait sketch done in the days following his first stroke, Jung is unable to notice any change in style or signs of neglect. Jung examined Thiel after his third and subsequently fatal stroke and described a left-sided hemiplegia and hemianopia.

(4) Lovis Corinth

Lovis Corinth (July 21, 1858 to July 17, 1925), who certainly had the most interesting patient history of this case series, is the subject of a separate chapter by Bäzner and Hennerici (pp. 30–43).

(5) Wolfgang Aichinger-Kassek

Wolfgang Aichinger-Kassek is an Austrian artist who suffered a right-hemisphere stroke on the basis of arterioarterial embolism from a severe carotid stenosis in 1995 [Aichinger-Kassek, 1997]. When he recovered slowly from his stroke he noticed that he was unable to continue working on his sculptures which he had constructed using heavy materials, cut from metal-welded iron. As a reaction to this drawback, he produced a series of 'neurological folios' comprising 30 colored graphics (fig. 3). His daughter, a consultant in neurology, writes in the preface to this collection: 'As soon as the acute stage of the apoplectic fit was over, it gave way to thoughts about the how of his future artistic career. They all ended in the question whether creative activity would still be possible. For many long months, the phases of depression and despair seemed to hold the upper hand. The paralysis of thought and inspiration outweighed all other problems. The artist's dependency on his ideas obliged [him] to assume the role of waiting in uncertainty of his fate. But then, from one day to the next, feelings and inspirations forced their way to the surface. It became possible to represent pictorially the phases of depression, fear, of incursions into his own body, the hospital

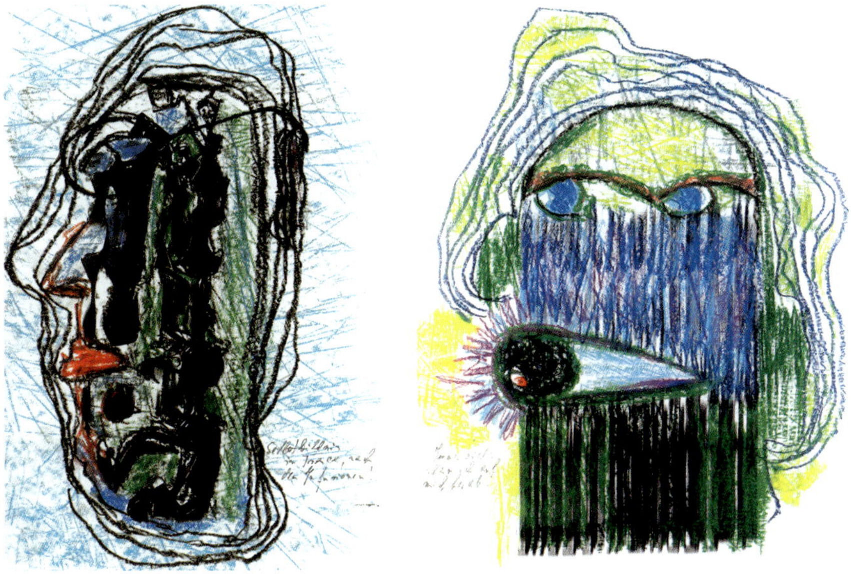

a *b*

Fig. 3** **a, b. Wolfgang Aichinger-Kassek, an Austrian artist suffered a right-hemisphere stroke in 1995. As a reaction, he produced a series of 'neurological folios'. According to the artist's daughter, they represent 'pictorially the phases of depression, fear, of incursions into his own body, the hospital environment' (private collection).

environment. Most of the works in this cycle were created within a few days. The person W.A. now sees prospects for his future once again.' Aichinger-Kassek himself comments on his stroke as follows: 'Apoplexy – that's a stroke of lightning in life's thunderstorm! It attacks you! And fells you like a blossoming tree. The stroke is the insidiousness of an unexpected menace. It's danger and warning. The stroken [sic!] one is defeated by a depressive attack while his life is passing before his eyes like a trashy movie. Apoplexy – that's also a determination of life-positions consisting in bygone past and uncertain future. At all, uncertainty is a serious component of insidiousness.'

(6) Federico Fellini

The case of the famous Italian movie director and skilled painter and cartoonist Federico Fellini (1920–1993) was reported extensively in 1998 [Cantagallo and Della Sala, 1998; Chatterjee, 2004]. The authors followed the artist for 2 months after a CT-documented right temporoparietal ischemic stroke leaving the artist with a severe sensorimotor hemisyndrome and left inferior quadrantanopia. Fellini was examined in detail for his left visuomotor hemineglect syndrome, including neglect dyslexia as well as some evidence of implicit processing of the neglected parts of the stimuli. The artist was aware of his motor and attentional deficits; however, he was unable to functionally compensate for them. The documents of visuomotor neuropsychological testing are reproduced in the paper and demonstrate besides the pure neuropsychological deficit a remarkable introspective analysis of the artist's own situation including some quite ironical and sometimes provocative though charming personalized performances. Federico Fellini is presented in detail in the chapter by Dieguez et al., pp. 44–74.

(7) Reynold Brown

Reynold Brown (1917–1991) got his first art education in the Alhambra High School in California. The following information was obtained through the web site designed and maintained by his son Franz (www.geocities.com/chapulinas). He illustrated and drew a comic strip, did illustrations for service manuals, several magazines and pocket books. In the 1950s Brown decided to go back to free-lance illustration, and took a teaching position at the Art Center College of Design. There, he would teach figure and head drawing for 26 years. At that time, he started a series of movie posters for the large movie companies and of record jacket covers. From the 1970s on Brown concentrated on fine arts painting with western themes as his preferred subject, where he succeeded and sold about 250 oil paintings including portraits, harbor scenes and landscapes.

In 1976, Brown suffered a severe stroke together with a myocardial infarction leaving him with a severe left-sided hemiparesis and hemineglect syndrome. Compared to his colleagues suffering from right-hemisphere damage, Brown was hit by the stroke in a even more devastating manner, since the paralyzed left arm was his 'drawing arm', and his doctors' prognoses as to future artistic work were pessimistic. His doctors were wrong: similar to Corinth and his wife Charlotte, Brown was helped to retrain his physical abilities and during his first steps back into arts by his wife Mary Louise, who was an artist as well. She was working with him day by day, so that he first started to draw and then to paint again. Emphasis was put on the effort to teach the 'good' right arm. Brown had to battle further a very dense left lower quadrantanopia; he would tend to leave the lower left portion of the canvas unpainted, started each painting session from the right side of a painting which resulted in canvasses heavily worked on to the right and thinly painted on the left. His portraits were disorganized with a marked distortion of facial structures, similar to Corinth's and Räderscheidt's (self-)portraits. Franz Brown comments on a stretching effect present from the upper right to the lower left, which decreased with time. The same effect can be seen in several of Corinth's portraits and self-portraits and in the series of Räderscheidt's self-portraits. A further source of frustration was the limited use of his previously dominant left hand, due to a severe reduction of

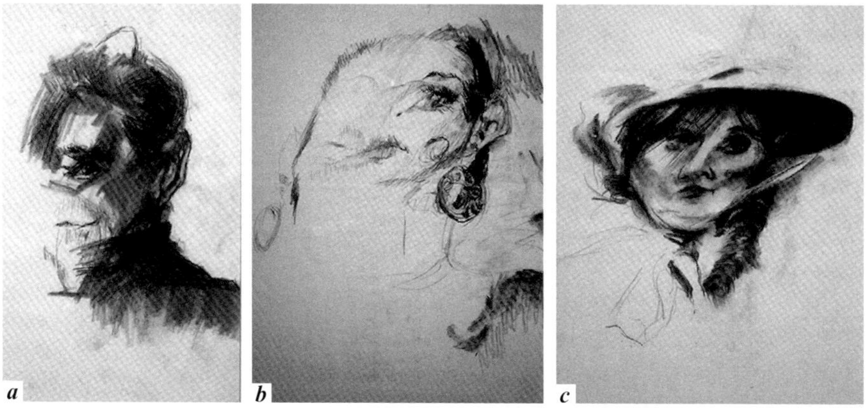

Fig. 4 a–c. Reynold Brown's drawings and paintings produced in the period after his right-hemisphere stroke resemble strikingly the early poststroke artwork by Lovis Corinth and Anton Räderscheidt. His drawings show a severe left-sided hemineglect, which is improving throughout the following years (reproduced with permission of the Tejeda-Brown family).

his tactile sense. In summary, according to his son, he was subsequently unable to do the highly representational work of his prestroke years, but 'was nonetheless able to produce some powerful drawings and beautiful landscape paintings of Nebraska, where he settled in 1983 and remained until his death in 1991. Franz Brown states that his portraits 'for some... carry a greater emotional impact than the more realistic work of his earlier years. His landscapes became looser and more painterly' and he 'seemed to see the world on different, more intense colours'.

In a striking similarity to the early poststroke artwork by Lovis Corinth, Brown's poststroke drawings show a severe left-sided hemineglect, which is improving through the following years but never perfectly resolved as far as can be told (fig. 4).

(8) Tom Greenshields

Tom Greenshields (1915–1994), an accomplished and well-known painter and sculptor, was 75 years old, when he had a right-hemisphere stroke in August 1989 [Halligan and Marshall, 1997]. His symptoms included a mild sensorimotor hemisyndrome on the left side, left lower quadrantanopia and left visual neglect. Already 8 years earlier, he had lost the use of his right painting arm in an accident. Therefore, he had learned to transfer his artistic skills to the left hand and continued to work as a painter and sculptor and to sell and exhibit his artwork. After his stroke, despite good physical recovery of his left arm and hand function, he became frustrated facing poorly constructed and less elaborate drawings compared to prestroke creations. He concentrated on the right side of his drawings and sculptures and neglected the left parts. Moreover, his artwork showed distorted, exaggerated or deformed figures. On neuropsychological examination, visuospatial neglect was confirmed. Similar to Reynold Brown, he would ignore food on the left side of the plate. A photograph of a sculpture in the paper of Halligan and Marshall (fig. 1, bottom) shows a clay sculpture with intact facial proportions on the right side of the face and very incomplete modeling of the left parts of the face. Similar disturbances can be noticed in figure 2, a drawing of a sitting man with a missing left face, left shoulder and left parts of the chair. According to Halligan and Marshall, residual traces of neglect were still discernible until the death of the artist in 1994. This is the only case of a sculptor with a severe neglect described so far who reflected the difficulty of the right-hemisphere-damaged individual to detect and depict the third dimension.

(9) Unnamed Swiss Artist

Schnider et al. [1993] described the case of an unnamed Swiss artist who suffered a CT-documented large ischemic infarct in the right temporoparieto-occipital region. Poststroke drawings differed markedly from prestroke ones with changes reflecting both behavioral and mood disturbances. Their artist exhibited hemispatial neglect, hallucinations, hyperverbalization (he would include much text in his early poststroke sketches), and a rapid cycling bipolar disorder. His drawings became simplified, more sketch-like, although the technical characteristics seemed similar to the premorbid artwork. Remarkably, the severity of neglect expressed in his drawings was highly variable and might change within hours.

(10) Artist with Right-Hemisphere Stroke

Vigouroux et al. [1990] published the case of an artist with right-hemisphere stroke. This unnamed 'well-known French painter' exhibiting a large variety of stroke risk factors presented with a severe left-sided sensorimotor hemisyndrome including a severe homonymous hemianopia to the left. Shortly after the stroke he experienced a severe depressive episode, apparently reflected in his drawings, which, according to the authors were of minor quality at that point although particularly expressive at the same time. This period was followed by a phase of rich pictorial production. Remarkably, these drawings and paintings showed no alteration of figural shape or volume, no change in style and unchanged artistic topics compared to the premorbid period but a variably severe hemineglect.

(11) 71-Year-Old Artist with Mild Left Neglect

Recently, Blanke et al. [2003] published the case of a 71-year-old artist with mild left neglect as the consequence of a right parietal hemorrhage. Drawings showed evidence of neglect to the left. Within these drawings, she used color minimally on the left whereas she colored the right side completely and evenly. Hence, she was able to produce the correct forms of images in the left visual hemifield but not the colors.

(12) Guglielmo Lusignoli

Guglielmo Lusignoli (born in 1920) was hit by a right-hemisphere stroke in 1987 at the zenith of his creativity and artistic production [Mazzucchi et al., 1994]. He suffered from hemineglect and left-sided paresis; however, he resumed his work and was enormously productive after the stroke.

(13) Kurt Schwitters

As far as can be told from his biography [Orchard et al., 1998], the famous German Dada artist Kurt Schwitters (1887–1948) suffered a right-hemisphere stroke in 1944 with a subsequent paresis of his left arm. A second stroke (presumably a hemorrhage) occurred in February 1946. In December 1945 he writes: 'I am [now] painting smaller formats and do some very small modelling, pocket format. My sculptures are a new experience for me; they are my best works now' [Orchard et al., 1998]. Further evidence for any alterations in artistic expression is scarce.

Conclusions

This series of 13 visual arts professionals with right-hemisphere stroke illustrates the consequences of stroke for their artistic creation. The painters reported had a mean age of 66 years at stroke onset and survived their first stroke for more than 6 years.

(1) Not surprisingly, the immediate reaction to the devastating and unexpected stroke 'attack' is very often a period of depression and despair. A stroke may lead to sometimes very severe episodes of depression and even to suicide attempts. Valuable introspective comments on their disease can be found in the reports of Lovis Corinth [Bäzner and Hennerici, pp. 30–43] and Wolfgang Aichinger-Kassek [1996].

(2) The stroke influences the painting in the vast majority of artists to a relevant degree. Whereas in some cases the stroke ended the artistic career (Fellini) [Dieguez et al., pp. 44–74], the majority of the painters reported resumed artistic production although they had to overcome various degrees of disability.

(3) Reynold Brown, a previously left-handed artist, suffered a right-hemisphere stroke and had to learn to use his previously nondominant right hand. His artwork was further altered by severe visual disturbances.

(4) Visuospatial neglect is common in right-hemisphere stroke. Noticeable degrees of neglect can be deferred from the poststroke artwork of virtually all of the right-hemisphere patient-artists. This severe problem for the visual artist is often compensated in paintings of the wider scenery of landscapes and large figural compositions, but is commonly detectable in self-portraits due to the necessity of strong fixation in the center of the visual field.

(5) The finding of facial distortion in at least 6 of the right-hemisphere patients hints at the representation of both facial recognition and spatial organization in the right hemisphere. Also the striking loss of self-resemblance in the self-portraits of Corinth, Dix, and Räderscheidt points to a certain degree of prosopagnosia in these right-hemisphere stroke victims.

(6) Spatial organization is disturbed in several of the right-hemisphere painters with disturbances of perspective or of third dimension in sculptural creation. In the poststroke artwork by Corinth, Räderscheidt, Dix, Greenshields and Brown, anatomical exactitude is altered, details are misplaced.

(7) Hallucinatory episodes, delusions, and dream-like optical sensations can be found in the case histories of several of the right-hemisphere stroke painters such as Räderscheidt, Corinth, Aichinger-Kassek, and Schnider's case.

References

Aichinger-Kassek W: Neurological Folios. Kranj, Gorenjski Tisk, 1997.

Blanke O, Ortigue S, Landis T: Colour neglect in an artist. Lancet 2003;361:264.

Butter CM: Anton Raederscheidt's distorted self-portraits and their significance for understanding balance in art. J Hist Neurosci 2004;13:66–78.

Cantagallo A, Della Sala S: Preserved insight in an artist with extrapersonal spatial neglect. Cortex 1998;34:163–189.

Chatterjee A: The neuropsychology of visual artistic production. Neuropsychologia 2004;42: 1568–1583.

Gardner H: The pathology of art; in The Shattered Mind. London, Routledge & Kegan Paul, 1977, pp 291–349.

Halligan PW, Marshall JC: The art of visual neglect. Lancet 1997;350:139–140.

Herzog G: Anton Räderscheidt. Cologne, DuMont, 1991.

Jung R: Neuropsychologie und Neurophysiologie des Kontur- und Formsehens in Zeichnung und Malerei; in Wieck HH (ed): Psychopathologie musischer Gestaltungen. Stuttgart, Schattauer, 1974, pp 29–88.

Kinkel H: Einleitung; in Karsch F (ed): Otto Dix, Das graphische Werk. Hannover, Fackelträger, 1970.

Mazzucchi A, Pesci G, Trento D: Cervello e pittura: Effetti delle lesioni cerebrali sul linguaggio pittorico. Rome, Fratelli Palombi, 1994.

Orchard K, Schulz I, Brogden J: Kurt Schwitters: Werke und Dokumente. Verzeichnis der Bestände im Sprengel Museum Hannover. Hannover, Sprengel Museum, 1998.

Richter H: Anton Räderscheidt. Recklinghausen, Bongers, 1972.

Schnider A, Regard M, Benson DF, Landis T: Effects of a right hemisphere stroke on an artist's performance. Neuropsychiatry Neuropsychol Behav Neurol 1993;6:249–255.
Schubert D: Otto Dix. Reinbek, Rowohlt, 1980.
Vigouroux RA, Bonnefoi B, Khalil R: Réalisations picturales chez un artiste peintre présentant une héminégligence gauche. Rev Neurol (Paris) 1990;146:665–670.

Hansjörg Bäzner, MD, PhD
Department of Neurology, University of Heidelberg
Universitätsklinikum Mannheim, Theodor Kutzer Ufer 1-3
DE–68135 Mannheim (Germany)
Tel. +49 621 383 3555, Fax +49 621 383 3807, E-Mail baezner@neuro.ma.uni-heidelberg.de

Bogousslavsky J, Hennerici MG (eds): Neurological Disorders in Famous Artists – Part 2.
Front Neurol Neurosci. Basel, Karger, 2007, vol 22, pp 14–29

I and Me: Self-Portraiture in Brain Damage

Olaf Blanke

Laboratory of Cognitive Neuroscience, Brain Mind Institute, Ecole Polytechnique Fédérale de Lausanne (EPFL), Lausanne, and Department of Neurology, University Hospital, Geneva, Switzerland

Abstract

Human bodily experience is characterized by the immediate feeling that our body is localized at a certain position in space and that the self is localized within these body borders (embodiment). Recent research from cognitive neuroscience and neurology suggests that embodiment is of major importance for neuroscientific models of self and self-consciousness. This is suggested by illusory own body perceptions (such as autoscopic hallucinations, heautoscopy, and out-of-body experiences) during which the self may be experienced as being localized outside one's body borders. I have previously argued that self-portraiture may rely on similar brain mechanisms and have proposed a classification of self-portraiture based on neurological classifications of illusory own body perceptions. Here I extend this model focussing on three types of self-portraits: visual self-portraits, disembodied self-portraits, and corporeal self-portraits. This is followed by a discussion of visuospatial, linguistic, and mnestic mechanisms in self-portraiture that are examined in selected painters.

For my part, when I enter most intimately into what I call myself, I always tumble, on some particular perception or other, of heat or cold, light or shade, love or hatred, pain or pleasure. I can never catch myself at any time without a perception, and never can observe anything but the perception.

David Hume

Self in Philosophy, Neurology, and Neuroscience

In the above statement Hume claimed that when he introspected, he was unable to catch his self without a perception and was unable to observe 'anything but the perception' itself. He concluded that the self (or the observing introspective subject) is nothing but a bundle or collection of different perceptions. The struggle of Western philosophy with the body was also exemplified in Descartes' effort to separate mind and body. Today there is a renewal of scientific interest in how bodies think, how conscious thought is embodied in the body as subject. Most discussions of embodiment draw on Maurice Merleau-Ponty's philosophy in *Phenomenology of Perception*, who was fascinated by our 'being-in-the-world' and the way our consciousness is incarnated in the world. For Merleau-Ponty and later Gibson and Neisser [1988] cognition is embodied and functions as part of the unity between subjects and objects that is the direct result of having a body. Recent years have seen increasing research in philosophy and cognitive science on embodiment and how the human mind and consciousness is ultimately linked to own body perception in the brain [Bermudez et al., 1995].

This has led to the development of neurocognitive theories on embodiment and own body perception and its relevance for the self and self-consciousness. This research investigated own body recognition of body parts (arm, face) or own action recognition [for review see Blanke and Mohr, 2005]. These studies focussed on how certain body parts and actions of humans are embodied or recognized as belonging to the self and how they are distinguished from those of other humans. A different line of research has investigated mechanisms of embodiment for the entire body and these seem especially relevant for self processing, self consciousness, and self-portraiture [Blanke, 2005]. For this a well-defined group of own body illusions in neurological patients that are characterized by different levels of embodiment have been investigated [Brugger, 2002; Blanke et al., 2004; Blanke and Mohr, 2005]. I have previously suggested that phenomenological and neurocognitive characteristics of these own body illusions can also be found in the pictorial phenomenology of self-portraits [Blanke, 2005].

Own body illusions are reduplicative experiences during which the subject has the impression of seeing a double in extrapersonal space either from an embodied or disembodied visuospatial perspective. They include out-of-body experience, autoscopic hallucination, and heautoscopy. In an out-of-body experience, subjects feel that their 'self' is located outside the physical body and somewhat elevated. It is from this elevated extrapersonal location that subjects experience seeing their body and the world. An autoscopic hallucination is defined as the experience of seeing a double of oneself in extrapersonal space without leaving one's body (no disembodiment). As compared to out-of-body experiences, individuals with autoscopic hallucination experience seeing the world from their habitual visuospatial perspective and experience their 'self' as embodied. During heautoscopy subjects also have the experience of seeing a double in extrapersonal space (as in autoscopic hallucination). However, it is difficult for the subject to decide whether he is disembodied or not and whether the self is localized within the physical body or in the double.

I have previously suggested that some of the phenomenological and neurocognitive characteristics of these own body illusions can be found in the pictorial phenomenology of self-portraits [Blanke, 2005]. I proposed to describe self-portraits as reduplicative phenomena since self-portraits contain the painter twice: as the painting painter and the painted painter [Bonafoux, 2004; Pächt, 1991]. This comparative analysis revealed that some of the neurocognitive mechanisms of own body illusions might also be employed by artists of self-portraits and beholders of such paintings. Based on this analysis a division of the genre of self-portraiture in three major types of self-portraits was proposed that reflects the characteristics of autoscopic hallucination (*visual self-portraits*), out-of-body experience (*disembodied self-portraits*), and heautoscopy (*corporeal self-portraits*). This is reviewed below and followed by neurological and neuropsychological findings in self-portraits of painters with neglect, aphasia and dementia.

Embodiment and Disembodiment Self-Portraiture

Jung [1974] remarked that '[a]n influence of brain damage... can especially be seen in... self-portraits'. This seems to be the case because of the more constant situation between painter and painted object in self-portraiture as compared to other genres and the possibility to analyze chronic effects [Blanke, 2005; Crutch et al., 2001]. The cognitive neurologist and neuroscientist – interested in painting – prefers to analyze painting situations as in self-portraiture that are rather stable with respect to its thematic and spatial content, thus relying on a specific subset of visuospatial and perceptual mechanisms. Other differences need to be mentioned. Whereas artists generally paint portraits of other people (objects and scenes) by direct inspection, the painter of a self-portrait cannot inspect himself (or can at least not inspect his entire body and his face) directly only with his eyes (but see the work of the American artist Tim Hawkinson). To paint their self-portraits painters throughout time have often relied on mirrors as well as mental imagery pointing to the possibility of functional differences between portraits of other people and portraits of oneself. To reiterate, self-portraits contain the body and self that interest the cognitive neuroscientist twice: as the painted painter and as the painting painter.

From Embodiment in the Self-Portraits of Rembrandt to Disembodiment in Velazquez and Schiele

Albrecht Dürer (1471–1528) is generally thought of as the first artist to have drawn a series of self-portraits for himself as well as the public: Bell [2000]

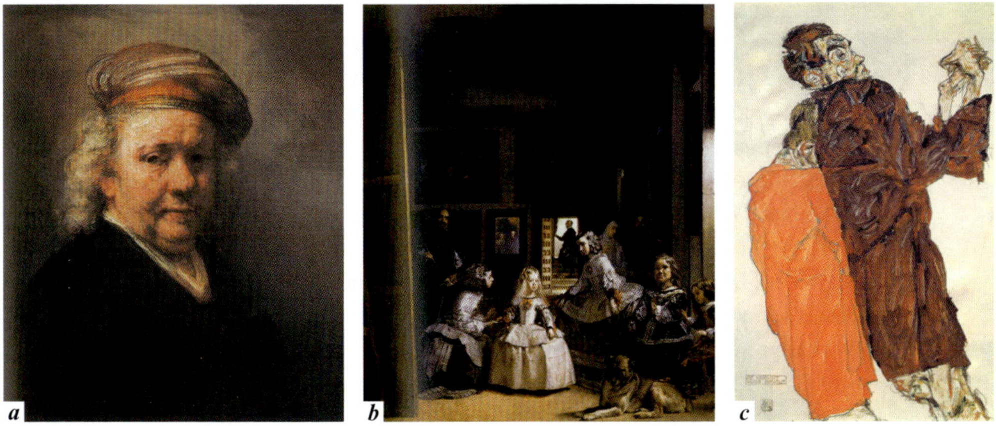

Fig. 1. Visual, disembodied and corporeal self-portraits. A visual self-portrait by Rembrandt focusing on the visual aspects of his face depicted from a short distance (***a***) and a disembodied self-portrait by Velazquez focusing on the spatial scene and the painter's entire body that is several meters away (***b***). A corporeal double self-portrait by Egon Schiele (***c***) reduplicates explicitly the painter's painted body (***c*** courtesy Wolfgang Werner KG, Bremen).

speaks of 'Dürer's pictorial discovery of the modern self'. Dürer's self portraits may be called visual self-portraits as they reflect visual mechanisms that can also be found in autoscopic hallucinations [Blanke, 2005]. They are the most frequent self-portraits and the painter draws himself as if he were seeing himself in the mirror (as if he were somebody else). Nothing in Rembrandt's *Self-Portrait* from Glasgow (1632; fig. 1a) could tell the beholder that the artist has drawn a picture of himself. Frequent instances of right-left reversals in visual self-portraits reveal not only the painter's concentration on his mirror reflection, but also highlight that the reflected person is seen as another person, as an image, disconnected from the painter. These visual characteristics appear in most of Rembrandt's self-portraits [Blanke, 2005] and in the majority of self-portraits shown in Bell [2000].

There is group of 'nonvisual' self-portraits that are less frequent and characterized by a distanced (third person) visuospatial perspective and disembodiment and might reflect mechanisms of out-of-body experiences (disembodied self-portraits). A famous example is *Las Meninas* (1656, Madrid; fig. 1b) by Velazquez (1599–1660). Many other examples are 'the artist in his studio' paintings and the great number of disembodied self-portraits of Caspar David Friedrich [Blanke, 2005]. In *Las Meninas* Velazquez paints himself as painting and as standing in front of a large canvas. By inverting the classical visuospatial perspective and thus imagining seeing the entire scene from the position and visuospatial perspective of the King and Queen, Velazquez turns the portrait of the emperors and their daughter into a portrait of himself.[1] The disembodied painter imagines or looks at his own body and person from a third-person perspective, notably of the King and Queen [see Blanke, 2005].

Next to visual and disembodied self-portraits, corporeal self-portraits (reflecting mechanisms of heautoscopy) directly depict the reduplicated body of the artist and may in explicit instances depict the painter twice or even more often. Any self-portrait may arouse the question in the beholder whether the location of the painter's self is on the canvas (and thus painted) or in front of the canvas (and thus painting) [Blanke, 2005]. Nevertheless, this is most explicitly expressed in corporeal self-portraits. Egon Schiele frequently drew doubles of himself or the painter on the same canvas, in similar body postures, and often as staring at the beholder [Schröder, 1999]. In a particularly striking example (*The Truth Unveiled*; 1913, private collection; fig. 1c), Schiele drew his double (in orange) that is shown as coming out of (or is entering) his own body's back (brown) stressing the physical connection between both bodies. It is impossible to say which body belongs to Egon Schiele and where the painter's (embodied) self is localized. This can be seen in other double self-portraits by Schiele and those of other painters [Blanke, 2005].

These observations suggest one way of linking self-portraiture with the field of cognitive neuroscience. I argued that neurocognitive mechanisms of three own body illusions [Brugger, 2002; Blanke and Mohr, 2005] may be relevant for analyzing and understanding the cognitive mechanisms involved in self-portraiture. While painting a self-portrait the artist is in a similar mental situation as neurological patients experiencing autoscopic hallucination, out-of-body experience, or heautoscopy.[2] Whereas the painter may voluntarily depict himself using visual, disembodiment-related, or corporeal brain mechanisms,

[1]I should also briefly mention Velazquez' masterly play with the mirror at the back of the painting where a reflection of the King and Queen of Spain can be seen who he should actually be in the process of portraying [Blanke, 2005]. The result is a portrait of the young princess Margarita who is shown in the center of the painting. Velazquez masterly plays and inverts a theme that had been introduced into portraiture by Jan van Eyck in his *Portrait of the Arnolfini Marriage*. In this latter painting Van Eyck had included his miniature self-portrait in a mirror at the back of the painting. By inverting the visuospatial perspective Velazquez draws and imagines himself, the Princess Margarita, and the rest of the visuospatial scene from the position and visuospatial perspective of the Spanish King and Queen. Both royals are 'only' depicted as small reflections in the mirror at the back of the room (corresponding to the position of Van Eyck 200 years earlier), whereas he paints himself large and in the foreground of the painting!

[2]When looking at a self-portrait the beholder of such art works is in a very similar situation.

these brain mechanisms related to visual, disembodiment-related, or corporeal processing are also activated in the brains of neurological patients leading to hallucinated self-portraits.

Neuropsychological Mechanisms in Self-Portraiture

How can findings from neurology and neuropsychology further be helpful to understand art and self-portraiture? The preceding considerations are speculative and based on the analysis of verbal and pictorial phenomena. In the remaining part of this article I will review empirical data on the influence of brain damage on self-portraiture. Importantly, the dramatic effects on artistry after brain damage differ after acute damage to the right (leading to neglect) or left brain (leading to aphasia) and during progressive damage to both hemispheres (leading to dementia). There is now an increasing body of clinical studies on the effects of brain damage on the works of internationally and locally known painters [Alajounaine, 1948; Jung, 1974; Chatterjee, 2004; Bäzner and Hennerici, 2006; Zaidel, 2006; Blanke, 2006; Blanke and Lenggenhager, in press]. As Jung [1974] and more recently Zaidel [2006] argue, these observations are probably the most direct empirical data that allow the examination of brain mechanisms in visual arts. It is hoped that these neuropsychological analyses will evolve into rich study material for art historians and philosophers of art.

The Effects of Neglect on Self-Portraiture

Neglect is a common neurological condition following right posterior brain damage. It may be defined as an attentional disorder characterized by disregard of sensory information in the part of space to the left of the midline [Robertson and Halligan, 2001; Blanke and Lenggenhager, in press]. The drawings of patients with visuospatial neglect classically show left-sided omissions and spatial deformities whereas the right side of the picture is more completely done [graphic neglect; Halligan and Marshall, 2001; Robertson and Halligan, 2001]. In addition, graphic neglect may be characterized by loss of spatial contours, difficulties in appreciating depth and three-dimensional objects, and enhancement of the right side of the picture. Left-sided neglect is in the large majority of cases due to right temporoparietal brain damage. The influence of neglect on painting has been analyzed in Otto Dix, Lovis Corinth, Anton Räderscheidt [Jung, 1974], and other painters [Vigouroux et al., 1990; Heller, 1994; Halligan and Marshall, 1997; Cantagallo and Della Sala, 1998; Blanke et al., 2003]. These analyses showed that independently of the premorbid style of

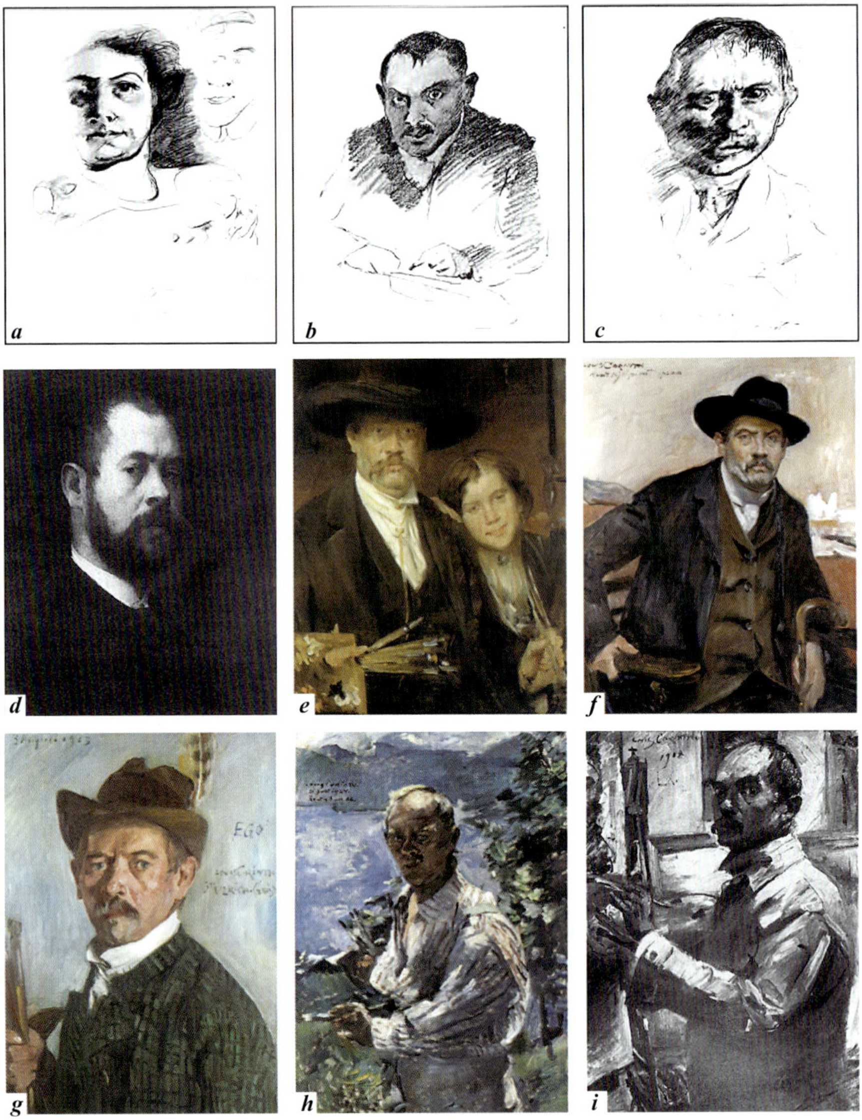

Fig. 2. Self-portraits by Lovis Corinth. ***a–c*** Graphic left-sided neglect with left-sided omission and deformities in drawn self-portraits of Lovis Corinth. ***d–i*** Positional change in the painted self-portraits of Lovis Corinth after and before 1912. Three self-portraits that were created before 1912 are shown: 1887 (*Selbstbildnis*, Museum Georg Schäfer, Schweinfurt, Germany) (***d***), 1901 (*Selbstporträt mit Modell*, Kunstmuseum Winterthur, Switzerland) (***e***), and 1911 (*Selbstbildnis mit schwarzem Hut und Stock*, Kunstmuseum, St. Gallen, Switzerland) (***f***). Compare with Corinths stance in self-portraits carried out after

the affected painter, neglect-related signs or style elements can be found in the works of these painters [Chatterjee, 2004; Bäzner and Hennerici, 2006; Blanke and Lenggenhager, in press].

Several neglect signs are present in self-portraits of Lovis Corinth (1858–1925). Corinth is one of the great individualists in the history of painting who transcended both his own time and conventional classifications [Kuhn, 1925; Schröder, 1992]. Corinth's productive years spanned nearly half a century and he studied at the academies in Königsberg, Munich, and Paris. By 1901 he had emerged as one of the most eminent German painters. Art historical labels, however, are not easily applied to Corinth's works [Kuhn, 1925; Schröder, 1992]. He painted naturalistic portraits, slaughterhouse scenes as well as interiors, still lives and landscapes that link him to Impressionism. At the same time he produced history paintings illustrating biblical and mythological scenes upon which his reputation in the last decade of the 19th century was based. Although he rejected Expressionism, some of Corinth's later works place him among the Expressionists [Schröder, 1992]. His work thus defies easy categorization and most people have failed to categorize this artist and his oeuvre. Two major periods have preoccupied art historians: Corinth's mature, 'impressionistic' period or style (1900–1911) and his late 'expressionistic' style (1912–1925) coinciding with a right hemispheric stroke in December 1911.

As described by Jung [1974] (fig. 2a) Corinth's postmorbid self-portraits reveal left-sided omissions: the central portrait depicts his wife Charlotte to which Corinth has added two portraits – probably of himself [Jung, 1974] – on each side of Charlotte's portrait. Many examples of left-sided omissions can be seen in Charlotte's face, her forehead and her hair. Her left shoulder was replaced by a small self-portrait. Although her left hand and arm are drawn both show signs of spatial deformities and are less precisely drawn than the corresponding right body parts. Her left hemiface is less wide and drawn with less spatial detail and nuances. Corinth's self-portrait on the right side also shows left-sided neglect suggesting the presence of object-centered graphic neglect [Halligan and Marshall, 2001]: despite placing this self-portrait in his preserved right spatial field, Corinth omitted left facial features (eye, hair, left facial contour). The left self-portrait also shows left-sided graphic neglect (left eye and other left facial features are missing). In a later self-portrait from 1912 further left-sided omissions can be found (fig. 2b). Here, the outer contour of the left arm is missing. The left arm is smaller than the right arm. In addition, the diagonal hatching of

1912: 1913 (*Selbstbildnis mit Tirolerhut*, Museum Folkwang, Essen, Germany) (***g***), 1918 (*Selbstbildnis im weissen Kittel*, Wallraf-Richartz-Museum, Cologne, Germany) (***h***), and 1924 (*Grosses Selbstportrait vor dem Walchensee*; Bayrische Staatsgemäldesammlungen, Munich, Germany) (***i***).

the left arm is missing whereas it is more complete for the right arm. Finally, the left hand is only roughly rendered without the depiction of individual fingers. This is not the case for the right hand, which is well modeled and completely drawn. Although Corinth's painted self-portraits do not reveal clear signs of left-sided spatial neglect, I have argued previously that Corinth changed his body position in front of the mirror when painting self-portraits. He thus deviated from his customary stance and that of his much admired Dutch masters Frans Hals and Rembrandt [Blanke, 2005]. In his self-portraits before 1912 Corinth depicts his body as turned rightwards (or facing straight ahead; fig. 2c–e), yet after 1912 Corinth depicts himself mostly as turned leftwards (or facing straight ahead; fig. 2f–h). The same analysis of 20 painted self-portraits of Rembrandt (who was right-handed as Corinth) revealed that Rembrandt positioned himself in front of the mirror as did Corinth before his stroke. I have argued that this change in stance was necessary in order to look at his mirror reflection in his preserved right visual field and not his left neglected visual field. Many of these changes have also been described in the painter Anton Räderscheidt [Jung, 1974] who carried out many self-portraits in the first year after his right-sided brain damage in 1967. Analysis of Räderscheidt's self-portraits reveals that he also changed his postmorbid stance in front of these paintings: analysis of postmorbid self-portraits [illustrated in Herzog, 1991] shows that he painted himself with his head and body turned to the left,[3] whereas this was not or less frequently the case in his premorbid self-portraits.

The Effects of Aphasia on Self-Portraiture

Aphasia is generally associated with damage to the left cerebral hemisphere and changes that have been observed in professional painters with aphasia are more variable and opinions diverge whether any postmorbid style changes can be observed or not. Aphasia due to acute left hemisphere brain damage and its influences on the work of several painters has been summarized previously [Chatterjee, 2004; Bäzner and Hennerici, 2006; Blanke and Lenggenhager, in press]. Bonvicini [1926] describes the consequences of left hemisphere stroke and aphasia in the works of Daniel Urrabieta y Vierge (1851–1904) and could not find any changes in style. Yet, Chatterjee [2004] and Bäzner and Hennerici [2006] suggested that painters with aphasia seem to use more vivid colors and seem to change their preferred genre or the content of

[3]This was found in 28 of 35 self-portraits in Herzog [1991].

their paintings. Often painters with aphasia – due to associated right-sided hemiparesis or hemiplegia – have to change the hand they use for drawing (from the right hand that is paretic or plegic to the unaffected left hand) [Zaimov et al., 1969]. Thus the paintings and drawings of those still painting with their paretic right hand may show signs of tremor [Kirk and Kertesz, 1989]. Interestingly, most painters rapidly acquired the same manual and drawing skills with their non-dominant hand in only a few months' time [Zaimov et al., 1969].

Few self-portraits of the Polish painter R.L. [Kaczmarek, 1991] have been published in the medical literature. In addition, Kaczmarek [1991] argued that R.L.'s paintings revealed a profound change in style following damage to the left hemisphere. R.L. was Professor of Art at Lublin University. His art was strongly inspired by war themes and included frequently verbal material in the form of letters, names or numbers that he integrated into his paintings (i.e. *Quo Vadis*) (fig. 3a). For his paintings *Requiem* and *Exhumed* (fig. 3b) he received major national prizes. At the age of 51 years he suffered a stroke leading to Broca aphasia and right-sided hemiparesis. He was unable to reproduce a sequence of events of a story. In addition, difficulties in action planning and control, emotional lability, and confabulations were noted. He did postmorbid drawings with his right hand and started 6 months after the stroke. Two postmorbid self-portraits reveal remarkable skill with his paretic hand 5 months after his stroke (fig. 3c, d). Although verbal and symbolic material was one of the key elements of his premorbid art, he did not include these elements in his postmorbid art [Kaczmarek, 1991]. Over the first year, he continued to paint portraits and landscapes and only started to paint more symbolically after the first year. It is important for the considerations of self-portraiture that left hemisphere damage associated with aphasia in this artist seems to leave the artist's capacity to draw and paint self-portraits relatively unaffected although his art shows major changes.

The Effects of Dementia on Self-Portraiture

The most famous painter who suffered from Alzheimer's disease is probably the abstract expressionist William de Kooning (1904–1997), who was diagnosed as suffering from Alzheimer's disease in 1989. Since the beginning of the 1980s several art critics noted major changes in his style and some suggested that these might have been due to neuropsychological changes related to Alzheimer's disease [Espinel, 1996]. Yet, there is disagreement on whether de Kooning's style change was due to neurological mechanisms, other causes, or a natural evolution of his art [Crutch et al., 2001]. There is much debate over the relevance and significance of his later paintings, which have been described as clean, sparse, and almost graphic compared to his dynamic and rich earlier

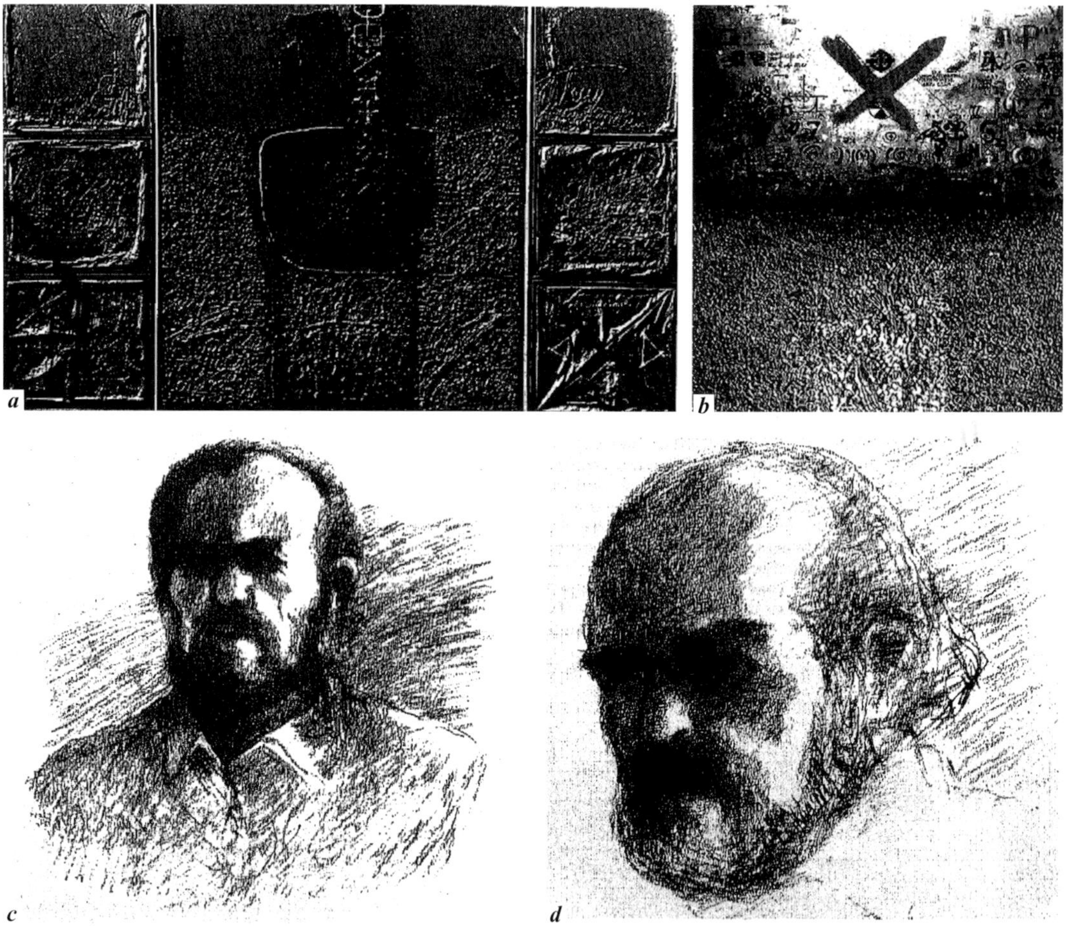

Fig. 3. Self-portraits by a Polish painter (Richard L.). Two premorbid paintings with verbal and symbolic elements of the Polish painter R.L. who suffered from aphasia are shown: *Quo Vadis* (***a***) and *Exhumed* (***b***). ***c***, ***d*** Two postmorbid self-portraits are shown [Kaczmarek, 1991] (with kind permission of Psychology Press, www.psypress.co.uk/journals.asp, 2007).

works. Some say his mental condition and/or attempts to recover from a life of alcoholism had rendered him unable to carry out the mastery of his early works, while others see these late works as prophesizing the clean, surface-oriented painters of the 1990s. Still others who knew de Kooning personally claim that his late paintings were being taken away and sold before he was able to finish them. Detailed medical data on de Kooning are sparse and MRI, neurological, or neuropsychological data are not available.

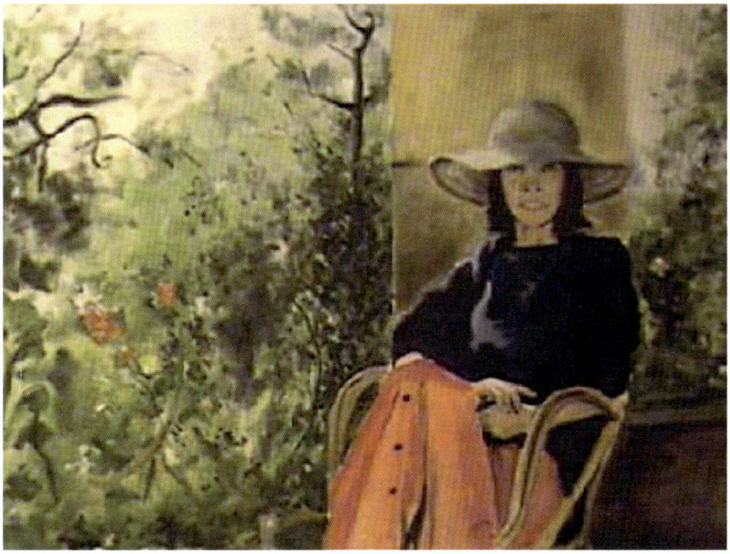

Fig. 4. Self portrait of Danae Chambers (1999) who suffered from Alzheimer's disease [Fornazzari, 2005] (with kind permission of Blackwell Publishing).

In another painter who suffered from Alzheimer's disease, Danae Chambers (born 1941), neurological and neuropsychological data as well as a self-portrait have been analyzed. In 1996 (3 years after diagnosis), Chambers' art is undergoing minor changes in the depiction of form and space, but still has a well-conserved overall structure [Fornazzari, 2005]. Self-portraits do not seem to have been affected at this point. In 1999, Chambers' self-portraits started showing more irregularities and overlapping structures characterized by frequent reworking and overpainting of certain image parts. These changes were especially prominent in faces and were analyzed by Fornazzari [2005] in a self-portrait (fig. 4). An MRI revealed a cyst in the left temporal lobe and moderate brain atrophy. The neurological examination was normal [for neuropsychological data, see Fornazzari, 2005].

Similar changes in many of his self-portraits have also been observed in William Utermohlen (born 1933) [Crutch et al., 2001]. Alzheimer's disease was diagnosed at the age of 61 years and his self-portraits were followed for a period of 6 years, from the age of 60 to 66 years (fig. 5) and were in addition also frequent objects of his art prior to symptomatic disease onset [Crutch et al., 2001]. MRI revealed general brain atrophy and the neurological examination was normal [for neuropsychological data, see Crutch et al., 2001]. Crutch et al. [2001] describe less accurate brush strokes, overlapping lines, frequent

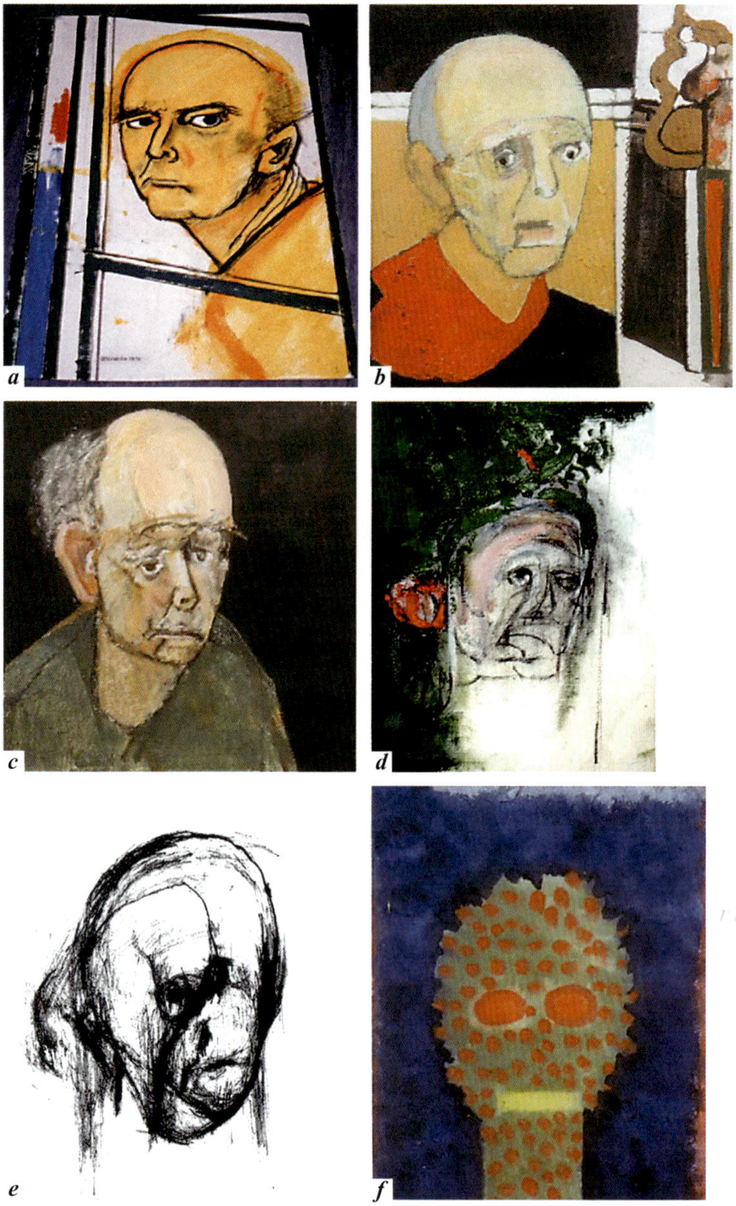

Fig. 5. Several self-portraits of William Utermohlen who suffered from Alzheimer's disease [Crutch et al., 2001]. ***a*** Premorbid self-portrait that was done at the age of 60 years. ***b–e*** Carried out at the age of 62–66 years. ***d***, ***e*** Increasing difficulties to capture his own face become prominent. ***e***, ***f*** Change from oil painting to crayon and aquarelle can be seen (with kind permission from Elsevier).

overpainting and reworking of lines, as well as rougher planes that increased progressively. They also pointed out his progressively increasing difficulties in depicting the human face, especially his own face.[4]

Conclusion

Postmorbid self-portraits in painters who suffer from neglect, aphasia and dementia differ in several aspects that are relatively independent of the painter's premorbid style, epoch and country. Self-portraits of painters with neglect reveal the acute signs of left-sided omissions, deformities, loss of color, and shifting of the overall scene to the right of the picture. Moreover, the painter seems to change his preferred position in front of the drawing mirror (Corinth; Räderscheidt), the preferred direction of light (Corinth) and tends to use more verbal material in his art than in premorbid paintings (Corinth; Alder, Swiss painter from Geneva).

This is different in painters with aphasia who – due to their left-sided brain damage – often have to switch the hand they use for drawing from their paralyzed right hand to the normal left hand. It is remarkable that left-handed postmorbid skill returns to premorbid levels within several months in most painters. Latter self-portraits have no or very minor right-sided minor omissions and are characterized by more harmonious or vivid colors, are less stylized, more imaginative, and more symmetrical. In a Polish painter a loss of verbal material and symbols has been observed. Although these signs may occur in the acute phase after brain damage, due to aphasia and right paralysis, the painter with aphasia generally starts to paint later than painters with neglect.[5]

Analysis of self-portraits painted by artists suffering from dementia reveal the progressive appearance of style changes over many years. These are initially more subtle than those in painters suffering from neglect or aphasia, but may – over the years – lead to an incapacity to paint which is never the case in painters with neglect or aphasia. These self-portraits are characterized by less accurate brush strokes, overlapping lines, frequent overpainting and reworking of lines, as well as rougher planes that can be found on both sides of the painting. These changes are especially prominent in the depiction of the painter's own face (Utermohlen; Chambers) leading in later stages of the disease to unrecognizability (Utermohlen).

To summarize, self-portraits of artists with neglect are characterized by *new spatial elements* affecting the global structure of the canvas, but can mainly

[4]Unfortunately no portraits of family members were shown or analyzed in comparison.

[5]Unfortunately, there are only few published self-portraits of artists suffering from aphasia.

be found on the left side of the picture and painted person. In self-portraits of artists with dementia *new form elements* are found leading to changes of contours and lines over the entire canvas, but predominantly in the center of self-portraits. Self-portraits of artists with aphasia are carried out with the nondominant hand and are characterized by *new verbal/symbolic elements* affecting the content and use of verbal material. These findings in artists suffering from brain damage should be compared with neuropsychological data on drawing ability (1) in nonartist patients after unilateral brain damage [Kirk and Kertesz, 1989] and Alzheimer's disease [Kirk and Kertesz, 1991], (2) painters without neurological disease, and (3) other visual artists with neurological disease (sculptors, architects, choreographers, video and installation artists, etc.). Findings from painters with other neurological disease such as epilepsy [especially temporal lobe epilepsy: Vincent van Gogh; Gastaut, 1956] and migraine [Giorgio de Chirico; Podoll et al., 2001; but see Blanke and Landis, 2004] and their effects on self-portraiture should also be analyzed and integrated.

These comparisons – for self-portraiture and other genres – will be necessary for the development of neuropsychological art theories that are based on the empirical principles of neuropsychology and neurology. As mentioned earlier – and briefly elaborated with respect to the neurocognitive mechanisms of own body illusions and self-consciousness – findings from cognitive neuroscience may further be integrated into an interdisciplinary field trying to elucidate the intricate and manifold relations between brain and visual arts in painter and beholder. It is hoped that collaborations can be established between art historians, art critics, neurologists, and neuropsychologists in order to build a bridge between art history and neuroscience that already exists between philosophy and neuroscience.

References

Alajounaine T: Aphasia and artistic realization. Brain 1948;71:229–241.

Bäzner H, Hennerici H: Stroke in painters. Int Rev Neurobiol 2006;74:165–191.

Bell J: 500 Self-Portraits. London, Phaidon Press, 2000, pp 5–10.

Bermudez JL, Marcel A, Eilan N: The Body and the Self. Boston, MIT Press, 1995.

Blanke O: Perception and experience of the self in autoscopic phenomena and self-portraiture. Swiss Arch Neurol Psychiatry 2005;156:173–188.

Blanke O: Visuo-spatial neglect in Lovis Conrinth's self-portraits. Int Rev Neurobiol 2006;74C: 193–214.

Blanke O, Landis T: Giorgio de Chirico: intricate links between spiritual fevers, metaphysical art, and the interictal temporal lobe syndrome. Eur Neurol 2004;51:186–187.

Blanke O, Lenggenhager B: Neuropsychologische Grundlagen der Malerei; in Bormuth M, Podoll K, Spitzer B (eds): Pathographie. In press.

Blanke O, Mohr C: Autoscopic phenomena of neurological origin. Implications for corporal awareness and self consciousness. Brain Res Rev 2005;50:184–199.

Blanke O, Ortigue S, Landis T: Colour neglect in an artist. Lancet 2003;361:264.

Blanke O, Spinelli L, Landis T, Seeck M: Out-of-body experience and autoscopy of neurological origin. Brain 2004;127:243–258.
Bonafoux P: Moi! Autoportraits du XX siècle. Milan, Skira Editore, 2004.
Bonvicini G: Die Aphasie des Malers Vierge. Wien Med Wochenschr 1926;76:88–91.
Brugger P: Reflective mirrors: perspective taking in autoscopic phenomena. Cogn Neuropsychiatr 2002;7:179–194.
Cantagallo A, Della Sala S: Preserved insight in an artist with extrapersonal spatial neglect. Cortex 1998;34:163–189.
Chatterjee A: The neuropsychology of visual artistic production. Neuropsychologia 2004;42:1568–1583.
Crutch SJ, Isaacs R, Rossor MN: Some workmen can blame their tools: artistic change in an individual with Alzheimer's disease. Lancet 2001;357:2129–2133.
Espinel CH: De Kooning's late colours and forms: dementia, creativity, and the healing power of art. Lancet 1996;347:1096–1098.
Fornazzari LR: Preserved painting creativity in an artist with Alzheimer's disease. Eur J Neurol 2005;12: 419–424.
Gastaut H: La maladie de Vincent van Gogh envisagée à la lumière des conceptions nouvelles sur l'épilesie psychomotrice. Ann Méd Psychol 1956;114:196–238.
Halligan PW, Marshall JC: The art of visual neglect. Lancet 1997;330:139–140.
Halligan PW, Marshall JC: Graphic neglect – more than the sum of the parts. Neuroimage 2001;14: S91–S97.
Heller W: Cognitive and emotional organization of the brain: influences on the creation and perception of art; in Zaidel D (ed): Neuropsychology. New York, Academic Press, 1994, pp 271–292.
Herzog G: Anton Räderscheidt. Cologne, DuMont, 1991.
Jung R: Neuropsychologie und Neurophysiologie des Kontur und Formensehens in Zeichnerei und Malerei; in Wieck HH (ed): Psychopathologie musischer Gestaltungen. Schattauer, Stuttgart, 1974.
Kaczmarek B: Aphasia in an artist: a disorder of symbolic processing. Aphasiology 1991;5:361–371.
Kirk A, Kertesz A: Hemispheric contributions to drawing. Neuropsychologia 1989;27:881–886.
Kirk A, Kertesz A: On drawing impairment in Alzheimer's disease. Arch Neurol 1991;48:73–77.
Kuhn A: Lovis Corinth. Berlin, Propyläen Verlag, 1925.
Neisser U: The five kinds of self-knowledge. Philosophic Psychol 1988;1:35–59.
Pächt O: Das Selbstbildnis; in Rembrandt. Munich, Prestel Verlag, 1991, pp 65–78.
Podoll K, Robinson D, Nicola U: The migraine of Giorgio de Chirico. 1. History of illness. Neurol Psychiatr Brain Res 2001;9:139–156.
Robertson IH, Halligan PW: Spatial Neglect: a Clinical Handbook for Diagnosis and Treatment. Hove, Psychology Press, 2001.
Schröder KA: Nähe und Ferne: Faktur und Ausdruck im Schaffen Lovis Corinths; in Schröder KA (ed): Lovis Corinth. Munich, Prestel, 1992, pp 8–35.
Schröder KA: Egon Schiele. Eros and passion. Munich, Prestel Verlag, 1999.
Vigouroux RA, Bonnefoi B, Khalil R: Pictorial creations of a painter presenting with left-sided neglect (in French). Rev Neurol (Paris) 1990;146:665–670.
Zaidel DW: Neuropsychology of Art. Neurological, Cognitive and Evolutionary Perspectives. Hove, Psychology Press, 2006.
Zaimov K, Kitov D, Kolev N: Aphasia in a painter. Essay on the analysis of certain elements of the work of the Bulgarian painter Z.B., before and after hemiplegic aphasia. Several comparisons with the Vierge case (in French). Encephale 1969;58:377–417.

Prof. Olaf Blanke, MD, PhD
Laboratory of Cognitive Neuroscience, Station 15
Ecole Polytechnique Fédérale de Lausanne (EPFL)
CH–1007 Lausanne (Switzerland)
Tel. +41 21 6939621, Fax +41 21 6939625, E-Mail olaf.blanke@epfl.ch

Bogousslavsky J, Hennerici MG (eds): Neurological Disorders in Famous Artists – Part 2.
Front Neurol Neurosci. Basel, Karger, 2007, vol 22, pp 30–43

Lovis Corinth: Integrating Hemineglect and Spatial Distortions

H. Bäzner, M.G. Hennerici

Department of Neurology, University of Heidelberg, Universitätsklinikum Mannheim, Mannheim, Germany

Abstract

Lovis Corinth suffered a right-hemispheric stroke at the age of 53 years, but died only 14 years later. The huge number of artworks that he produced after this life-threatening disease allows a detailed analysis of his poststroke artwork in comparison to his prestroke artwork. When performing this analysis as a neurologist, an enormous diversity of subtle stroke sequelae can be discovered, which can mostly be explained by a left-sided hemineglect. These findings clearly go far beyond pure psychological processes. Moreover, Corinth is a good and motivating example for patients suffering disability after a stroke, because he was able to produce great artwork after his stroke. Lovis Corinth was struggling against motor disability that admittedly was not severely affecting his artistic production but he also had to fight against severe neuropsychological deficits that did have clear consequences for his artistic production. Corinth's credo was 'true art means to use unreality'. Taken together with the often cited phrase of 'drawing means to [details]', there will be a clear-cut interpretation for the neurologist that can be derived from the understanding of a right-hemisphere lesion and subsequent left-sided neglect.

The interpretation of diseases in famous people will always be debatable. The case of the painter Lovis Corinth, however, is truly intriguing. On the one hand, numerous art experts define the year of his stroke in 1911 as the turning point of his artistic development, and claim that the illness did not cause a change in artistic style. On the other hand, biographical sources and the study of his artwork before and after the stroke suggest to the neurological art lover quite a clear impact on his artistic production through a right-hemisphere lesion caused by a stroke in 1911. In 1974, the German neurologist Richard Jung made the first attempt at such an interpretation [Jung, 1974]. Jung, however, had provoked severe annoyance in Corinth's son Thomas, when he confronted him with the idea that his father's stroke might have led to certain omissions in paintings and drawings due to a spatial hemineglect: 'A doctor has claimed, that certain omissions in Corinth's drawings are caused by his stroke . . . this very theory is . . . disputable, because Corinth rendered homage to the maxim of: "Drawing means to omit details" ' [Corinth, 1979]. The painter's family was always rather reserved as to his diseases. This may partly be due to the fact that Corinth was featured in the Munich exhibition Entartete Kunst (degenerate art) organized by the Nazis with almost three hundred of Corinth's late works, including some of his greatest masterpieces. The organizers of this most infamous exhibition suggested that his stroke was responsible for 'inadequate craftsmanship and artistry'. Hence, neither the extensive collection of biographical sources published by Lovis Corinth's son Thomas in 1979, nor the biographical sketches by his wife Charlotte [Berend-Corinth, 1958a, b], nor the autobiographical novel by his daughter Wilhelmine [Corinth, 1980] contain clear hints of a further stroke event between 1911 and the painter's death in 1925, as had been suggested by some authors. However, a careful and detailed analysis of Lovis Corinth's enormous artwork from the neurological point of view leads to the conclusion that his cerebrovascular events are not only an accidental biographical occurrence on the way to a changing style but rather a consequence of the right-hemisphere stroke which the painter had suffered in 1911. Therefore, the above-mentioned phrases which Lovis Corinth [1926] had cited in his memoirs, shortly before his death: 'Drawing means to omit details' and 'true art means seeking to capture the unreal' indeed allow a different interpretation: Corinth was forced to intensively struggle with a spatial hemineglect, which obviously handicapped him with variable severity for the long period of 14 years. Slowly, he was able to compensate for this handicap, which probably unmasked a new artistic principle.

Biographical Sketch

Lovis Corinth was born on July 21, 1858 in Tapiau (Eastern Prussia). After years of study in Königsberg, Antwerp, and Paris, he visited Berlin for the first time in his life in 1887/1888, returned to Königsberg after his father had died in 1889 and went back to Berlin in 1890. He then moved to Munich, where he stayed between 1891 and 1900 and became a founding member of the Munich 'Secession'. After establishing contacts to several leading members of the Berlin 'Secession' including Max Liebermann, Walter Leistikow and Paul Cassirer, he finally decided to move to Berlin, where he settled in 1901, to work as a painter and teacher of arts. In Berlin, Corinth rapidly succeeded in becoming a leading member of the Berlin Secession. There, he founded the first women's painting school of Berlin in 1902. His first pupil, Charlotte Berend, 22 years younger than him, became his preferred model. In March 1903, he married her. His wife and children Thomas (born in 1904) and Wilhelmine (born in 1909) frequently sat as models for portraits. He started to write his memoirs in 1906. In 1910, he was at the crest of his fame and participated at the Venice Biennale. Together with Liebermann and Slevogt he formed the triad of German impressionism. On December 11, 1911, a right-hemisphere stroke reportedly caused a left-sided hemiparesis. Several weeks after the stroke Corinth and his wife traveled to the Italian Riviera. There, his recovery was hampered by fierce debates about the control of the Secession, which finally led to Corinth's resignation from the executive committee. For instance, Paul Cassirer was spreading the rumor that the painter had become mentally incompetent, and that the stroke had left him insane. On the occasion of his 60th birthday, a large exhibition of Corinth works was held at the Secession and he was appointed Professor of the Berlin Academy of Arts. However, Corinth retired more and more from roaring Berlin. Starting in 1919, he spent the summers in the newly built house in Urfeld at the Walchensee in Bavaria. During a trip to Amsterdam in 1925 with the intention to study the paintings of Rembrandt and Frans Hals, he died of pneumonia in the 68th year of his life. Nowadays, paintings by Lovis Corinth are exhibited in many important museums all over the world, and record prices are paid for his works at auction.

History of His Illnesses

In his younger years Lovis Corinth was famous for his ability to binge drink and for his impulsive and extroverted character. 'No student was considered competent', Corinth wrote in his memoirs, 'unless he was also a notorious drinker. We soon developed great mastery in the consumption of alcohol.... All my new friends drank... until we could no longer tell which one of us could hold the most.' His wife describes Lovis when she met him fort he first time as a 'quite strange looking man. A fresh, somewhat ruddy face, an enormous neck and part of his chest sticking out of his half-open flanel shirt' [Berend-Corinth, 1958b]. Thomas Corinth cites Karl Schwarz: 'His face was... bronzy and full of stubbles.' Furthermore: 'he was tall and his stature was strong, but his posture was stooped... He was unsociable, i.e. that he was closing himself against strangers and appeared grumpy and unapproachable' [Corinth, 1979]. As to a putative risk factor profile, he definitely was a heavy smoker. Arterial hypertension cannot be proven, but might have been the case following the characterizations of his contemporaries. Furthermore, he suffered from repeat attacks of gout, which were treated with 'radon' cures.

In the night of December 11, 1911, Corinth sustained a right-hemisphere stroke with a left-sided hemiparesis and hemineglect and a subsequent severe depressive episode. In his memoirs, he writes: 'Often during this night the deceased appeared and seemed to wave to me, while from above a brute force oppressed me, deeper and deeper. "It's neck or nothing" I said to the nurse, and the doctor, to whom I expressed the same suspicions, answered to me: "with a heart like yours, there is no dying"' [Corinth, 1926]. His wife Charlotte reports: 'I had just dozed off, when I heard sounds and shouts from his room. At the same moment, I was standing next to his bed; he was lying on his left side and groaned.... Very quickly, the doctors came, I was told, that he would survive.... He was given a Morphium injection, and the ungovernable power was calm' [Berend-Corinth, 1958a]. From the documentation by his son Thomas, we learn that Dr. Paul Strassmann came immediately, 'although he was in a bad physical condition himself'. Strassmann, a gynecologist running a women's hospital in Berlin was a friend of the family. The then 7-year-old boy remembers that his father was afraid to die, because his own father had died of the same disease (Corinth's father died on January 10, 1889 of a stroke) [Corinth, 1979]. In the days immediately following the stroke, Corinth describes dream-like optical sensations and states further that he had come face-to-face with death: 'My entire life passed before me, a life which in this lonely battle seemed more precious now than when I was young and strong. I was forced to reckon with myself. Job called to me: Gird up thy loins like a man for I will demand of thee, and answer thou me! "Where wast thou when I created thee?" Thus my path was to be illuminated once more. But time seemed so very short' [Corinth, 1926].

On December 22, 1911 Corinth wrote to Heinrich Keitel: 'Adieu-Adieu-Adieu, it hurts very much... Bad news, that I am feeling lousy. Lots of pain, very dreadful.' Some days later, Corinth writes: 'For more than 8 days I was bedridden and suffered lots of pain' [Corinth, 1979]. The interpretation by Thomas Corinth that he developed 'neuritis' does not seem plausible. Rather an episode of his recurrent gout might have been the cause of the pain. Alternatively, we can speculate that Corinth's pain might be related to his stroke: apart from a stroke localization in the territory of the middle cerebral artery as proposed by Jung, the documented symptoms such as hemianopsia and hemineglect might have been caused by a posterior cerebral artery stroke, which could explain a thalamic lesion and a consecutive thalamic pain syndrome. Still on January 30, 1912, more than 6 weeks after stroke onset, Corinth apologized for not receiving any visitors at his sickbed because of a 'health-related indisposition' [Corinth, 1979].

Alfred Kuhn, a contemporary critic who edited an early Corinth monograph in 1925, reports that Corinth was bedridden for many months. Here, we read that 'while still on the sickbed, Corinth asked for pencil and paper and sketched a series of horrible monsters and strange ghost-like images of famous figures from history' [Kuhn, 1925]. According to Uhr [1990]: 'apparently, none of these drawings has survived'. Kuhn had noted a marked change in Corinth's temper: 'When Corinth arose from the sickbed, he was a new person. He had become prescient for the hidden facets of appearance' [Kuhn, 1925]. Obviously, Corinth suffered a severe depressive episode at that time, which recurred several times afterwards, especially after 1912. Charlotte Berend-Corinth writes: 'Maybe his illness has aggravated his grief; however, it was not its cause. He was not melancholic, because his hand had become heavier and his life could no longer be as wild as before... If he was very depressed, which was the case almost every second day, I decided not to console him at all, but ridiculed him come hell or high water.... We had tested which reactions would help him the most. For instance, when his nerves came across, or he was full of anger, or nervous and prone to explode, I used to agree always' [Berend-Corinth, 1958]. Lovis Corinth [1926] made the following remark in his memoirs: 'People will have to thank [Charlotte] if in my later days I still managed to produce a few good things.' He used to express his bad mood quite drastically: 'I could scream. All painting disgusts me. Why shall I keep on working? Everything is trash. This dreadful effort to keep on working is enough to make me sick. I am in my sixty-seventh year and this summer will begin my sixty-eighth. What is there still to come of it? Old age takes hold of me more and more; my physical strength declines. Senility? I always pray that I do not become senile. The fear of it is horrible.'

On February 19, 1912, Corinth left Berlin with his 'faithful nurse' Charlotte for Bordighera at the Italian Riviera which was intended to be a kind of rehabilitation stay. There, Charlotte further detailed the sequels of his stroke. She described her husband's anxiety and depression and the exhaustion following the slightest physical exertion [Berend-Corinth, 1958b]. The course of the disease was certainly not uncomplicated, which we learn from an impressive documentation of contemporary stroke rehabilitation: 'Now, 9 p.m. Lovis is sleeping – he is always very tired here, and the doctor, who is very sincere and thorough, has told me that his condition is alarming. He found that he needed a lot of rest and told me lots of things that I had never heard before from the Berlin doctors. His day is exactly planned by the doctor: Lovis drinks caffeine-free coffee.... He is allowed to walk for half an hour twice daily. Half past 12 he has lunch, individually prepared for Lovis. At 4 p.m. a light tea..., at 7 p.m. dinner.... Lovis is very calm and pensive, infinitely nice and grateful for every little encouragement or help.... I don't want to leave Lovis alone at all, and the doctor agreed with me. In the beginning, I was desperate, to stay here in such beautiful surroundings virtually housebound, but since I have talked to the doctor, I have changed my point of view' [Corinth, 1979]. The very drastic diet was described by Corinth: 'The doctor has forbidden any alcoholic drink. I have a swelling of my liver, the doctors claim from too much of cognac. Now, I am behaving well, and drink three bottles of Fachinger (mineral water) daily' [Corinth, 1979]. Only in April 1912, 4 months after the acute stroke, Corinth wrote to his friends that he felt that his health was improved now. He was not quite sure of a complete recovery, however, because he wrote on August 1, 1912 to his good friend Hermann Struck: 'Concerning my state of health, the newspapers say that I am completely recovered, and I dare not suggest anything else' [Corinth, 1979]. His contemporary Karl Schwarz described Corinth at that time quite drastically as a 'gruff man' whom illness had turned into a 'wreck' [Corinth, 1979]. He expresses his astonishment about Corinth's energy while painting: 'When he stood before the easel, it was as if a volcano erupted. He flung the paint at the canvas, groaned and moaned, cursed and thundered, totally oblivious to the world around him.' And Rudolf Grossmann, who was portrayed by Corinth in 1924, writes: 'He knows how to take advantage of his diminished locomotive powers.... His hand gropes about on the palette and gradually turns as red as madder.... At the end, after two and a half hours of uninterrupted work,... he lowered his hands; they were as red as blood, as if he had burrowed into my intestines' [Uhr, 1990]. Finally, Alfred Kuhn [1925], who had met Corinth for several times while preparing a monograph featuring the artist, characterizes him as a 'stooped man' with an 'emaciated body,..., a shuffling walk, and trembling, red, swollen hands'. In this description, we hear of a further medical problem: a hand tremor. Most reports speak of a tremor of his right hand, his painting hand. Some confusion arose after his stroke caused by reports based on insufficient research, claiming that the painter Lovis Corinth was no longer able to move his right hand, which was definitely not the case. However, it is correct that Corinth himself and many contemporaries described a tremor of his right hand. According to Thomas Corinth, this was only present 'at times', but was occasionally very prominent. To the surprise of eyewitnesses, the tremor stopped at the moment when the hand with the paint brush touched the canvas or the pencil was put to paper. This was further documented in a short movie sequence dating from 1922. Corinth commented that 'an awful tremor of the right hand had been aggravated by effortful work with the [etching] needle and had been caused by earlier alcoholic excesses' [Schuster et al., 1996]. Phenomenologically, there is a tremor with action and during postural tasks, possibly meeting the criteria of an essential tremor.

Remarkably, Charlotte writes in her memoirs on several occasions of her husband's 'first' stroke, although a definite description of a second stroke is never given. On the occasion of his 60th birthday, Corinth had a syncopal attack as far as can be gathered from his wife's diary [Berend-Corinth, 1958b].

In later years, he limped when tired; his gait became shuffling, and small-stepped ('his gait is shuffling, such as it has been for years, unfortunately. Alas, how he struggles to walk as fast as I do') and his left hand no longer obeyed when he tried to perform intricate tasks [Berend-Corinth, 1958b]. Later photographs show a spastic posture of his left arm and hand, but his wife states that he used his weak left hand to press the copper plate to his body while engraving [Schuster et al., 1996; Uhr, 1990]. 'As a consequence of his disease, his left hand remained clumsy, although he could do any movement he intended to do. He has never mentioned this handicap – he just went on working... This left hand was clumsy in fine movements such as untwisting tubes, buttoning shirts; however, he didn't need any personal assistance. Only a little help at times for these small things' [Berend-Corinth, 1958b]. On the other hand, Charlotte Berend-Corinth makes the following remark later in her memoirs: 'Following Corinth's disease, I did no longer have a lot of support through him.' And his son writes: 'After the attack of 1911, this [paresis] had improved to a marked and satisfactory degree. But still, it remained deplorable enough for the artist' [Corinth, 1979].

Poststroke Artwork

Other than might be expected, Corinth's productivity was even growing after his recovery. Close to 500 paintings, over 800 prints, and scores of water colors and drawings – more than half of all his works – date from this period [Uhr, 1990]. However, he focuses on self-portraits, family portraits, and landscapes and produces large series of lithographs and etchings, partly as illustrations to books. 'My entire life passed before me, a life which in this lonely battle seemed more precious now than when I was young and strong. I was forced to reckon with myself.... But time seemed so very short' [Corinth, 1926].

The first written evidence by Lovis Corinth after the stroke is a pencil draft of a payment order dating from December 18, 1911. The first artistic products after his stroke are very fascinating: Thomas Corinth remembers that his father was drawing some pencil sketches displaying a skeleton with the Greek word 'Thanatos' (death) [Corinth, 1979]. When Charlotte accompanied him on returning to his studio for the first time, she watched as he gazed long into the familiar large mirror.

In her diary-like memoirs, she writes: '[Corinth was walking upstairs] indifferently, although cumbersome, step by step.... Again and again he moaned in despair, black thoughts attacked him... I had no more ideas to console him.... Then suddenly, he reached for palette and paint, sat down and quickly dashed off this first of a long series of sorrowful self-portraits' [Berend-Corinth, 1958b]. In fact, this self-portrait shows the painter wearing a coat over the pajamas from his sickbed.

The self-portraits following his stroke show a continuous process of confrontation with his declining physical constitution and focused on his physical

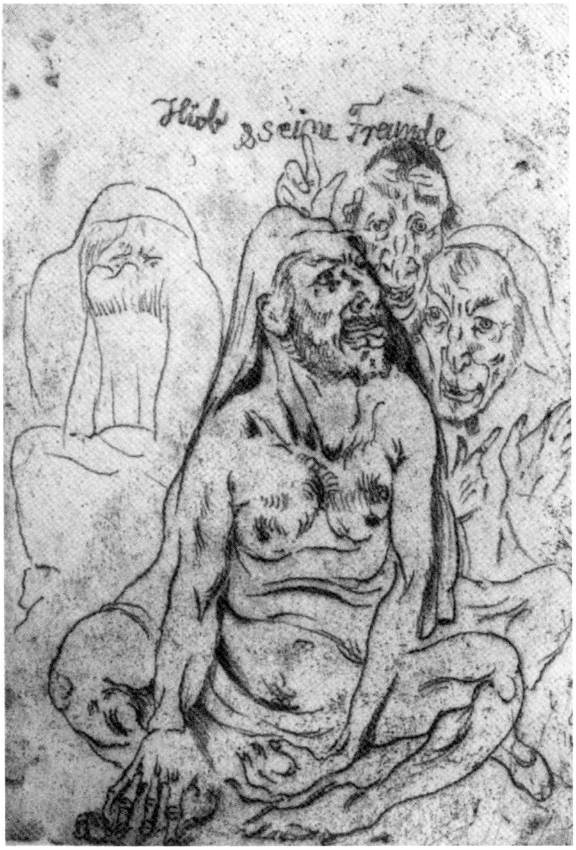

Fig. 1. Lovis Corinth's self-portraits following his stroke show a continuous process of confrontation with his declining physical constitution and focused on his physical frailty and mental anguish. In early February 1912 he made a small engraving showing the sick painter as 'Job with his friends' (copyright Kupferstichkabinett, Staatliche Museen zu Berlin – Preussischer Kulturbesitz, Inv. 2-1965, Schwarz 85).

frailty and mental anguish. In early February 1912, using the 'vernis-mou' technique he made a small engraving showing the sick painter as 'Job with his friends' (fig. 1). His son, Thomas, remembered that Hermann Struck, a friend of Corinth, assisted with the preparation of the printing plate [Corinth, 1979]. 'I saw him painting in his sickroom drawing on a plate covered by a sort of tissue paper.' In the print, Job is depicted while sitting on the floor with crossed legs, his right hand is placed on the right foot, the supinated and palmar-flexed lame and atrophic left arm is resting on the floor, his right foot is supinated. Job is wearing a cape like the one Corinth had used in earlier self-portraits. The title of the etching contains a small mistake in the mirrored text with a twist of the character '&'.

In Bordighera, during his rehabilitation stay in February 1912, he completed a small self-portrait in pencil that hardly resembles the painter. With larger-scale paintings, according to Horst Uhr, his wife Charlotte 'laid out the colours before him, placed palette and brushes in his encumbered left hand, and removed them from his stiff and swollen fingers when he had finished painting. When his own hand failed to provide adequate support, she gently and tactfully helped to steady his sketchbook' [Uhr, 1990]. Several drawing studies at this time show a left-sided neglect with missing parts of right upper extremities. A pencil drawing of his wife also finished in Bordighera grossly lacks texture, her dress looks lifeless; the lack of plausible anatomical articulation results in a strong sense of compression, his wife appearing ill at ease [Schuster et al., 1996]. In contrast, a very appealing balcony scene in Bordighera shows his wife on the balcony of the hotel at the moment when she unfolds a small parasol. Following Horst Uhr, this painting lacks correct perspective with the vertical lines of the hotel's facade not matching and the building appearing to lean to the left [Uhr, 1990]. Later Bordighera paintings, however, seem to reflect his ongoing recovery. The first large painting of 1912 shows *Samson Blinded* as a martyred and desperate figure, grasping in the direction of the observer, insecure, and not yet relying on his regained forces [Uhr, 1990]. In a preparatory pencil study for *Samson Blinded*, the biblical figure is grotesquely distorted [Schuster et al., 1996]. Still in October 1912, 11 months after the stroke, a small pencil study of his wife still shows a marked neglect with missing contours of the left face (fig. 2) [this very detail of a larger sketch was reproduced in the autobiography of Corinth, 1926]. We agree with Jung [1974], who finds the neglect compensated after 1913 in landscape paintings but notices several occurrences of uncertainty in the reproduction of left-sided facial aspects in his self-portraits. Here, the artist has to fixate strongly on his face in the mirror. In doing so, a visual field defect focused in the parafoveal region might become apparent. Interestingly and other than famous colleagues, Corinth never corrected the mirror effect in that the right-handed painter holds the pencil in the left hand in all his self-portraits (however, this can also be noticed prior to his stroke!).

Change in Style – Psychological or Physical Consequence of Stroke?

According to Uhr [1990], Lovis Corinth's poststroke artwork bears the mark of him having come close to death during the first hours and days after stroke onset. He refers to the stroke as 'an experience that ultimately led him to a new freedom of expression'. In this sense, many critics agree that Corinth's

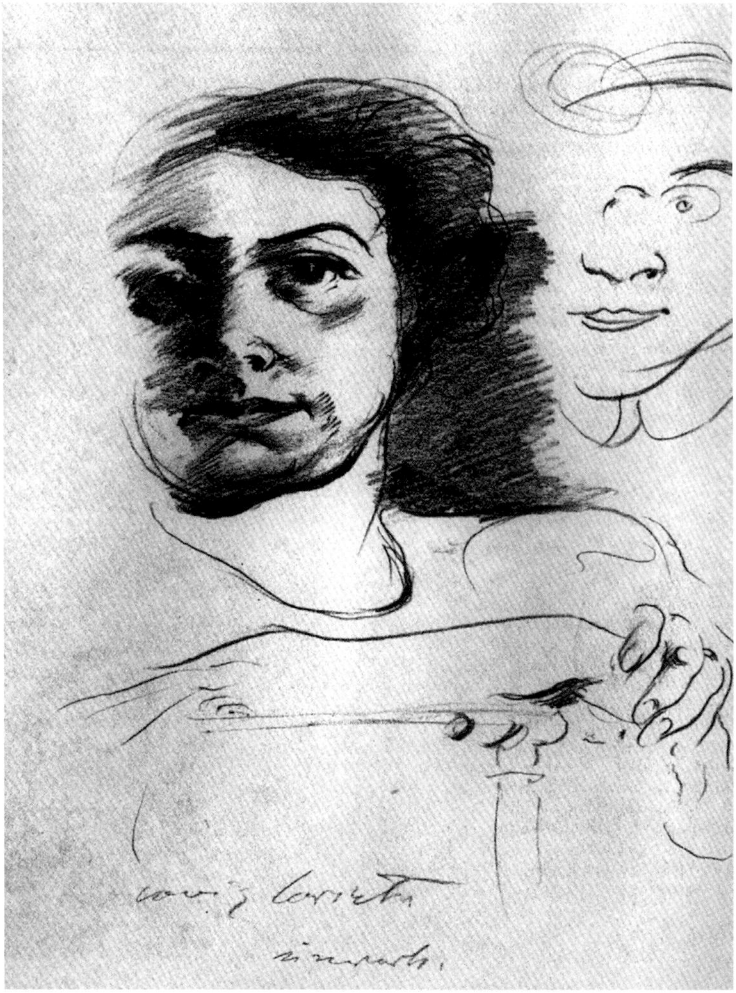

Fig. 2. Portrait of Charlotte Berend-Corinth with omissions on the left side of her face and body (detail of a larger sketch) [reproduced in his autobiography, Corinth, 1926].

work underwent a change of style, but they are unanimous in attributing this change to purely psychological factors such as depression and intensified awareness of the fragility of human life, increasing preoccupation with death, and heightened capacity to seize the essence of objects and experience. Lovis Corinth himself stated in the preface to a large retrospective exhibition in 1913: 'My most recent pictures... were initially hard to do because of many a fateful affliction, but I hope that I have overcome these impediments, and I intend to continue on my path' [Uhr, 1990].

Christoph Vitali, in his preface to the large Corinth Retrospective in 1996, doubts whether the stroke had a definite influence on Corinth's late style. '[Following the stroke] his painting technique is changing fundamentally once again, his style is decisively radicalised. The pure physiological explanation for his metamorphosis is unquestionably too short-minded…His experience to come close to death and to suffer severe illness may have accelerated and intensified its development, which has its fundament in the preceding works, but not any more' [Schuster et al., 1996]. Alfred Kuhn describes the change in style more detailed: '…the contours disappear, the bodies are often as if ripped asunder, deformed, disappeared into textures…also the faithfulness of portraits had ceased almost entirely…all detailed execution came to nothing. With wide stripes the person is captured in essence. Characterization is now exaggerated, indeed, often to caricature…models, no matter who they are, are now just objects to be painted…Indeed, the models must suffer every deprivation. Corinth always seems to be painting a picture behind the picture, one which he alone sees…at this point Corinth shifted from the ranks of the great painters to the circle of great artists' [Kuhn, 1925].

This is further supported in the report of the session for his own portrait in 1923: 'For the old Corinth the world was only a shell inhabited by a slowly disintegrating body, only an opportunity to receive new inspirations for visions of colour. When one sat opposite him during these last years and talked to him, one soon became aware that the conversation did not interest him in the least, that his gaze, so firmly fixed, was not intended for anyone in particular, and it could happen that Corinth would suddenly say such things as, "Hold still, that yellow forehead interests me", or "What a strange colour there is in your eyes right now"' [Kuhn, 1925].

Certainly, the judgment of an art critic or art historian, who is used to observe stylistic changes during the career of an artist, will be different from that of a neurologist familiar with the consequences of right-hemisphere damage. Of course, the artist reacts to the 'stroke attack' with thematic changes and may be obliged to do stylistic variations. Richard Jung was the first to describe the typical signs of visuospatial neglect in Lovis Corinth's poststroke works. Unilateral spatial (hemi-)neglect is a clinical term used to describe a number of different clinical symptoms which have in common the patient's failure to attend to, respond adequately to, or orient voluntarily to people or objects in the contralesional space. Unilateral spatial neglect is most often observed following brain lesions affecting the right hemisphere, and in particular the right inferior parietal cortex (angular and supramarginal gyrus) and right temporoparietal junction. Importantly, the term hemineglect cannot be meaningfully used if the target behavior is explained by primary sensory or motor deficits only. Typically the patient's deficit is supramodal: patients with hemineglect fail to respond to novel or meaningful stimuli irrespective of whether they are presented in the visual, auditory, and somesthetic (somatosensory) domain. Drawings by patients with left-sided hemineglect show typical omissions and spatial distortions on the left side of the drawing, the right half, however, will be drawn correctly. Furthermore, such drawings show often missing spatial contours, spatial depth is missing and three-dimensional objects will not be recognized as such in the left half of the drawing [Blanke, 2006]. Further details of Lovis Corinth's hemineglect have been pointed out by Gardner [1977]. Gardner finds Corinth's neglect essentially compensated for after several months (he mentions the occasional placement of persons in portraits on the right part of the painting or the less accurate execution of left parts of paintings in some works) [Gardner and Winner, 1981]. Interestingly, descriptions of poststroke paintings by art historians such as for instance the following text by Uhr [1990] concerning the painting *The Interior before the Mirror (1912)* contains several findings that are typical for right-hemisphere damage: 'This painting rephrases a picture from 1911 showing Charlotte Berend in her boudoir attended by a hairdresser. The later work shows an astonishing change. The high-keyed tones of the earlier painting have given way to colder hues of greater opacity; the fields of colour are separated by large areas of black; the brushstrokes have been applied flatly, with little variation in accent or direction . . . the features of both their faces are so generalized that the two figures appear virtually faceless. This results in a marked psychological distance, especially in comparison with the earlier, erotically charged, double portraits.' After an own detailed analysis of Lovis Corinth's works after the stroke [Bäzner and Hennerici, 2006], specific symptoms of right-hemisphere damage can be detected both in smaller graphic works but also in large-scale paintings. The altered features are striking:

- Loss of contours can be exemplarily shown in the *Portrait of the Painter Bernt Grönvold* (1923) or in *Frauenraub* (1918)
- Misplacement of details, such as in an etching of *Knecht Franz* (1919, with marked asymmetry of arm length)
- Neglect and obscuring of texture such as in *Susanna and the Elders* (1923) and in *Birth of Venus* (1923)
- Loss of emotional closeness and, hence, marked alteration of emotional distance such as in the portrait of his son *Thomas with a Hat in His Hands* (1922)
- Increased subjectivity such as in the last portrait of his wife as *Carmencita* (1924) (fig. 3b), compared with a prestroke painting of a similar subject, *The Black Mask* (1908) (fig. 3a)
- Idiosyncrasy, coarsening of structure, such as in *Still Life with Flowers, Skull, and Oak Leaves* (1921)

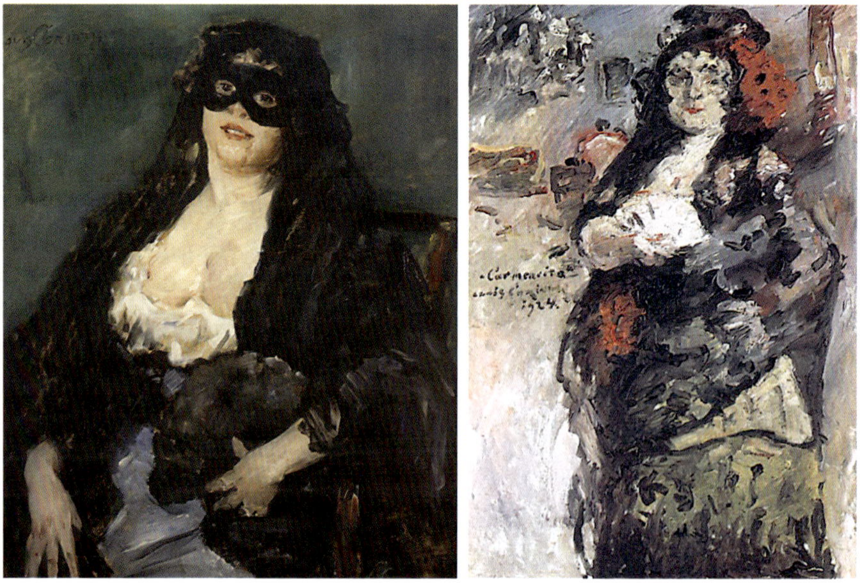

a b

Fig. 3. Lovis Corinth's poststroke paintings show a marked increase in subjectivity. ***b*** A good example for this feature is the painting *Carmencita* (1924) (courtesy of Städel Museum, Frankfurt am Main, Eigentum des Städelschen Museums-Vereins e.V.), the last portrait of his wife Charlotte. ***a*** In contrast, a prestroke painting of a similar subject, *Die schwarze Maske* (woman with a black mask), dating from 1908 (courtesy of Staatliche Museen Kassel), is much more realistic.

- Obscurity and blurriness, such as in several Walchensee paintings of 1924 and 1925
- Dissimilarity of familiar faces in portraits, for instance in a portrait drawing of his wife (1920), compared to a prestroke portrait (1911), possibly as a correlate of mild prosopagnosia
- Asymmetry and distortion of faces in portraits and self-portraits
- Lack of correct perspective, for example in the painting *On the Balcony in Bordighera* (1912) and in *Berlin unter den Linden* (1922)
- Anatomical curiosities and the lack of anatomical exactitude such as in a preparatory study for *Samson Blinded* (1912) and in *Pieta* (1920).

Maybe these examples could be completed by a more thorough analysis of Corinth's total oeuvre, but to be fair, large parts of his late work are simply superb products of a great artist and do not bear any 'pathological features', either from the point of view of a critical neurologist and ambitious pathographer. On the other hand, Corinth's immense number of artworks allows a detailed study of some very subtle consequences of his cerebrovascular disease.

True Art Means Seeking to Capture the Unreal

In the last year of his life, Lovis Corinth [1926] wrote in his memoirs: 'I have discovered something new. True art means seeking to capture the unreal. This is the highest goal!' According to Uhr [1990], Corinth had 'long ago abandoned conventional verisimilitude'; thus, this new discovery is probably not alluding to a pure technical artistic aspect, but might merely reflect a matter of conception. As Corinth came close to abstraction in his late work, though 'never yielding to it', this had merely prompted this recognition. Together with the maxim of 'drawing means to omit [details]', a phrase that has been ascribed to Corinth's friend Max Liebermann and which he had cited at the same place in his memoirs, there is suddenly the option to interpret these mottoes in the context of Corinth's stroke and its sequels. One might conclude that Corinth – deliberately or not – had invented a novel artistic principle on the basis of left-sided visuospatial hemineglect. At least, this may add to a most interesting debate regarding the 'late' Corinth that has not come to an end so far.

References

Bäzner H, Hennerici M: Stroke in painters; in Bradley RJ, Adron Harris R, Jenner P (eds): International Review of Neurobiology. Amsterdam, Elsevier, Academic Press, 2006, vol 74.
Berend-Corinth C: Lovis. Munich, Langen-Müller, 1958a.
Berend-Corinth C: Mein Leben mit Lovis Corinth. Munich, List, 1958b.
Blanke O: Visuospatial neglect in Lovis Corinth's self-portraits; in Bradley RJ, Adron Harris R, Jenner P (eds): International Review of Neurobiology. Amsterdam, Elsevier, Academic Press, 2006, vol 74.
Corinth L: Selbstbiographie. Berlin, Hirzel, 1926.
Corinth T: Lovis Corinth. Eine Dokumentation. Tübingen, Wasmuth, 1979.
Corinth W: Ich habe einen Lovis, keinen Vater. Munich, Langen Müller, 1980.
Gardner H: The pathology of art; in The Shattered Mind. London, Routledge & Kegan Paul, 1977, pp 291–349.
Gardner H, Winner E: Artistry and aphasia; in Sarno MT (ed): Acquired Aphasia. New York, Academic Press, 1981, pp 361–384.
Jung R: Neuropsychologie und Neurophysiologie des Kontur- und Formsehens in Zeichnung und Malerei; in Wieck HH (ed): Psychopathologie musischer Gestaltungen. Stuttgart, Schattauer, 1974, pp 29–88.
Kuhn A: Lovis Corinth. Berlin, Propyläen, 1925.
Schuster PK, Vitali C, Butts B: Lovis Corinth. Munich, Prestel, 1996.
Uhr H: Lovis Corinth. Berkeley, California University Press, 1990.

Hansjörg Bäzner, MD, PhD
Department of Neurology, University of Heidelberg
Universitätsklinikum Mannheim, Theodor Kutzer Ufer 1-3
DE–68135 Mannheim (Germany)
Tel. +49 621 383 3555, Fax +49 621 383 3807, E-Mail baezner@neuro.ma.uni-heidelberg.de

Bogousslavsky J, Hennerici MG (eds): Neurological Disorders in Famous Artists – Part 2.
Front Neurol Neurosci. Basel, Karger, 2007, vol 22, pp 44–74

Visconti and Fellini: From Left Social Neorealism to Right-Hemisphere Stroke

Sebastian Dieguez[a], *Gil Assal*[b], *Julien Bogousslavsky*[c]

[a]Brain Mind Institute, Laboratory of Cognitive Neuroscience, and [b]Chauderon 38, Lausanne, and [c]Department of Neurology, Valmont Clinic, Genolier Swiss Medical Network, Glion-sur-Montreux, Switzerland

Abstract

The acclaimed Italian directors Luchino Visconti and Federico Fellini had very different life trajectories that led them to become major figures in the history of cinema. Similarities, however, can be found in their debuts with the neorealist genre, their personalities, creative styles and politicocultural involvement, and ultimately in the neurological disease that struck them at the end of their careers. Both suffered a right-hemispheric stroke that left them hemiplegic on the left side. We review their life and career to put that event into perspective, and then discuss its aftermath for both artists in the light of our current knowledge of right-hemispheric functions. Visconti showed a tremendous resilience following the accident and managed to direct several films and plays as an infirm, whereas Fellini had to put an end to his career but still was able to display his talents to the neuropsychologists that treated him. A speculative account is given of the links between right-hemispheric symptomatology and the premorbid personality of these highly prolific patients.

Lumping Luchino Visconti and Federico Fellini together in a single chapter might foster the illusion that these two acclaimed film directors had comparable careers. Nothing could be farther from the truth. Although they were compatriots and contemporaries – the beginning and end of their respective careers were separated by about a decade, Visconti starting first – they never worked together and shared few actors and topics. Their backgrounds were enormously different and anyone who has seen their movies can attest to their wide stylistic contrast. However, in a book that concerns itself mainly with neurological disease, the analogy between both artists should not shock fans and scholars. It so happens that both of them had a stroke on the same side of the brain, the right side. Fellini was struck at age 73 and would die 3 months later from a second stroke, Visconti was 66 and would die 4 years later of influenza. And to clear up that relevant fact from the outset, both were right handed. Starting with these facts, one might feel entitled to delve into the past, taking a look, and comparing their lives and works. What we now know of their histories and symptoms could then be compared, leading to a discussion of patient variability and premorbid determinants of right-hemispheric symptomatology. We might as well also say, from the beginning, that our conclusions will be highly provocative. In the meantime, however, we will have to introduce both directors' lives and works separately, providing an account of each neurological casuistic. Before we go into this, it would also be important to devote some time to their common background in the history and cinema of Italy.

Italy had the misfortune of being the first European nation under a fascist government, from 1922 to 1945. Indeed, the very word 'fascism' was created at the incipience of this period, by the perpetrators themselves (by grouping fasci di combattimento as contrived by Mussolini). During that era, the cinema was obviously a tool of propaganda, or at best closely supervised and thereby harmless entertainment for the masses, as exemplified by the vapid 'telefono bianco' movies. It is in this context of dictatorship, anticommunism, media control and muzzled popular culture that the emergence of the neorealist movement immediately following the war must be understood. This will become relevant once we introduce Visconti's and Fellini's work, as both started their careers as neorealists.

For starters, what exactly is neorealism? Unfortunately, answering this question is rather like trying to capture what is or what became of structuralism or deconstructionism, a close to impossible task. Briefly, neorealism was construed as a response to the aforementioned, deplorable state of cinema and culture in postwar Italy, with a clear social and political intent. Story lines depicted everyday life for the working class as they struggled with difficult economic conditions and their moral aftermath. Italy was not in good shape in the 1940s: defeated, poor and still oppressed. These films hence had a Marxist feel to them, as they tried to embody social reality through the eye of the camera. Ideologically, their emphasis was on the need for democracy, a nonjudgmental attitude towards the working classes and the importance of authentic emotions and morality. Fascism was not so much directly denounced as subtly mocked throughout artistic choices. Stylistically, neorealist films were close to documentaries and often staged nonprofessional actors. These films were shot almost exclusively on location, obviously with an emphasis on realism, that is, plausible stories, characters and events. An absence of artificial devices gave the movies a certain 'organic' feel.

The two films most representative of the genre, which were not form the directors discussed here, are Roberto Rossellini's *Roma, Città Aperta* (1946) and Vittorio De Sica's *Ladri di Biciclette* (1948). Though neorealism per se enjoyed a short life span, it left a broad and durable impact on cinema as a whole. Its influence can still be seen in genres such as the spaghetti westerns of Sergio Leone, the French Nouvelle Vague, the documentary movement in the USA, and more recently the Danish Dogma school.

For the postwar left, a film's value was based mainly on whether an honest depiction of societal issues had been rendered, while hinting at a revolutionary solution. Directors who followed their own imperatives, whether artistic, historical or psychological, were immediately labeled conservative or reactionary, traitors of the 'cause'. As we shall see, this is a critique that would follow Visconti and Fellini throughout their entire careers, and their staunch resistance to being commandeered by any ideology or dogmatic framework may not be irrelevant to their reaction to disease.

Luchino Visconti

Life and Work

Visconti's life could arguably be a topic for a great movie. From his prestigious familial origins to the combative ending of his career, we revisit a uniquely strong character filled with fascinating contradictions. Count Don Luchino Visconti di Modrone was born November 2, 1906 in Milan. He is the descendant of a noble family that ruled Milan back to the Middle Ages. His grandfather, Duke Guido Visconti, was the director of the famous opera house La Scala and his second son, Don Giuseppe, married the immensely rich Carla Erba, heiress of an important pharmaceutical company. Luchino, the fourth son of these two, was thus raised in an environment of outstanding wealth and style, surrounded by famous figures of the cultural and social scene. A strikingly handsome young man, he became a womanizer and paid little attention to any formal education, going from private school to private school. He also discovered his homosexuality very early on, and remained quite ambiguous about this for the rest of his life. Before he became an acclaimed director, Visconti's main passions were horses and driving fast cars. The former came from his experience in the army cavalry and led him to become a successful race-horse breeder. The latter resulted in the death of his chauffeur in an accident where Visconti was at the wheel, and in his subsequent, temporary retirement to the Tassili region of the Sahara desert, a period we know little about and, during which his view of life apparently changed profoundly. The aristocrat then traveled in Europe and America.

In France, Visconti met Coco Chanel, who introduced him to Jean Renoir, a successful French film maker in the 1930s. Visconti became his assistant during the period of the Front Populaire in Paris. From Renoir, he imbibed a spirit of realism and the sense of refined lavishness, which are really antinomic concepts but, nevertheless, would end up characterizing the new Italian cinema. Contrary to the pure standards of neorealism, Visconti would never sacrifice estheticism for realism, as was also true of Fellini. Favorite topics were the disintegration of the family and the decadence of aristocracy and the bourgeoisie, which he knew first hand. His family had split up in 1924 following the separation of his parents, who would never see each other again. His sister, Uberta, was to transmogrify into his replacement mother.

His first movie was *Ossessione* (1943), a transposition of James Caine's novel *The Postman Always Rings Twice* to fascist Italy, which many argued would truly launch the neorealism movement. Showing the reality of misery in low social classes was quite revolutionary at the time, as was any portrayal of homosexuality, or openly challenging traditional institutions such as marriage. The movie was immediately condemned by the Catholic Church. It was even said that holy water was spread on screens where it had been shown. Visconti was just beginning to discover that he was a scandalous man and this movie was an extraordinary debut for him.

Visconti filmed poverty again in *La Terra Trema* (1948), a movie funded by the Italian Communist Party, with which he would remain affiliated. He then departed from the strict purity of neorealism with *Senso* (1954), where he began to display his taste for the theatrical and grandiose, and for the first time in color. The films which followed are among his best known works: *Rocco and his Brothers* (1960), *The Leopard* (1963), *The Damned* (1969), *Death in Venice* (1971), and *Ludwig* (1972). However, the editing of Ludwig was interrupted by a stroke. As we will describe in the next section, he made two more films afterwards: *Conversation Piece* (1974) and *The Innocent* (1976), which was posthumously shown as a premiere at the Cannes Film Festival. Most of his films were derived from famous literary works, but Mendes Sargo (1963–1964) notes that: 'He approached these works as a pretext, as it were, to make films that stand on their own feet and not to make films as mere illustrations or adaptations of books.' Indeed, he mixed the most scrupulous faithfulness to texts with wild liberties of his own. However, this proved completely impossible for what he saw as the project of his life: adapting Proust's *A la Recherche du Temps Perdu* to the screen. The project was disproportionate and he seemed to have abandoned it even before his stroke, as the problems he faced seemed insuperable [as others after him would also learn, see Ifri, 2005].

Dirk Bogarde, one of Visconti's favorite actors, asked himself: 'Was he decadent? I never witnessed that. Homosexual? Though I never held him the candle, I always supposed he was. Cruel? Sometimes. And arrogant? Seriously. Generous? Very so. Amusing? I don't think so. I rarely heard his laughter. Only a few times, I saw him vaguely smile, an eyebrow raised. This was generally in front of a good cook, as he was himself fond of cookery. I heard a loud laughter, like a dog barking, then he quickly spoke in the cook's own dialect. But I never knew anyone like him, certainly not in the world of cinema, who could speak of Klimt, Karajan, Proust, "Peanuts", Mozart and Mantovani (he liked the Eurovision song contest), Duse and Doris Day' [Bogard, 1990].

Politically, Visconti was criticized for 'voting left and living right'. Salvador Dali sneered that 'he was a Communist who only liked luxury'. Indeed, his productions were increasingly lavish and created an ever-heightened sense of melodrama. His late films explored the nature of high-society's decadence. For a time, he had some curiosity and admiration for fascism. He even went to Germany to see the nascent Nazi displays. But soon, especially as he gradually came to terms with his homosexuality, he was repelled by the whole thing. He kept, however, a taste for the notion of social order and revolution, frequently visited in his movies. As he told an American reporter in 1961, 'I believe in life, that is the central point… I believe in organised society. I think it has a chance.'

Critics have often emphasized the inconsistencies of the social and political involvements in Visconti's works. One wrote: 'Born on the barricades, the work dies on the sofas' [in Criqui, 1982]. The frequent use of the word 'melodrama' by activist critics shows quite well the pejorative view held of the late Visconti. There certainly is an evolution to that effect in Visconti's career; a Marxist observer could readily see that the proletarian and revolutionary content of his movies went 'from fire, to embers, to ashes' [Criqui, 1982]. But this is to acknowledge the uniqueness of an unclassifiable man: he would enjoy more than anything to be seen as a radical threat by his fellow aristocrats while being denigrated as a pompous grand bourgeois by activists on the left. However, the evolution from the neorealism of his beginnings to the operatic impressionism of his last movies should not be seen as a change in his political opinions. His allegiance to the left was sincere, but his career was long. He was first forced to deal with fascist censorship, then with that of the Christian Democrats. As the social scene changed enormously so did the movie industry and his priorities. As he grew older it was eventually infirmity that caught him, not the intransigence of age [Criqui, 1982]. While certainly not guilty of changing his colors, one has to recognize that Visconti was in a cumbersome position from the beginning. As Criqui [1982] wrote: '[Here] appears the big problem with Visconti, his inability to reconcile contradictory aspirations: aristocrat and Marxist, individualist and humanist, aesthete and activist, the descendant of the dukes of Modrone has a hard time finding his way between his passion for the beautiful and his revolutionary ideal, between poetry and realism' (p. 839). Indeed, his defiance of black and white categorizations was visible up to his open bisexuality, which could also be seen in the underlying homoeroticism of many of his movies, if one's attention were not entirely captured by the stunningly beautiful actresses he liked to film.

Disease

Asked by a worried friend how many cigarettes he smoked per day, Visconti sneeringly answered: 'About three thousand, you think that's enough?' That was a bit of an exaggeration of course, as Visconti merely smoked about 80 cigarettes a day, up to 120 when stressed. That would safely count as a risk factor for stroke. Another less publicized compulsion of Visconti's was his frenetic consumption of coffee. Not any coffee though, he made it himself and it was said that if a naïve collaborator drank a single cup, he would find no sleep for a whole week. This man also put too much into his work, this is certain. Also, conditions at shoots did not help either: the shooting of *Ludwig* took place in the cold mountains of Bavaria. After finishing some extra scenes at Cinecittà, he spent some days under the overwhelming sun of Tunisia. Back to Rome, on July 27, 1972 – a 'perfectly ordinary day', that is, another carnival of work, meetings, coffee and cigarettes – his favorite scriptwriter, Suso Cecchi d'Amico, found him unusually pale [all the following quotations in this section are from Schifano, 1987, pp. 431–456]. As he brought a glass of champagne to his lips, he said, 'it seems to me it is not cold enough' and, putting the glass on the table, he was hit by a stroke. He bent forward and grasped his armchair, without falling or losing consciousness. He was 66 years old. He would later say that he remembered the episode entirely: 'There was not a moment where I wasn't perfectly lucid.' His friends brought him into a room and took his shoes off. Visconti remembers having thought, upon seeing his 'electric blue' socks: 'How could I have made such a visual mistake?' Visconti seemed embarrassed by the whole spectacle, Suso remembers: 'One of his legs was moving of its own will, it was absolutely uncontrolable… I have never seen anything like that; it seemed like a leg gone crazy. And Luchino kept excusing himself, so much so that, in the end, I had to leave the room, so as not to bother him too much.'

Visconti was brought to a clinic in Rome that he disliked, his room was too hot and too small. He had innumerable visitors there, all of whom he engaged in conversation and reminisced, even a Professor Lopez who came expressly from Madrid to see him. The left side of his body was completely paralyzed; he had to spend 15 days in bed, totally immobile. The blow was very hard, but it seems that he was spared mentally, as he could think, reason, and enjoy music on a little tape player. Indeed, he was quite aware of the explanations the doctors gave him: 'Luckily, I got it on the right side, if it were the left side that would have been tough, because on the left there's the centre for speech and intelligence, if in my case there ever was one…' There certainly was no damage to his sense of humor. But he became increasingly frustrated and felt guilty: 'I recognized at once that all this was my own fault, because I didn't follow any advice I should have followed, because I went on smoking despite the warnings, because I didn't take any rest... It has been said that the cardiovascular collapse has been caused by the cigarettes. It is true, I smoked a lot, 70 or 80 cigarettes a day, certain days up to 120. It became an automatism, I hardly noticed I was even smoking anymore. When one is working, one doesn't notice one is smoking that much.' When his condition permitted him to be transferred, he was taken to the University Hospital of Zürich, in Switzerland, where the great neurologist and neurosurgeon, Hugo Krayenbühl, took care of him[1].

Of course, there was not much to be done for Visconti's condition, except for physiotherapeutic exercise in which he would engage with tremendous energy and courage. The master now needed help with the simplest activities, a cruel humiliation for a man of domination and liberty like him. He had a hard time even standing by himself on a chair. Maybe more than other patients, he hated his disease: 'Before, I was free. I used to mistreat my body as if that were the most natural thing to do... And suddenly, the blow, the revision. The improvised discovery that I could not do certain things anymore... That liberty has run away forever... That's why I hate my disease: because it has deprived me of my freedom. Because it has humiliated me and continues humiliating me... Because I must learn to walk again, to move my hands, to use them again... And the need to be assisted ... It's so degrading.'

More than anything, Visconti hated the word 'patience', which the doctors kept repeating to him. Tons of letters reached him everyday during the 2 months of his stay in Zürich, and friends came to see him from all over the world. However, Visconti was far from finished. Being hemiplegic and in a hospital is strong motivation for the arrest of many professional lives, but Visconti had work to finish. *Ludwig* was yet to be edited and the sound needed synchronization: 'the will to work even more than the will to live', as he would say, '... The fear of not finishing *Ludwig*... I couldn't stop worrying about *Ludwig*, not a minute. To the contrary, I must say that it is this worry which gave me the strength to fight the disease, the strength to make strenuous physical exercises every day.... That is why *Ludwig* is the film I love the most.'

Professor Krayenbühl understood the kind of patient he was dealing with. He said: 'Visconti, you don't have to stay. Go away, leave the hospital and go on with your work.' As soon as possible, he left for his villa in Cernobbio, by the Lake Como, where an editing room had been installed especially for him. Not

[1]These were the 1970s, the reader should take good note that there was something prestigious about 'Swiss clinics' at that time.

only did he manage to finish *Ludwig*, but already other projects popped in his mind. Thomas Mann's *The Magic Mountain* was foremost, as it is the story of a sick man, the author of which died in the same hospital where Visconti was a patient. The director, only 2 months after his stroke, was back into the game. His determination seemed indestructible: 'I *must* bring all my projects to an end. I cannot renounce. I must do it.' However, *Ludwig* was mutilated beyond recognition by commercial directives and was a commercial failure. Perhaps Visconti was too vulnerable at this time to defend what he wanted to be his masterpiece. Far from discouraged, he continued fighting the disease and the difficulties to set up his projects. Though he could hardly move his left leg and arm, and needed a cane to walk, he seemed very lucid and did not, for one second, think of retirement. He could sensibly have done so, however. Visconti had nothing more to prove, except perhaps to himself. His last years are a vibrant lesson in resilience; it is almost as if the stroke was nothing but a mere obstacle in his career: 'If I didn't work, I would be so bored that I'd throw myself out of the terrace. Someone who, like me, has worked unremittingly during 30 or 40 years, cannot stay inert. It would be like removing morphine from a drug addict.'

Almost immediately, Visconti began to consider future possibilities. He set up *Old Times*, a play by Harold Pinter. However, Visconti was, by then, 'like a surgeon who cannot operate with his own hands'. Nevertheless, a journalist wrote: 'Many came ... to see how he was reduced by disease. Well, I hope they took note that he is still the best.' However, almost immediately, an infuriated Harold Pinter turned up to denounce the 'obscene' treatment of his work by Visconti. It seemed that the master, hapless as many would like to see him, was more scandalous than ever. Unhindered by his persisting paresis, he then set up another theatrical play, Puccini's *Manon Lescaut*, while continuing his own, exhausting 'therapeutic exercises'.

One year after his stroke, Visconti decided to go back to the camera. The project was *Gruppo di famiglia in un interno* (*Conversation Piece*). He had not fully recovered, but he managed to direct while standing upright. The film is a kind of counterpart to *The Leopard*, this time approaching the political climate of his time. He was, by then, unable to manage the gigantic proportions of his earlier, sumptuous displays, so quite aptly he decided to direct a contemporary *huis clos* which allowed him to address the social changes of the early 1970s. This film, though often seen as autobiographical, should rather be considered his testament. Again, Visconti managed to stir a scandal, this time because the film was funded by a right-wing publisher, which outraged his fellow leftists. Instead of simply replying that no one else at this time would put money into a movie directed by an invalid, Visconti created a polemic by saying: 'Where does the money of other film-makers come from? From workers' unions perhaps? I know of no single left-wing entrepreneur. I never knew one, I never saw

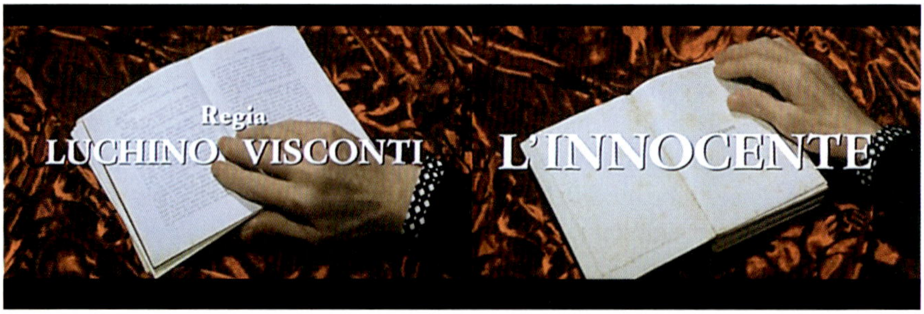

Fig. 1. Visconti's right hand is seen in the opening credits for *The Innocent*, his last movie. He uses it without help from the left hand, and fumbles on some occasions. Was the left hand too handicapped or did he prefer to keep it hidden for cinematic purposes?

one.... Films are made with money, the producers bring in that money, and these really are no ascetics tormented by the problem of social injustice.' Again, the master gives evidence of his perfectly realistic frame of mind.

Other projects did not make it, though. Like Thomas Mann's *The Magic Mountain*: 'Yes, this one will be an autobiographical film', he frequently said, 'because it's the story of a disease and you know my current condition...'. However, Suso Cecchi said: 'No producer would hear about it. Indeed, the story of an ill man, shot by an ill man...' [Schifano, 1987, p. 448]. Besides, filming in the cold winter of Davos would have been absolutely impossible in his state.

His last film was *The Innocent*, adapted from a novel by Gabriele d'Annunzio (fig. 1). By the spring of 1975 Visconti had mostly recovered his previous vigor. He was even able, in his state, to convey the inherent eroticism and cruelty of d'Annunzio's novel. He insisted on directing the movie upright, without his cane. Everyday he practiced walking, alone in his room. The result was calamitous: on April 3, he fell and broke his right (nonparalyzed) leg. Back to the hospital and back to frustration. He blamed his life, which until now 'had been a friend and became the cruellest of his enemies'. That 'life which he had always dominated and now dominates him' [quoted in Schifano, 1987, p. 451]. Indeed, now his two legs had gone. All was ready for the movie to roll, but Visconti was reluctant to show up in his diminished state. In the end, he accepted his role as director in a wheelchair. His doctors were quite sure that directing this movie under the tedious heat of the summer would destroy him, but they reasoned that maybe it was the best thing for him to continue his work anyway. He seemed resolute and indestructible. To the journalists, he boasted: 'Despite this wheelchair, here I am, ready to direct another movie. Next time, maybe I will do so from a stretcher, but I will never give up.'

Visconti worked harder than ever, directing and preparing for the next day, staying up late, resuming his frenetic smoking. Many people were involved, and whenever someone moved him in his wheelchair, he would quip: 'Lets move the cadaver!' All along, he seemed perfectly aware that this was going to be his last movie. Doing it seemed to be enough to keep him alive for the time being. He used to say, 'The day I will not be able to work anymore I will shoot myself in the head.' The surest sign that one is dead is to have one's movies displayed on television, he thought: 'It will be my turn soon.... It's logic; but it is the sign that you are done.'

In the first months of 1976, Visconti was struck by influenza. On March 17, in his bed with flu, surrounded by flowers, his dogs and the pictures of Helmut Berger and Marlène Dietrich, he listened to the Second Symphony of Brahms in the company of his sister, Uberta. When the music ended, he looked at Uberta and said in Milanese: 'That's it. I'm tired.' After that, he died.

Luchino Visconti's funeral was attended by President Giovanni Leone and Burt Lancaster. That day, the walls of Rome were covered with the following notice: 'Luchino Visconti. A man of great culture whose work has enriched, for more than thirty years, the history of art, of cinema and of theatre in our country, Europe, and the world. We will not forget Luchino Visconti, antifascist activist of the resistance who always showed a deep and truthful solidarity with workers and fighters.'

In many of his movies, the intrigue revolves around the notion that the end of something is really the beginning of something else. Remember the words of Tancredi in *The Leopard*, played by the young Alain Delon: 'If we want things to stay as they are, things will have to change.' Visconti's work was a new beginning, and presumably the end of something. As for any direct influence from his stroke on his last two films, there are absolutely no right-hemispheric 'symptoms' to be detected (one would indeed be surprised to see a movie made by a director with unilateral neglect). There is certainly a change in style, if one compares *Conversation Piece* and *The Innocent* with earlier movies, but we are quite sure that this is due both to the personal evolution of the author and to the adjustments required by infirmity, which rather than 'symptomatic' are perfectly voluntary. The main character of *Conversation Piece*, an ageing professor often seen as the counterpart of Visconti himself, aptly explains this notion by invoking: 'the terrible knowledge that is given by all disease, less by the suffering it causes than by the strange novelty of the definitive restrictions it imposes to life. One sees oneself dead, in that case, not at the precise moment of death, but months, sometimes years before, from the moment the disease comes hideously to dwell inside of us.'

Anosognosia?

The extraordinary fighting spirit of Visconti following his right-hemispheric stroke raises the legitimate question of a possible anosognosia in the director. After all, perhaps he somehow failed to entirely realize the severity of his condition. Though it may well be the case that the stroke was primarily subcortical – as apparently there were no higher cortical impairments such as unilateral neglect, delusions or visuospatial disorders – subtle cognitive deficits may also appear in those types of strokes, presumably due to diaschisis. Obviously, he was well aware of his impairment. But anosognosia can be described as a more subtle disorder than plain denial of hemiplegia. Right from the beginning, Babinski [1914] distinguished between anosognosia (unawareness and denial of hemiplegia) and anosodiaphoria (awareness of hemiplegia with inappropriate emotional impact) [see also Critchley, 1957]. What is more, Marcel et al. [2004] have recently proposed a fine-grained analysis of anosognosia, where the 'unawareness' of such patients may be quite specific, for example involving only a lack of appreciation of the consequences of the stroke. It has also been proposed that anosognosia may involve a decrease in negative emotions, thereby inducing overly optimistic thoughts and actions in right-hemispheric patients [but see Turnbull et al., 2005].

However, Visconti was also quite realistic. He had been told that it would be 1 year before he recovered: 'However', he said, 'I think it would be much longer. One needs patience and will. I never had much patience, but I have lots of will.' Besides, his last films are evidently not devoid of 'negative emotions', rather the contrary. His treatment of the scripts shows how lucid and sharp his mind was, as *Conversation Piece* and *The Innocent* involve highly complicated psychological ploys between the characters, which, by the way, indicates that there was surely no impairment of 'theory of mind' [the human ability to represent, understand and manipulate other minds has been theorized as a function of the right hemisphere, see Griffin et al., 2006]. Besides, these two movies have a sense of psychological realism that seems to preclude altogether a delusional, impaired or overoptimistic frame of mind from their director. It is therefore safe to reject anosognosia to any degree in Visconti.

Federico Fellini

Life and Work

Federico Fellini was born in 1920 in the seaside town of Rimini, on the Adriatic coast of Italy. Of his childhood, he would say that: 'Although I am often described as the "filmmaker of memory", I really remember very few things [from childhood]' [Fellini, 1984]. He quit the provinces for Rome at age 18 to make his debut as a journalist, scriptwriter and cartoonist. A gifted drawer since his school days, he also became a wandering caricaturist and was hired in 1939 by *Marc'Aurelio*, a widely read humorous magazine. In 1944, after the fall of Mussolini, he even opened a shop where he would draw caricatures of American marines. It is in this shop that he met Roberto Rossellini. He would work with the famed director (for *Rome Open City*, 1945 and *Paisà*, 1946) and with other neorealists on various scripts, though he had no formal technical training in his profession. As for his influences, Fellini preferred Chaplin, Buster Keaton, Laurel and Hardy, and the Marx brothers to more 'respectable' intellectual names. Fellini's formative influences can be traced back to the popular Italian culture of the period, and not primarily the cinema. Cartoons, caricature sketches, and radio comedy brought him to the cinema as a gagman and scriptwriter. The caricature and the grotesque would always be an obvious visual influence on his later works [Stubbs, 1993]. Fellini was trained 'on the job', so to speak: over 10 years of scriptwriting and an on-the-set apprenticeship equipped him with practical skills and valuable insights.

Also, Fellini began his career at the heart of the postwar neorealist movement, which would be the first inspiration for his early films. However, his work would soon depart from the strict, neorealist standards and he would begin to develop his own, inimitable style. In the words of the journalist Jonathan Jones: 'One of the ways in which he rejected Marxism was by dwelling on the true scale and depth of Italy's history, the ghosts of baroque Rome, and most of all Roman Rome. Like Julietta talking to the spirits, Fellini prophesied wonders and terrors. He created the most original visual images that cinema has produced in the sound era. He demonstrated the space and range and life of which film is capable' [Jones, 2004]. Indeed, Italian neorealism ended in 1948. Postwar Italy was quickly changing, liberal and left wing parties were defeated at the polls, levels of income were increasing. American films became the big thing and the vision of a desolate, poverty-stricken country was simply too depressing for a newly emerging democracy that aimed at prosperity. Federico Fellini's films perfectly captured this move, from social and political concerns to the new self-fulfilled individual, with individual anxieties about happiness and success. In his book *Fellini's Films: from Postwar to Postmodern*, Burke [1996] extensively deals with Fellini's evolution. He traces in his works the rise and fall of individualism, 'the movement from a relatively realist cinema, generally concealing the act of filmmaking itself, to a highly self-conscious examination of cinematic and narrative technique'.

While it is true that Fellini's first films were clearly in the neorealist tradition, (*Luci del Varietà* (1950), *Lo Sceicco Bianco* (1952), and *I Vitelloni* (1953)), he displayed, from the beginning, a concern for 'character subjectivity', which he treated with great humor in his portrayals of eccentrics and clownish personalities. After working on the script of Rosselini's *Paisà*, he redefined his artistic credo as 'looking at reality with an honest eye – but any kind of reality; not just social reality, but also spiritual reality, metaphysical reality, anything man has inside him' [in Bondanella and Gieri, 1987, p. 217]. Quite like Visconti, Fellini was also trashed by the left for betraying his neorealist origins and notably for introducing religious undertones about salvation in *Il Bidone* (1955) and *La Strada* (1954) – the film Fellini called 'the complete catalogue of my entire mythological world. *La Strada* is indeed an important transitional movie in the history of Italian film. The larger social concerns of humanity, treated by neorealists, gave way to the treatment of more individual needs and the difficulties of human communication. However, this idea of salvation should by no means be seen as a dogmatic ideology in Fellini. Quite to the contrary, he had very little patience with the Church, as he showed in *Le Notti di Cabiria* (1957). In that tale of a prostitute looking for love, Fellini shows the shrine to be ineffective for a crippled man who falls flat while trying to walk, and the prostitute's prayers go hopelessly unanswered.

La Dolce Vita (1959) – arguably his most famous movie – points to Italy's economic boom of the late 1950s and the rise of consumerism and celebrity worship. We follow Marcello Mastroianni as a photoreporter in Rome, accompanied by his assistant Paparazzo, a name that will stick in common parlance. Over three hours long, the storyline gives way to an emphasis on the visuals and a 'jumpy' narration which gave rise to unforgettable – if rather unrelated – images, like the buxom Anita Ekberg capriciously enjoying the Trevi Fountain. This highlight, unfortunately, might easily obscure other great moments such as the sarcastic coverage of a sighting of the Virgin by two children, the hilarious, vapid intellectualizing of the high society, the pathetically decadent orgy in a borrowed apartment and the mystical stumbling upon a monster fish on the beach at dawn. The story revolves around a tabloid account of sterile love affairs, behind which the disillusioned Marcello will engage in a quest for purity and truth. This is shown symbolically as a failure in the last scene, where Marcello cannot hear the words of the only innocent and authentic person of the movie. Fellini's increasing genius and pessimism earned him a worldwide reputation with this movie. From his next movie on (*Eight and a Half*, 1963), he will devote much more effort to his fantasies and memories (*The Clowns, Fellini's Roma, Amarcord*). His last films will go further in the analysis of the ploys of authorship and the baroque (*Satyricon, Casanova, City of Women, E la Nave Va, Ginger and Fred, Intervista, La Voce della Luna*). His favorite topics, nascent in his earlier films, will be constantly expanded until the end of his career: authorial self-consciousness, dreams (in his own words, 'I make a film in the same manner in which I live a dream…'), imagination and memory. Causal relations and logical connections in storylines would increasingly give way to further interplays between fantasy and reality. It has been said that his whole career could be summarized as follows: from simplicity, to complexity, to self-parody [Stubbs, 1993]. Fellini, by then, has not merely buried neorealism but all rules of what cinema was supposed to be. 'Why must it have a simple story, clear idea, lucid images? Is that really like life?', asks journalist Jonathan Jones [2004]. Esotericism and the unconscious would be explored in *Roma, Intervista* and *Giulietta degli Spiriti*, where the author's images and subjectivity keep replacing the storyline. All his films dramatize the clash between a character's social 'role' or 'mask' and the more authentic 'face' of his true aspirations. *Satyricon* (1969) portrays a labyrinth and Minotaur as the director's own unmanageable unconscious. In *Amarcord* (1973), exploring what he called his 'invented memories' (see Pettigrew's award-winning feature documentary, *Fellini: I'm a Born Liar*), he goes back to his childhood and teenage years in the Rimini of the fascist era, conveying, in his dreamlike fashion, a more honest account of fascist Italy than in many early neorealist movies.

Fellini's politics were ambiguous. We have seen that he was considered a traitor by the left, which was very much in accordance with Visconti's experience. Indeed, in various movies he shows little patience for serious and grave activism. But he always sided with the underdog in times of police repression. Jones [2004] writes that: 'Fellini rightly sees that "post-fascist" popular culture is not innately virtuous, but might even be fascistic itself. In reality, postwar Italy was consumerist, media-saturated and glamour-obsessed, and Fellini reflected all of this accurately.' Doctrinal leftism, in the guise of Pasolini's violent diatribes, was obviously too serious for him.

> Fellini was criticised at home for betraying or perhaps never having supported the left. However, the superficial difference between his early 'neorealist' films and his later visual feasts vanishes on closer inspection. Fellini never made films about the working class. He made films about people who are far more desperate than that – misfits, classless fantasists. Fellini made films that uniquely combine acerbic realism and unhinged poetic fantasy, about things you can barely put into words: the extremes of cruelty and innocence, the madness and authority of love. He was never a neorealist. He was the greatest realist of all [Jones, 2004].

Exposing the means of the creative act in filmmaking (in contrast to the neorealist posture of delivering an unmediated story with newsreel esthetics), Fellini, in line with the compatriots Pirandello and Calvino in the same period, uncovers the 'ploy' of authorship. *Intervista* (1988) concentrates all the issues reflecting on cinema itself, in the form of an amalgamated film that includes its author's present and past, or what Fellini called a 'live' film. In one of his rare interviews, he said: 'I make the film as if I were escaping from something, as if I were in flight, to get rid of it, to get it off my back. Like getting rid of an illness. I don't want to exaggerate the pathological aspects of the creative act, but deep down, that's what it is.... I am...a puppeteer, a marionettist, a storyteller.... I recognize that this is my life' [Bachmann, 1994].[2]

[2]This is a collection of conversations held *before* the stroke.

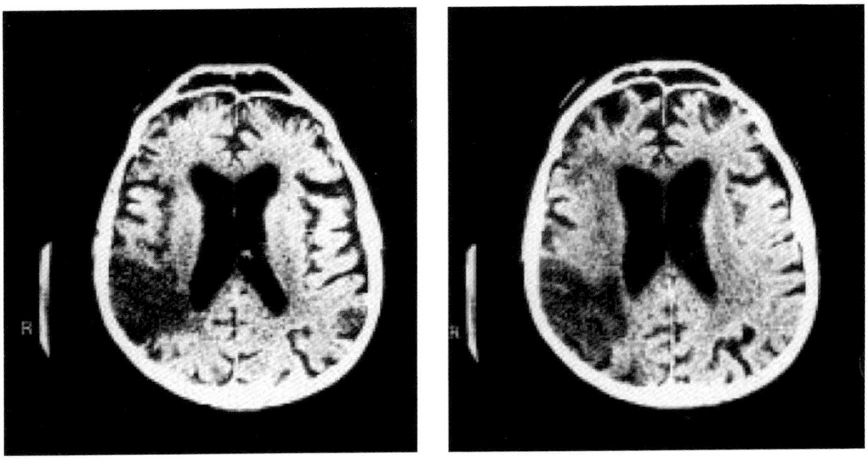

Fig. 2. CT scan of Fellini 1 week after the stroke showing the large lesion encroaching upon the temporoparietal regions of the right hemisphere. The CT scan was performed at the Hospital of Rimini [from Cantagallo and Della Sala, 1998, with kind permission].

At the Academy Awards Ceremony in March of 1993, Fellini received a special Oscar for lifetime achievement in filmmaking. The statuette was added to a quartet of Best Foreign Language Film awards for *La Strada* (*The Road*, 1954), *Le Notti di Cabiria* (*The Nights of Cabiria*, 1957), *Otto e Mezzo* (*Eight and a Half*, 1963) and *Amarcord* (*I Remember*, 1973). In August of that same year, Fellini suffered a stroke (see below for details) and succumbed, at the end of October, to a second, massive, stroke. After his death at age 73, on October 31 – one day after he and his wife (who was to die of cancer less than 5 months later) celebrated their 50th wedding anniversary – tens of thousands of people packed the narrow streets of Fellini's hometown of Rimini, applauding as the director's casket was carried from the main piazza to the cinema where Fellini had watched his first films as a child.

Disease

At 73 years old, shortly after having received his Oscar for his lifetime achievement, Fellini suffered a stroke in the territory of the right middle cerebral artery (fig. 2). As we shall see, even at his worst Fellini managed to teach us an important peculiarity of the human mind. True, the stroke ended his career, but he was still very creative as a patient, and his specific symptoms seemed like an invention of his own. Indeed, his case raises the most confusing questions about the nature of self-awareness. Usually, patients who, like him, suffer from left unilateral neglect have poor insight into their condition. Patients with this condition behave as if their left visual space simply no longer existed. What is more, they simply do not *notice* that something is lacking in their experiential field. But this was not the case for Fellini. In what follows, we draw extensively from the very detailed report of the neuropsychologists Anna Cantagallo and Sergio Della Sala, who were able to examine the director at some length for 2 months following his stroke. This is in contrast to Visconti, for whom there is – to our knowledge – no neuropsychological exam available. Modern neuropsychology was already well on its way by 1972, so presumably Professor Krayenbühl would have detected anomalous cognitive features in Visconti if there had been any substantially obvious ones.

When Fellini was first examined, he presented with a severe sensorimotor left hemisyndrome and a left inferior quadranopsia. He had preserved eye movements and no head deviation, but showed florid, unilateral visuospatial neglect. The hemisyndrome itself showed little recovery in the 2 months he survived. From the beginning, it was clear that he was not anosognosic of his physical impairment. On the contrary, according to the authors, he displayed hints of misoplegia, i.e. negative feelings towards his paralyzed limb [Loetscher et al., 2006], which he called 'a bloated, damp bunch of asparagus'. He also showed some confusion at night, believing he was in his real home instead of the hospital (a nocturnal form of reduplicative paramnesia). He was otherwise alert and collaborative with the staff, with preserved language functions and general intelligence. Other than the neglect syndrome, which will be described below, he had no neuropsychiatric impairment (e.g. no prosopagnosia, visual agnosia, amnesia, depression or delusions).

Fellini's neglect profile was characterized by severe visual extinction (a left stimulus went unseen when another was presented in the right hemifield at the same time), and an extrapersonal visual neglect in classic paper-and-pencil tasks like target cancellation, geometric shape copying, and line bisection, all of which showed some improvement after 1 month. Fellini would not merely follow the instructions of the neuropsychologist docily by 'bisecting' lines or copying complex shapes, he would spontaneously add drawings that were not only very creative, but were also evidence that he was aware, at least implicitly, of the errors he made (see figs. 3–6). Neglect was also apparent in his reading: he would often 'forget' or 'confabulate' the beginning of the words. For example, 'disgrazie' became 'grazie', and 'giace' became 'piace'. This showed poor improvement after 1 month, but by this time reading an entire text correctly was possible. In contrast, Fellini never showed neglect signs for writing, neither spontaneously nor on dictation.

The apparent, implicit processing of his left hemifield, as shown by his drawings, was further studied by the authors. Using specific stimuli called

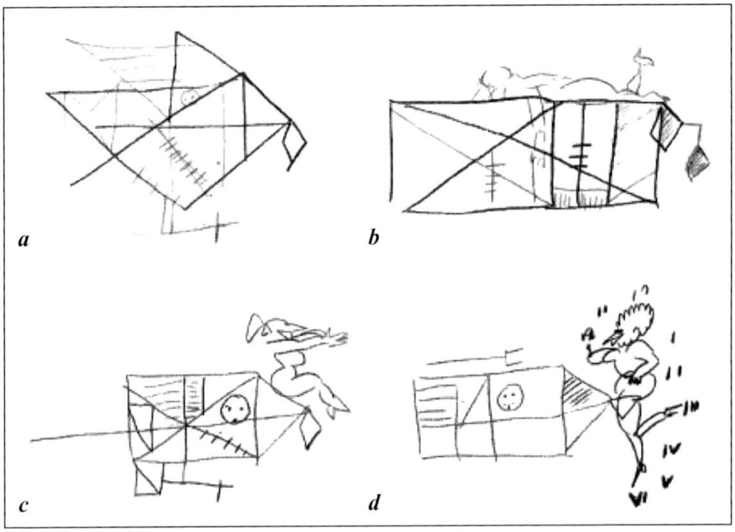

Fig. 3. Fellini's performance on the Rey's figure: first assessment: copy (***a***) and memory (***b***), and second assessment: copy (***c***) and memory (***d***). ***d*** Note the drawing of a clock with the Roman numbers from I to VI on the right and Arab digits from 10 to 12 on the left and anticlockwise [from Cantagallo and Della Sala, 1998, with kind permission].

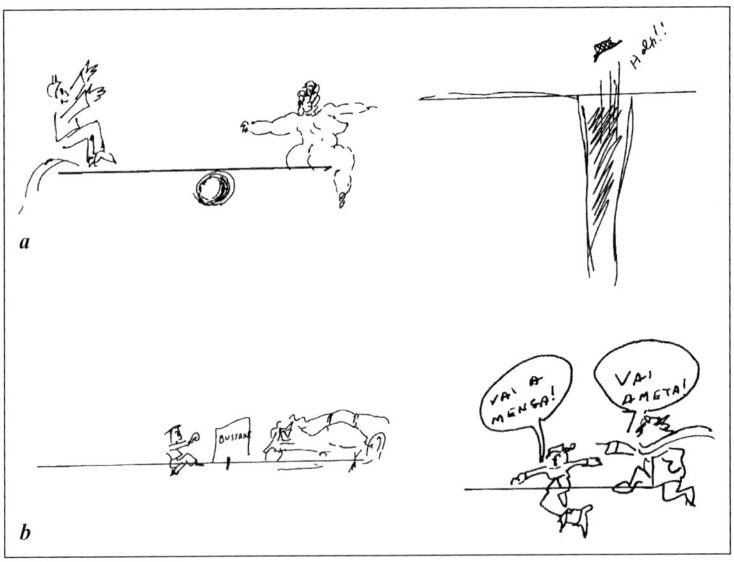

Fig. 4. Some examples of line bisection performances of Fellini. He often tended to personalize his performance (***a***). However, in so doing, some times he clearly showed that his perception of the stimulus reached the leftmost extremity (***b***) [from Cantagallo and Della Sala, 1998, with kind permission].

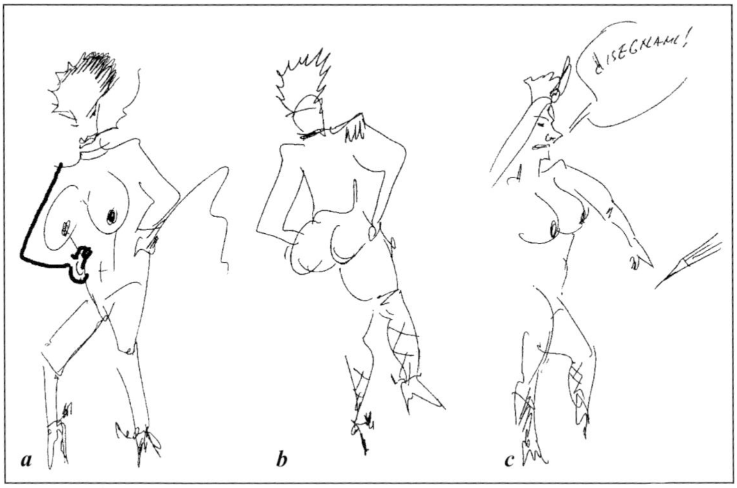

Fig. 5. Fellini's drawing from memory (25 days after the stroke) of a female human figure from three different perspectives on three separate sheets of paper, front (***a***), back (***b***) and in profile (***c***). In all three instances some details are missing from the left part of the human figure. ***a*** Fellini realized his omission, and made up for it adding in a second go with a red pencil the right arm of the woman he had drawn with a blue ballpoint pen. ***c*** He added the command 'draw me!' as if coming from one of the female neuropsychologists assessing him [from Cantagallo and Della Sala, 1998, with kind permission].

'chimeras', they were indeed able to gain some insight into this. For example, while Fellini was not able to consciously perceive the difference between a normal banknote and one torn on the left, he would 'prefer' the untorn one on the grounds that 'it is bigger' or, using his characteristic humor, that 'there is no Craxi' on it (Craxi being an infamous former Italian minister). Shown a trombone with a rifle butt on its left side, he did not see the incongruence but described it as a 'trombone to fire notes'.

While Fellini clearly had unilateral neglect for his left extrapersonal visual space, he showed no such impairment with regard to his own body. He could reach out with his left hand, point to and name body parts on both sides equally, and simulate bilateral combing and shaving. Thus, he had no so-called 'personal neglect'. He had no 'representational neglect' either; meaning his ability to visualize full maps mentally was spared. When asked to draw from his memory, for example a daisy, a bike, a table or a figure (figs. 7, 8), he showed rather mild signs of left neglect. Furthermore, he tended to collapse his drawings on the right side of the paper, which is a classic neglect symptom. However, 1 month after being tested, that is, 2 months after his stroke, his drawings were again comparable to an earlier one without neglect (fig. 9).

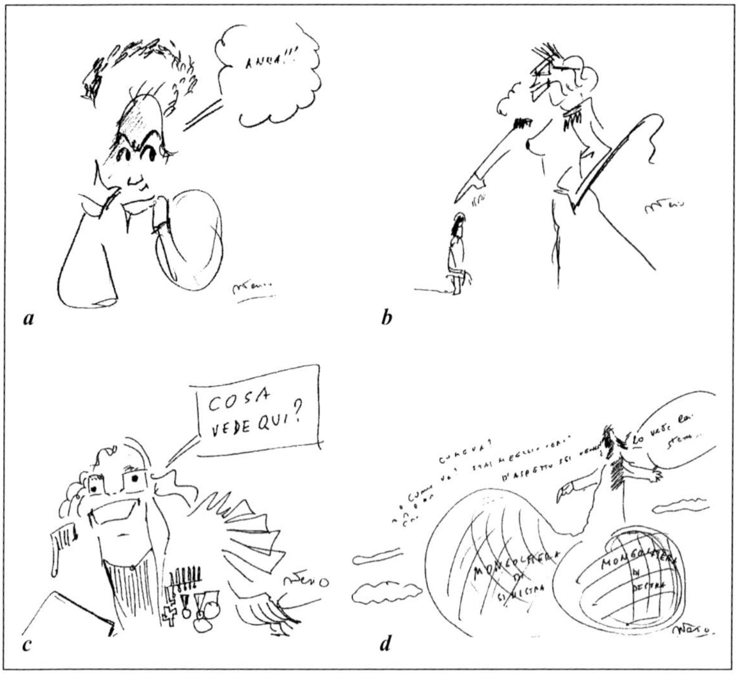

Fig. 6. Fellini's spontaneous drawings 3–4 weeks after the stroke. All drawings are well centered on the page. ***a*** A self-portrait with crown with laurels to indicate the virtues and the patience of a patient. ***b*** The relationship patient/examiner. ***c*** The neurologist seen as a general asking: 'What do you see here?' ***d*** His feelings towards all the people asking for news about his health ('How are you') and trying to reassure him ('You look exactly the same') [from Cantagallo and Della Sala, 1998, with kind permission].

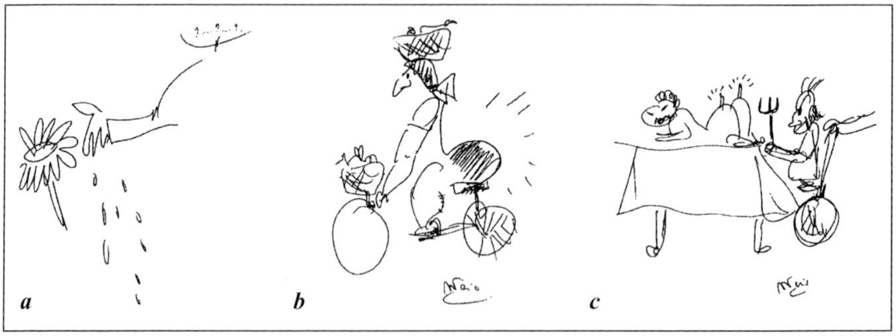

Fig. 7. Fellini's drawing from memory, 25 days after the stroke, of a daisy (***a***), a bike (***b***), and a table (***c***). Note the missing petals, the missing spokes on the left wheel and the uncompleted face of the cyclist. The laid table was drawn on the right side of the page, but there is no further evidence of neglect [from Cantagallo and Della Sala, 1998, with kind permission].

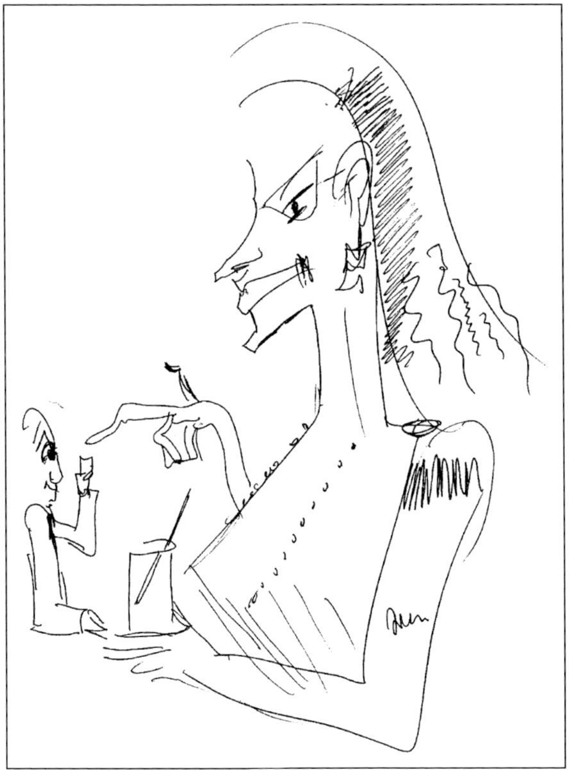

Fig. 8. Fellini's drawing from memory, 25 days after the stroke, of a human face. Some particulars are omitted, such as the forehead of the female examiner and the back of his head. Note that he expressed his feelings by depicting himself as a pygmy completely in the hands of his examiner [from Cantagallo and Della Sala, 1998, with kind permission].

All in all, as the authors summarize in their abstract, 'the neuropsychological profile of [Fellini's] neglect syndrome was characterized by left visuomotor neglect which persisted for two months. At onset, [he] also showed indications of neglect dyslexia as well as some evidence of implicit processing of the neglected parts of visual stimuli. However, there was no sign of personal and representational neglect, and [he] was well aware of his motor and attentional deficits. [Fellini's] neglect was characterised by several dissociations, of which the lack of functional carryover despite intact conceptual and semantic insight is the most relevant' [Cantagallo and Della Sala, 1998].

Another striking feature of the ill Fellini was his use of humor. Of course, he always had been a very funny man; remember that he started his career as a

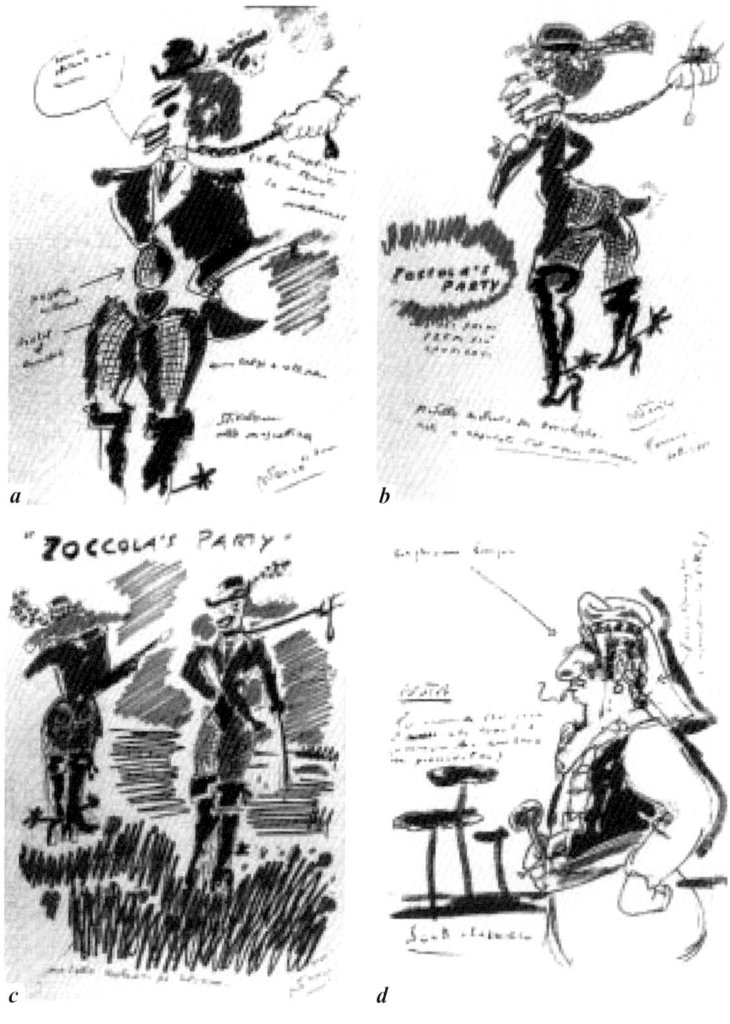

Fig. 9. Three spontaneous drawings (***a–c***) of Fellini 60 days after his stroke compared with one sketch (***d***) he produced before his brain lesion [illustration taken from De Santi, 1981, copyright 1976 by Diogenes Verlag, Zürich]. The style is equivalent and there are no signs of neglect (original in colors) [from Cantagallo and Della Sala, 1998, with kind permission].

caricaturist and a gag writer. Now, some studies indicate a right-hemispheric dominance for the understanding of jokes [e.g. Coulson and Williams, 2005; Heath and Blonder, 2005], but clearly there was no impairment of causticity in Fellini. He was very much appreciated by the therapists and his fellow patients.

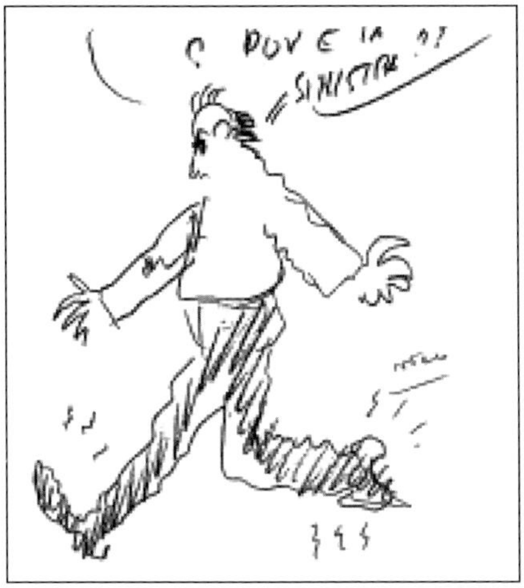

Fig. 10. Fellini asks himself: 'Where is the left?' [from Cantagallo and Della Sala, 1998, with kind permission].

To tease the clinicians, he humorously modified the tests to his benefit and in so doing, he showed at once that he knew what was wrong with him and that he could do nothing about it. For example, he added drawings and items on cancellation tasks, showing his awareness of his impairment in his drawings.

Insight in Neglect

As we have just seen, Fellini suffered from an extrapersonal neglect of which he was perfectly aware. This means that, despite his knowledge of a very specific disorder of spatial allocation of attention, he could not help succumbing to it (fig. 10). This should be expanded a little, in order to clearly understand why Fellini's case is so illuminating. One could ask, why in the first place should patients with neglect be unaware of their impairment? The fact is that they generally are and this has been of great interest to cognitive scientists and philosophers alike. In a nutshell, what unawareness of neglect shows is that these patients simply do not notice that something is missing from their available, visual phenomenal field. In other words, their world is 'complete', as is ours. Presumably, this is one reason why these patients are so hard to rehabilitate: it is hard to make them realize that something is actually wrong with them. Indeed, whereas anosognosia for hemiplegia is a well-known phenomenon that *adds* to the physiological fact of hemiplegia, it is widely accepted that somehow anosognosia *is part* of the phenomenon of neglect. For how could we explain that a part of the visual world is left unattended while at the same time *being aware* that it is unattended, all happening in the same brain? The deficit, hence, must run deeper than a mere inattention to the left space. To quote from a recent paper on precisely that issue: 'The lack of awareness must concern not only the left side of *space*, but its *absence*. The contralesional space is not merely neglected: its absence is indeed lacking.... In neglect, the left side of space is not merely not present: it is this "not present" that is lacking' [Becchio and Bertone, 2005, p. 488]. Philosopher Thomas Metzinger also insisted on the very same point, with an apt comparison to normal subjects:

> Patients with hemi-inattention...do not consciously experience the obvious discontinuity of available mental content from the first-person perspective. But how obvious is it really?...We do not *explicitly* experience the non-represented part of the world behind our backs as a phenomenal hole in our subjective model of reality.... As to many neglect patients, the world appears to us as complete in spite of this obvious deficit.... [Neglect shows that] an extended spatial restriction of the phenomenal model of the world does not have to be accompanied by an awareness of this deficit.... Large portions of this model may disappear by becoming functionally unavailable; they just drop out of existence, and in such situations the initiation of introspective, exploratory, or self-investigative behaviour becomes very difficult for systems like us – because, as it were, it assumes an impossible situation. How could a system search for something that is not part of *reality*, not even part of a *possible* reality? [Metzinger, 2003, pp. 223–224].

Yet, and this is the crucial point, Fellini *had* some insight into the incompleteness of his world. The peculiar fact is that his knowledge of a distortion in his visual awareness could not allow him to correct it. He not only knew that the left side was missing, he knew that its very *absence* in consciousness was missing.

Of course, therapists have known for a long time that higher cognition deficits cannot be cured by merely making patients aware of their problem, or even by trying to make them aware that they are unaware of their problem. Usually, this awareness comes progressively, paralleling the rate of function recovery. Nonetheless, Fellini was aware of his neglect even when the latter was at its most severe stage. He knew and understood the nature of his deficit, as the clinicians could observe this fact directly and by interviewing his relatives, friends and therapists. To a friend, he could explain the idea of 'unilateral neglect', a concept that is among the most counterintuitive things that could happen to someone. Then, obviously, it must be concluded that knowledge at a semantic level is not enough to overcome pathological performance, even for simple tasks such as bisecting lines or cancelling specific targets. Conversely, as the authors note, 'overt, extrapersonal neglect is possible even when the patient is conceptually aware of his left-sided deficits in exploration' [Cantagallo and Della Sala, 1998].

Fellini is not the first patient to show this pattern, but he certainly displayed it in the most spectacular and convincing fashion. Even more strikingly – and this is a fact that has been overlooked by Cantagallo and Della Sala – the case of Fellini not only shows that neglect and anosognosia for neglect can be dissociated, but also that *awareness* of neglect and *implicit processing* of neglected stimuli can coexist. Furthermore, these two processes need not be ccollapsed into one single mechanism, as this would be confusing a *reportable* level of consciousness with one that is merely *indexible* [Marcel, 2003].

As Fellini showed throughout his professional career, human consciousness and actions operate in a multilayered theater of astounding complexity and irony. In disease, he nailed the issue by showing to the scientific and philosophical community that awareness is not as straightforward or even as subtle as one might think. It is a package of apparent contradictions. Had he read the account of his own case in *Cortex* [Cantagallo and Della Sala, 1998], one might safely assume that he would not have been as puzzled as its authors. After all, he was urged on to make films by a devotional entanglement with, in his words, 'the expressions of the human creature in all its aspects, all its contradictions, all its elements' [Bachmann, 1994].

Personality and the Right Hemisphere

After discussing the lives, works and diseases of Visconti and Fellini, it is time to draw our conclusions. There are no immediately obvious reasons why we should link these two men in the single, speculative account that follows, and most certainly not because of the simple coincidence that the two most acclaimed Italian directors happened to have had a right-hemispheric stroke with left-sided hemiplegia. Nevertheless, we think that this is a good place to bring together a few ideas about the consequences of right-hemispheric damage, exploring some tentative hypotheses that are usually not approached in the scientific literature.

To summarize quickly, following his stroke Visconti apparently exhibited no cognitive deficits while Fellini displayed clear signs of unilateral extrapersonal neglect. Importantly, neither showed evidence of anosognosia. As Sherlock Holmes drew the attention of Watson to the 'curious incident of the dog during the night' – where, famously, the curious incident was precisely that the dog did nothing – we would like to say a few words about the lack of anosognosia in these two left-hemiplegic patients, which we argue may not be a trivial fact.

Neurologists are used to detecting and reporting anomalies, but unfortunately all too often these are *positive* in nature. A neurological anomaly may as well be *negative*, but the absence of symptoms is understandably often overlooked by clinicians. By the same token, we would also like to address the notion of influence from premorbid personality in the symptomatology of right-hemisphere strokes.

Absence of Anosognosia and of Other Symptoms

Of course, one could try to explain the absence of anosognosia in these two particular patients from a purely anatomical point of view. Unfortunately, the state of the matter is still very much unresolved: we simply do not know for sure what brain regions are precisely involved in anosognosia. This is not due to a lack of research, but rather to the multifaceted nature of the phenomenon itself, which still does not benefit from clear conceptual clarifications and straightforward assessment methods [Jehkonen et al., 2006].

Though we have no brain imaging for Visconti, we can assume from the apparent absence of cognitive impairment in his case that his stroke was restricted to motor or subcortical areas. For Fellini, we know that he suffered from a stroke in the territory of the right middle cerebral artery, involving large temporoparietal and underlying structure damage. Recent studies and meta-analyses have tried to elucidate the anatomical basis of anosognosic symptoms. We can use this information to see if Visconti and Fellini had been spared some localized damage that would have yielded anosognosia otherwise, keeping in mind the caveat mentioned earlier about the unresolved nature of this question. One thing at least is for sure: anosognosia is much more frequent after damage to the right hemisphere. Pia et al. [2004] found that anosognosia for hemiplegia can happen when damage is confined to frontal, parietal or temporal cortical structures and also after subcortical lesions, though the probability of its occurrence is highest when the lesion combines parietal and frontal structures. Karnath et al. [2005], distinguishing hemiplegic patients with or without anosognosia, pinpointed a specific role for the right posterior insula in anosognosia, while Berti et al. [2005], comparing patients with hemiplegia and neglect with or without accompanying anosognosia, found the involvement of a larger network of premotor, somatosensory and primary motor cortex in the former (with anosognosia). The latest study on this issue, however, found no specific location for anosognosia as compared to neglect [Appelros et al., 2007]. So clearly, from our current knowledge and by what we know of our two cases in point, it is simply impossible to say that the absence of anosognosia here was due to a specific sparing of brain tissue. One should add that, while neglect is often accompanied by anosognosia for hemiplegia, there have been many reported instances of a double dissociation between both, and different forms of anosognosia may also be dissociated from each other [see e.g. Jehkonen et al., 2006]. Hence, the absence of neglect in Visconti was no safeguard against anosognosia, and its presence in Fellini was no guarantee at all for its presence. However, the case of Fellini raises the question of the influence of different subtypes of neglect on anosognosia. Cantagallo and Della Sala [1998] propose that personal neglect, which was absent in Fellini, might be more closely linked to anosognosia than extrapersonal neglect. But

Table 1. Unilateral body schema disorders resulting from right-hemispheric strokes

- Depression or adequate reaction
- Unawareness or frank denial. When pressed, patients may admit to some degree their disability but frequently explain it away with some inadequate excuse (*anosognosia*)
- Downplaying the importance of impairment or joking about it, making inadequate comments, attribution to some benign cause, lack of concern (*anosodiaphoria*)
- Ignorance or forgetfulness of ownership, and even existence, of one's left body parts (*asomatognosia*)
- Spontaneous claim that the left limbs belong to another person, real or imaginary, alive or dead, or that the limb is a dead corpse, an animal, an object, a child, etc. (*somatoparaphrenia*)
- Feeling of increased strength, dexterity and usefulness in the unaffected limbs (delusion of enhancement of function – Enhanced concern about the affected limb (*acute hemiconcern*)
- Proprietary attitude, material or hostile, towards the paralyzed limbs (*personification* or the paralyzed member)
- Excessive aversion towards the disabled limb with hatred of paralysis and verbal or physical mistreatment of the paralyzed limb (*misoplegia*)

this is all we have at hand for a neurocognitive account of poststroke profiles for Visconti and Fellini.

Table 1 shows the many disturbances involving knowledge of the left body that are liable to occur after right-hemispheric damage. Despite the notion that Fellini had misoplegia, which we find unconvincing as it is based only on some derogatory comments directed at the left limb and signs of disgust,[3] it is apparent that neither Visconti nor Fellini had body schema disorders. Remember also that there was no impairment of 'theory of mind' in Visconti, and no loss of humor in Fellini, two characteristically human abilities thought to be mediated by the right hemisphere.

Premorbid Personality

Hence, Visconti and Fellini had none of the spectacular higher-level disturbances that not so infrequently affect, at least transiently, victims of right-hemispheric strokes. Current neurocognitive knowledge seems unable to satisfyingly account for these negative findings. Somehow, the lesions that inflicted severe left-sided hemiplegia in both of them did not affect their

[3]The whole idea of misoplegia might lose its appeal and relevance if it is used on every occasion on which a patient shows or expresses an understandable dislike for a paralyzed limb. Instead, we propose that misoplegia should stand for continuous, extreme, inappropriate or delusional behavior (verbal or otherwise) towards the contralesional limb [Dieguez et al., in preparation; Dieguez et al., 2007; see also Loetscher et al., 2006].

intelligence, awareness of impairment, personalities or belief systems. Yet, aside from visuospatial skills, these are usually the consequences of such damage that capture the attention of clinicians, researchers, therapists and lecturers when they deal with the higher-level functions of the right hemisphere. Of course, they do not pay much attention to the numerous negative cases, those patients who get on quite well with their previous selves after the damaging event. This is precisely what we intend to do here. We do not find it uninteresting or trivial that patients may actually *not* show the classical or expected symptoms after a stroke. Instead, learning more about them might give important clues as to the structure of the mind and even provide hope for future stroke survivors. Given that the current state of neurocognitive knowledge seems to fail to account for these negative cases, we may as well seek a speculative account in that very muddy field of early neuropsychiatry, namely the controversial idea that the premorbid personality might account for some consequences (or lack thereof) of brain damage. This was actually a widely accepted idea during most of the 20th century in early French, German, English and American neuropsychiatry (see the works of Lhermitte, Schilder, Goldstein, Critchley and Weinstein, who all did much to promote the idea that symptoms varied depending on who had them).

It is, of course, always hard to decipher what the important aspects of premorbid personality in neurological patients are, so the study of famous people, whose personalities are quite well known from works, writings and interviews, can help us. Obviously, there is always a risk in forming ad hoc hypotheses about aspects of personality we report later, to explain whatever aspect of a syndrome is at hand. This is indeed why such an approach lies in murky waters and why the claims of 'neuropsychoanalysis' are so poorly heard. This field, also called 'depth neuropsychology' has made some noise in recent years, mainly through a few of their most vocal proponents. While clinicians of this flavor do not deny the importance of lesion location in neuropsychiatric symptomatology, they insist on the relevance of intrapsychic processes, which always seem to involve some defense mechanism, the purpose of which is to protect the conscious self from excessively rough narcissistic blows and the specifics of which depend on the premorbid personality structure and the emotional reactivity of the patient [see Kaplan-Solms and Solms, 2002]. Hence, the same damage in the right hemisphere might lead to different disorders, depending on the nature of the preexisting emotional system implemented in the depths of the right hemisphere. 'Neuropsychoanalysts' are almost the only ones to acknowledge the importance of the patient's previous personality to his symptoms. While we entirely reject their wildest claims and interpretations, we also strongly feel that there might be 'something to it', if it is only for stressing the importance of actually listening to the patient and then describing him as accurately as possible, things that apparently have been lost with the massive appearance of semimagical technological devices.

So, what might these 'preexisting emotional systems' be, as they were implemented in Visconti and Fellini's right hemispheres? Despite the tremendous differences in their lives and works – as we hope we have made clear in our biographical sketches – and although word had it that they did not like each other very much,[4] they had a great deal in common. First, they shared a common zeitgeist, which was the emergence of a postfascist Italy. Then, they had a similar artistic trajectory: both started in the neorealist style, focusing on the sociopolitical background of the working classes, and both shifted progressively to an interest in the subjective and psychological. They also shared lucid insight into the decadence of high society, a constant appreciation of the role of the author and the work of the filmmaker (Fellini liked to portray his own creative process, Visconti reflected on the creations of writers). Both were smart, charming, witty, sarcastic, subversive and staunchly independent. In a word, they were *free* men. This was despite – or maybe because of – tremendous opposition, obstacles and difficulties. How do such people manage to accomplish astounding careers with disproportionate ambitions in the face of fierce competitors, vicious journalists, capricious actors, unreliable collaborators, an audience following fashion and inept, demanding producers? We opine that genius is not enough. It takes a special psychological profile to do that. Psychologists and neuropsychoanalysts alike are fond of unearthing 'defense mechanisms', but they would be hard pressed to find any in Visconti and Fellini. In a sense, their entire lives were defensive mechanisms. They had no need for a rationalizing left hemisphere or a mindset concerned too much with detail. They had confidence in their abilities, they lent no ear to disgruntled or skeptical critics, they only believed in themselves. Being somehow 'natural anosognosics', they seemed immune to 'acquired' anosognosia from the beginning.

Fellini, in his own terms, was a born liar. He was an expert at exploring and fabricating his own mind and world. What he meant by 'liar' was that he had very poor confidence in one's ability to faithfully report 'true' autobiographical events. In many interviews, he stated from the onset that he found it very bizarre that journalist might be interested in his accounts of his work and life, as he was known to merely invent anecdotes and contradict himself all along. He just did not care that much for reality. However, he had a strong notion of his possibilities.

[4]Claudia Cardinale was to experience first hand their enmity, as she worked with both at the same time during the shooting of Visconti's *The Leopard* and Fellini's *Eight and a Half.*

'If I cannot do what I feel like doing, I'd rather not do it', he said [in Pernot, 1987, p. 14]. All the difficulties he had to endure before he could begin a movie were creative strengths for him: 'The struggle helps me make a movie what it is. Without it, it would be different and most of the time less good. The stupidity, the mediocrity of the producers, in the end, helped me to become aware of the nature of my work…' [Pernot, 1987, p. 14]. His posture was that of a *dilettante* – even if a combative one, he knew himself to be 'too serious to be an amateur and not serious enough to be a professional'.

Visconti lived in an imaginary world from his boyhood on, cut off from all reality. An aristocrat, he created his own universe with no involvement of material worries. We might paraphrase for Visconti the famous Tancredi quote in *The Leopard*: this man strived all his life to 'make things change so that nothing will change'. This is exactly the attitude of the confabulating anosognosic. Remember that, at his worst, he said he would still direct if he was confined to a stretcher.

We have also seen that Fellini was a man of exquisite humor, even in illness. Visconti was probably less so, but he was quite sarcastic in his own manner. Mixed with their impressive strength of character and enormous ambition, humor and irony form a very robust defensive mechanism to confront the difficulties of life. While this may hint at anosodiaphoria in the eye of the clinician, we opine that their strong frames of mind and unique personalities not only allowed them to achieve successful careers but also helped them cope with disease and prevented them from falling under the unstable modifications of awareness that strike down so many patients who suffer right-hemispheric damage.

This idea is, of course, provocative, but then there are many things that we ignore with respect to how the brain works. We therefore dare to take a further step. There has been theorizing about the psychological bases of political beliefs. Conservatism has been associated with a fear of death, a denial of self-inconsistencies and fear of change [Jost et al., 2003]. At the same time, right-hemispheric syndromes have been seen as the display of defensive mechanisms linked to denial of negative consequences and a quest to preserve one's threatened self-integrity in the face of harm and risk of death. Arguably, Visconti and Fellini, in their lives and careers, escaped both accounts. Could there possibly be an influence of personality, political opinions and creativity on the symptomatology of a right-hemispheric stroke? Perhaps their leftist sensibilities, honed from neorealist beginnings, reemerged as they most needed them, helping them face the cruel reality of neurological impairment.

Finally, we must now confide that much of this conclusion has been made tongue in cheek, as a tribute to two provocative and sensual artists who were not afraid of new ideas.

Acknowledgment

We thank Mark Inglin for outstanding professional English editing of the manuscript, and Sergio Della Sala for his kind permission to reproduce Fellini's CT scan and wonderful drawings.

References

Appelros P, Karlsson GM, Hennerdal S: Anosognosia versus unilateral neglect: coexistence and their relations to age, stroke severity, lesion site and cognition. Eur J Neurol 2007;14:54–59.

Babinski J: Contribution à l'étude des troubles mentaux dans l'hémiplégie organique cérébrale (anosognosie). Rev Neurol 1914;27:845–848.

Bachmann G: A guest in my own dreams: an interview with Federico Fellini. Film Q 1994;47:2–15.

Becchio C, Bertone C: The ontology of neglect. Conscious Cogn 2005;14:483–494.

Berti A, Bottini G, Gandola M, Pia L, Smania N, Stracciari A, Castiglioni I, Vallar G, Paulesu E: Shared cortical anatomy for motor awareness and motor control. Science 2005;309:488–491.

Bogard D: Review of Schifano's book (excerpt). Daily Telegraph, November 24, 1990. http://emmanuel.denis.free.fr/visconti/texte/texte2.html (last access September 2006).

Bondanella P, Gieri M (eds): La Strada: Federico Fellini, Director. New Brunswick, NJ, Rutgers University Press, 1987.

Burke F: Fellini's Films: from Postwar to Postmodern. New York, Macmillan/Twayne, 1996.

Cantagallo A, Della Sala S: Preserved insight in an artist with extrapersonal spatial neglect. Cortex 1998;34:163–189.

Coulson S, Williams RF: Hemispheric asymmetries and joke comprehension. Neuropsychologia 2005; 43:128–141.

Criqui E: Pour une lecture politique de l'úuvre cinématographique de Luchino Visconti. Rev Fr Sci Polit 1982;32:837–847.

Critchley M: Observations on anosodiaphoria. L'Encéphalie 1957;46:540–546.

Dieguez S, Gonzales M, Bogousslavsky J: Chronic mistreatment towards the plegic limb: Critchley's misoplegia revisited. In preparation.

Dieguez S, Staub F, Bogousslavsky J: Asomatognosia; in Godefroy O, Bogousslavsky J (eds): The Behavioral and Cognitive Neurology of Stroke. Cambridge, Cambridge University Press, 2007.

Fellini F: Fellini par Fellini. Entretiens avec Giovanni Grazzini. Paris, Calmann-Lévy, 1984.

Griffin R, Friedman O, Ween J, Winner E, Happe F, Brownell H: Theory of mind and the right cerebral hemisphere: refining the scope of impairment. Laterality 2006;11:195–225.

Heath RL, Blonder LX: Spontaneous humor among right hemisphere stroke survivors. Brain Lang 2005;93: 267–276.

Ifri PA: One novel, five adaptations: Proust on film. Contemp French Francophone Stud 2005;9:15–29.

Jehkonen M, Laihosalo M, Kettunen J: Anosognosia after stroke: assessment, occurrence, subtypes and impact on functional outcome reviewed. Acta Neurol Scand 2006;114:293–306.

Jones J: Scene stealers. The Guardian, July 24, 2004.

Jost JT, Glaser J, Kruglanski AW, Sulloway FJ: Political conservatism as motivated social cognition. Psychol Bull 2003;129:339–375.

Kaplan-Solms K, Solms M: Clinical studies in neuro-psychoanalysis: introduction to a depth neuropsychology. London, Karnak Books, 2002.

Karnath HO, Baier B, Nägele T: Awareness of the functioning of one's own limbs mediated by the insular cortex? J Neurosci 2005;25:7134–7138.

Loetscher T, Regard M, Brugger P: Misoplegia: a review of the literature and a case without hemiplegia. J Neurol Neurosurg Psychiatry 2006;77:1099–1100.

Marcel AJ: Introspective report: trust, self-knowledge and science. J Conscious Stud 2003;10:167–186.

Marcel AJ, Tegnér R, Nimmo-Smith I: Anosognosia for plegia: specificity, extension partiality and disunity of bodily awareness. Cortex 2004;40:19–40.

Mendes Sargo T: Review of the Leopard. Film Q 1963–1964;17:35–38.
Metzinger T: Being No One. Cambridge, MA, MIT Press, 2003.
Pernot H: L'Atelier de Fellini, une expression du doute. Paris, L'Harmattan, 1987.
Pia L, Neppi-Modona M, Ricci R, Berti A: The anatomy of anosognosia for hemiplegia: a meta-analysis. Cortex 2004;40:367–377.
Schifano L: Luchino Visconti, les feux de la passion. Paris, Perrin, 1987.
Stubbs JC: The Fellini manner: open form and visual excess. Cinema J 1993;32:49–64.
Turnbull OH, Evans CE, Owen V: Negative emotions and anosognosia. Cortex 2005;41:67–75.

Sebastian Dieguez
Brain Mind Institute, Laboratory of Cognitive Neuroscience
EPFL, Dorigny, Station 15
CH–1015 Lausanne (Switzerland)
Tel. +41 21 693 1681, Fax +41 21 693 1770, E-Mail sebastian.dieguez@epfl.ch

Bogousslavsky J, Hennerici MG (eds): Neurological Disorders in Famous Artists – Part 2.
Front Neurol Neurosci. Basel, Karger, 2007, vol 22, pp 75–88

De novo Artistic Behaviour following Brain Injury

Thomas A. Pollak[a], *Catherine M. Mulvenna*[b], *Mark F. Lythgoe*[c]

[a]King's College London, [b]Department of Psychology, University College London and [c]RCS Unit of Biophysics, Institute of Child Health, University College London, London, UK

Abstract

The effect of brain injury and disease on the output of established artists is an object of much study and debate. The emergence of de novo artistic behaviour following such injury or disease, while very rare, has been recorded in cases of frontotemporal dementia, epilepsy, subarachnoid haemorrhage and Parkinson's disease. This may be an underdiagnosed phenomenon and may represent an opportunity to further understand the neural bases of creative thought and behaviour in man and those of cognitive change after brain injury. There is clearly an important role for hemispheric localization of pathology, which is usually within the temporal cortex, upon the medium of artistic expression, and a likely role for mild frontal cortical dysfunction in producing certain behavioural and cognitive characteristics that may be conducive to the production of art. Possible mechanisms of 'artistic drive' and 'creative idea generation' in these patients are also considered. The increased recognition and responsible nurturing of this behaviour in patients may serve as a source of great comfort to individuals and their families at an otherwise difficult time.

The images in figure 1 were painted by a 56-year-old housewife who, 5 years previously, had begun to take art classes, despite having shown no previous interest in art. During this period, she had become uncomfortable in social situations and had withdrawn socially. In the next 10 years her speech became disinhibited and then rambling, she gained weight, became incontinent and began to wander. At age 71 she died of advanced dementia [Miller et al., 1998].

The artworks in figure 2 were created by a 51-year-old ex-builder who, in the months following a subarachnoid haemorrhage, felt a compulsive urge to paint, draw, sculpt and write poetry using whatever materials available, even

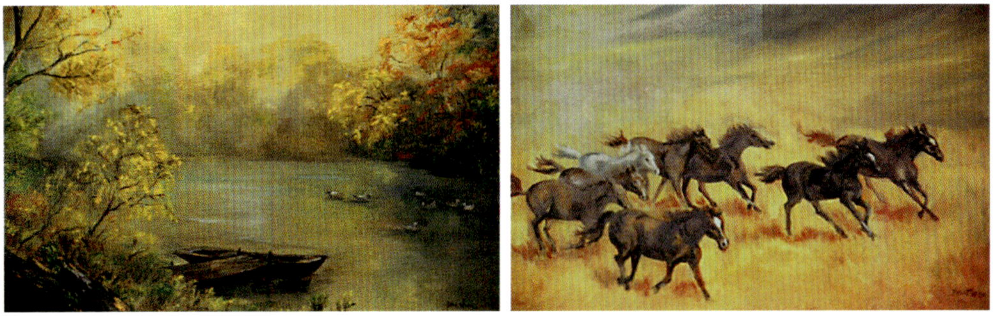

Fig. 1. The rural scene was painted by patient 2 in the series of FTD patients described by Miller et al. [1998]. It was painted approximately 6 years after she had started taking art classes. The painting of horses was made 8 years later, when the patient had become disinhibited (reprinted with permission from Lippincott Williams & Wilkins).

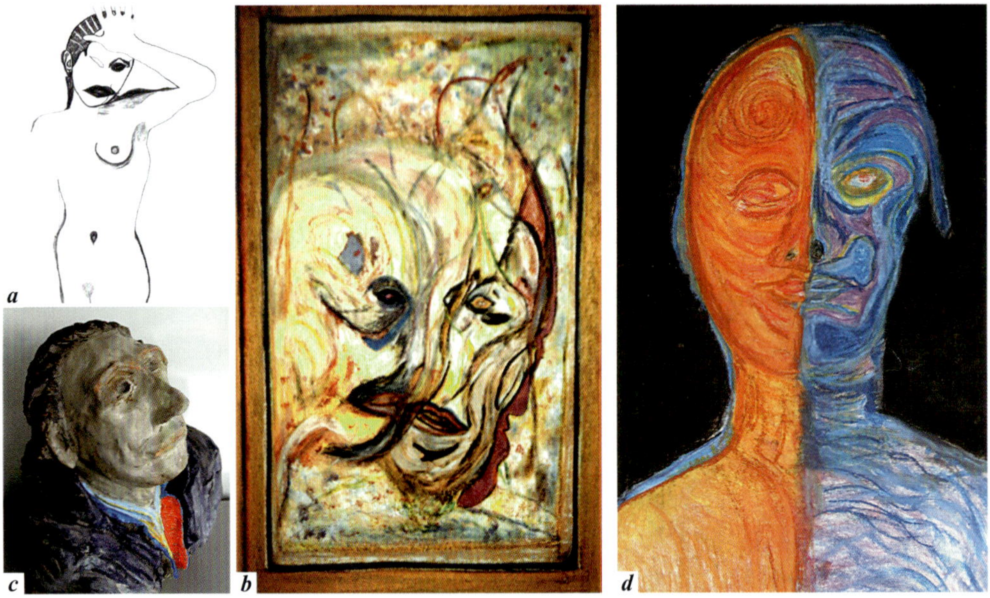

Fig. 2. ***a*** Suggestive of a left hemispatial neglect, the artist's earliest, hauntingly simple line drawings would frequently exclude one half of the subject. ***b*** His early works show naivety, colour and passion. The artist painted this, one of many representations of his 'split brain' on the inside wall of his house. ***c*** A later sculpture demonstrates a growing technical capability. This clay head shows a striking congruency and the features are more symmetrical and colours more naturalistic than found in his earlier work. ***d*** A sense of a cognitive 'split' represented in his paintings complements the sentiment of much of his poetry.

using the walls of his house as a giant canvas. He had shown no previous interest in art. He now exhibits his work in galleries throughout the United Kingdom [Lythgoe et al., 2005].

The effect of brain injury on the creative output of artists is a well-documented and intriguing topic that forms the basis for this collection of essays. Less well-known is the development of a previously non-existent artistic output in individuals who have sustained brain injury. This phenomenon is all the more remarkable for its occurrence across a variety of neurological conditions and at least three different artistic modalities (table 1).

Development of de novo Artistic Output in Particular Neurological Conditions

Visual Art and Music

The condition in which de novo artistic behaviours are encountered most commonly is frontotemporal dementia (FTD), a dementia that usually presents in the sixth decade with personality change and/or progressive loss of language function. Bilateral frontotemporal degeneration can occur, although frontal and temporal subtypes also exist and pathological load can be unilateral.

Miller et al. [1998] report on a series of 5 FTD patients who developed previously absent visual artistic skills following the onset of their dementia; 4 of 5 were found to have unilateral anterior temporal dysfunction together with significantly impaired language and social function. As with the case described above, the development of painting, sculpture or photographic skills stands in stark contrast to the increasing degeneration of function found in other domains. Two further FTD patients reported by the same group [Miller et al., 2000] developed previously absent musical abilities; one constantly whistled and sang musical songs, another composed classical music despite limited training, with both becoming progressively aphasic. Both had left temporal hypoperfusion revealed by SPECT.

The emergence or maintenance of visual or musical artistic talent found in some FTD patients has been conceptualized as a 'paradoxical functional facilitation' [Kapur, 1996], or functional disinhibition of the posterior right parietal and temporal cortices in the context of an impairment in 'language dominant patterns of thinking organized in the dominant frontal and anterior temporal regions' [Mell et al., 2003]. The right parietal and temporal cortices are associated with visuoconstructive skills: they are thought to be essential for accurate copying of images and drawing internally imagined images, as well as for representing the spatial relationships between parts of an image or visual array. A similar functional disinhibition of posteriorly located, right-sided musical

Table 1. Summary of studies of de novo artistic behaviour following brain injury

Study	Subjects[1] (age, sex, handedness)	Condition	Artistic behaviour	Lesion	Comments
Finkelstein et al. [1991]	27, M, right-handed	Epilepsy	Drawing	Left interictal frontotemporal EEG spikes	Drawing activity occurred during ictal state; 'psychodiagnostic tests' suggestive of left frontal dysfunction
Miller et al. [1998]	(1) 53, M, left-handed	FTD	Painting	SPECT: left frontotemporal	
	(2) 55, F, left-handed	FTD	Painting	Autopsy: right frontotemporal	
	(3) 38, M, right-handed	FTD	Photography, miniature carving	SPECT: right frontotemporal	
	(4) 45, F, right-handed	FTD	Craftwork	MRI and SPECT: left frontotemporal	
	(5) 58, M, right-handed	FTD	Painting	MRI and SPECT: bilateral temporal	
Miller et al. [2000]	(1) 44, M, right-handed	FTD	Whistling, composing songs	SPECT: left temporal	
	(2) 68, M, right-handed	FTD	Composing classical music	SPECT: left temporal	
Schrag and Trimble [2001]	44, M, right-handed	Parkinson's disease	Poetry	Symptoms began on left, suggesting initial right-sided pathology	Artistic behaviour began after initiation of dopamine agonist treatment; neuropsychology suggestive of frontal dysfunction
Thomas Anterion et al. [2002]	65, M, right-handed	FTD	Drawing	CT: frontotemporal atrophy SPECT: frontal hypoperfusion	

Table 1. (continued)

Study	Subjects[1] (age, sex, handedness)	Condition	Artistic behaviour	Lesion	Comments
Mendez [2005]	58, M, right-handed	Epilepsy	Poetry	Right interictal temporal EEG spikes; small strokes in right thalamus and right cerebellum on imaging	
Lythgoe et al. [2005]	51, M, right-handed	Subarachnoid haemorrhage	Visual art and poetry	Bilateral middle cerebral artery aneurysms; no focal injuries on CT 16 days postadmission	Neuropsychology suggestive of frontal dysfunction

Neuropsychological findings included if available whereas imaging results are unavailable or unremarkable.
[1]Age is that at which evidence of artistic skills emerges.

ability is postulated as an explanation for the emergence of musical creative output in FTD [Miller et al., 2000].

Consistent with this mode of explanation is a report of a 27-year-old right-handed man who would impulsively commence de novo drawing behaviour during seizures. Interictal EEG showed spikes in the left frontotemporal area, with psychodiagnostic tests suggesting left frontal dysfunction [Finkelstein et al., 1991].

Miller et al. [2000] point out that taken as a whole, the artworks of FTD patients are somewhat bereft of a symbolic element. That is, while many works are accurate reproductions, for example, of scenes recalled from earlier in life, there are relatively few whose elements are representationally symbolic. This is perhaps unsurprising, given the pathological involvement of the hemisphere dominant for symbol manipulation, but it also raises potential questions regarding the 'creativeness' per se of such works.

Although undeniably central to the production of works described as 'art', the issue of technical talent is not one that will be considered in detail here, despite recent interesting evidence that a temporary 'brain lesion' induced by transcranial magnetic stimulation of the left frontotemporal area can transiently lead to the adoption of a more complex visual artistic style or even of a savant-like visual assessment of objects within an array [Snyder et al., 2003, 2006]. Suffice it to say, however, that a baseline degree of technical proficiency (certainly present in the FTD patients described by Miller et al. above) may be a prerequisite for the continued development of art in brain-injured individuals. A left-sided lesion may then disinhibit premorbid right-sided drawing abilities to an extent that they are considered 'artistic'. It should also be considered, however, that a tendency on the part of family, friends and clinicians not to recognize the less technically accomplished productions of brain-injured individuals as 'art' may contribute to the relative paucity of these cases in the literature.

Poetry and Literature

If visual artistic output is associated with left-sided lesions and a relative impairment in language, what of literature and poetry, language-based art forms? 'Hypergraphia' is a term originally used to refer to the phenomenon, first described by Waxman and Geschwind [1974] wherein patients with temporal lobe epilepsy would, in an interictal phase, produce vast amounts of written material, associated with a compulsive drive to write. Although the content of this material may concern the individual's thoughts and feelings, often it is considerably more mundane, pedestrian or repetitive and unlikely to be designated as 'creative', let alone 'art'. Nonetheless, in some individuals a more truly creative output occurs. Mendez [2005] reports a patient with partial complex seizures who complained of words constantly rhyming in his head and the need he felt to write them down as poetry. EEG revealed right temporal spikes. The author suggested that the hypergraphia may reflect interictal hypometabolism of the right hemisphere and a subsequent disinhibition of left-sided language function.

Hypergraphia occurs in other disorders, notably in stroke, where the phenomenon also corresponds to right-sided injury, and in mania. Hypergraphia in the latter tends to be more creative in terms of content, while in the former it tends to be iterative on a lexical and/or lexicographemic level and hence is devoid of creative content [Van Vugt et al., 1996]. We consider it unlikely, however, that the content of hypergraphic writing (i.e. whether it is for 'artistic' writing, for nonsense, or for meaningful non-artistic written material such as personal, academic or journalistic writings) is determined solely by the nature of the lesion. Rather, it is possible that the lesion confers a drive and a mode of expression (i.e. the written word) and that the content of the writing is partly determined by premorbid and environmental factors. Further study of the determinants of creative content in hypergraphic writings is clearly required.

Schrag and Trimble [2001] report on a male patient with Parkinson's disease who developed previously non-existent poetic talents (leading to publication and prizes) within a month of starting dopamine agonist treatment at age 44 years. Interestingly, the patient's symptoms started on the left side, suggesting a right-sided brain pathology – hence again opening the possibility of right-sided pathology disinhibiting left-sided language function. The authors speculate that the drugs may have led to the development of either a cognitive enhancement, increased perception or a hypomanic syndrome, in addition to a selective frontal cortical dysfunction, leading to the unmasking of poetic talent. This speculation raises the question of the neurochemical basis of creative drive as well as the cognitive changes required for the creative process to flourish – both are considered in subsequent sections.

Poetry has existed in a verbally transmitted form for considerably longer and throughout many more locales and cultures than it has as a written tradition. However there has been little interest, to our knowledge, in the effects of brain injury (other than psychiatric illness) on the increased creative content of spontaneous speech. The remarkable, performative playfulness of speech found in various neurological (and psychiatric) groups may be interpreted as a kind of spoken poetry and may warrant consideration as a genuinely de novo artistic output.

Limitations of a Hemispheric Model

It is a satisfying symmetry that injury to the language-dominant hemisphere can produce de novo visual artistic or musical output, usually in the context of impaired language, while right-sided injury is associated with the development of increased written or verbal creative output. We have, however, reported on a patient who, in surprising contrast to the FTD patients described above, developed a prolific visual artistic output in the context of a preserved language function which also enabled a prolific written poetic output [Lythgoe et al., 2005]. A 51-year-old right-handed man with no previous artistic interest suffered a subarachnoid haemorrhage in 2001. On admission, brain CT showed blood in the anterior parts of the basal cisterns. Bilateral middle cerebral artery aneurysms were suggested by angiography. No focal injuries were detected on CT taken 16 days after admission.

Soon after recovery began, he started to write poetry about his mental state, which he described as like having a 'split mind', with his thoughts 'riding out on parallel lines'. He began also to draw, paint, and make sculptures obsessively, to the neglect and detriment of many social aspects of his life. He filled many notebooks with verse and would paint and draw on the walls of his house.

He drew hundreds of sketches of faces, all asymmetric. Early drawings suggested a left hemispatial neglect; he also reported difficulty shaving on the left. The patient now exhibits regularly at galleries and has continued to mature in his creative style and technical abilities. (see fig. 2).

On neuropsychological testing in 2004, verbal and performance IQ were within the normal range and although the patient was not grossly inappropriate in his behaviour he demonstrated a marked verbal disinhibition, with frequent punning and rhyming. The overall profile was one of a mild frontal deficit. It is possible that frontal damage has led to a disinhibition of both visual and verbal creative abilities localized to the right and left hemispheres, respectively. What is convincingly demonstrated nonetheless is that a disinhibition or facilitation of visual artistic areas can occur in the context of dysfunction of other areas than dominant areas specialized for language. That he showed some left hemispatial neglect may also be suggestive of a right frontal/parietal disconnection [Doricchi and Tomaiuolo, 2003].

This case suggests that the hemispheric model adopted thus far is at best a simplification. There are further unanswered questions: while in the vast majority of cases, hypofunction or dysfunction of one hemisphere would appear to lead to a functional disinhibition of abilities lateralized to the other hemisphere and thus dictates the medium of artistic expression, the source of creative drive and the means of idea generation remain unclear. Why do only some FTD patients paint or write music? Why do only very few hypergraphics show creativity in their writings?

Artistic Drive and Creative Idea Generation

The drive to create art may be usefully distinguished from the faculty by which 'creative' ideas are generated. Can the patients described above help our understanding of either?

Many of the individuals described above not only developed previously absent or nascent artistic tendencies, but they did so with such enthusiasm as to be variously labelled obsessive [Lythgoe et al., 2005], compulsive [Miller et al., 2000], impulsive [Finkelstein et al., 1991] or hypomanic [Schrag and Trimble, 2001]. In most, this enthusiasm was seen as part of a more general change towards behaviour that would be described as inappropriate or disinhibited. In addition the patient described by Mendez [2005] demonstrated behavioural changes which included anger and irritability. It may be, as suggested by Miller et al. [1998], that artistic or creative drive develops well in the context of a disregard for the constraints of society upon the behaviour of individuals. This picture certainly resonates with the popular image of the artist as an outsider or rebel in society. Disinhibited behaviour may appear very much like such a disregard for societal constraints or, indeed, such a disregard may be part of the general picture of disinhibited behaviour.

The disinhibited behaviour shown by these patients is typical of a frontal, particularly orbitofrontal, cortical deficit and in each of the cases described by Miller et al. [1998, 2000], Finkelstein et al. [1991] and Lythgoe et al. [2005] there is evidence, from either neuroimaging or neuropsychology, of frontal cortical dysfunction.

Some degree of frontal dysfunction may be conducive towards artistic behaviour via other means than by predisposing towards disinhibited behaviour. One characteristic shown by patients with even mild frontal cortical dysfunction that becomes evident in neuropsychological testing is a degree of perseveration or a failure of task disengagement. In terms of macroscopic behaviour it is certainly possible that perseverative tendencies are central to understanding these patients' drive and could be integral to their sustained and voluminous output of often thematically similar work. Nonetheless, if perseveration is very marked, as seen in patients with severe frontal dysfunction, the creative process may not even be able to get started. It may be that the emergence of de novo artistic behaviour after brain injury actually requires some mild frontal cortical dysfunction but is restricted by severe dysfunction.

What then of idea generation? The considerable psychological literature on creativity may hold some answers. One possible explanation of idea generation in creative individuals without brain injury posits a reduced level of latent inhibition as a causal factor [Carson et al., 2003; Flaherty, 2005]. Latent inhibition may be described as the capacity of the brain to filter from conscious awareness stimuli previously perceived as irrelevant [Lubow and Moore, 1959], as measured by various behavioural tests in humans and animals. The construct figures prominently in numerous theories of schizophrenia and it has been demonstrated that reduced latent inhibition is associated with psychotic states or psychotic susceptibility as well as high dopamine levels [Gray, 1998]. Much of the phenomenology of psychosis includes the formation of associations between unrelated or irrelevant stimuli and this has led some researchers to speculate that creativity, which involves 'original recombinant ideation' [Carson et al., 2003], may involve a reduction in latent inhibition.

Carson et al. [2003] measured creativity in a sample of high-IQ individuals using a range of indicators of creativity from divergent thinking scales to eminent creative achievement and found that high scorers showed reduced latent inhibition. They suggest that 'the results of these studies and analyses indicate a substantial and significant relationship between a variety of indicators of creativity and reduced LI'.

Is it possible that a brain injury-induced reduction in latent inhibition is responsible for the de novo artistic behaviours in the patients described above? It is of note that, subjectively, our patient described in Lythgoe et al. [2005] reported being 'flooded' with new associations, everyday perceptions triggering new mental imagery: 'Even when looking at my kitchen floor I see hundreds of different faces which I need to draw, paint or write about.' Might a similar failure of latent inhibition underlie the genesis of creative ideation in these brain-injured patients?

In the patient described by Schrag and Trimble [2001], creative activity became manifest after initiation of dopamine agonist therapy. Since dopamine agonism can reduce latent inhibition, it seems plausible that the patient's idea generation could be explained in this way. The case is more difficult to make in the other patients, however: there is evidence that lesioning frontal regions does not produce a reduction in latent inhibition [e.g. Lacroix et al., 2000] and there is no evidence on the effects on latent inhibition of lesioning the temporal lobes in areas other than medial temporal regions.

We may also question whether we would necessarily expect all of the patients under discussion to show much evidence of increased creative idea generation, or indeed any psychological marker, such as reduced latent inhibition, associated with it. In particular, that the output of FTD patients' art has been described as lacking in symbolism [Miller et al., 2000] may be suggestive of a somewhat *limited* 'original recombinant ideation' in these patients. One should perhaps be cautious in equating 'creativity', or any of its psychological synonyms, with whatever is being demonstrated when a patient engages in an activity which is nominally labelled as 'creative', such as painting. It is far from obvious that all the patients who exhibit de novo artistic behaviours are 'creative' in the sense that psychologists understand that term.

Nonetheless the latent inhibition hypothesis of creative ideation is an attractive theory as applied to normal subjects and might therefore usefully serve to inform future studies, particularly neuropsychological ones, into the precise nature of increased artistic behaviour in brain-injured individuals. In particular, the role of dopaminergic influences may be important. Flaherty [2005] has suggested a theory of idea generation and creative drive that incorporates frontal, temporal and limbic (primarily dopaminergic) influences. Increased activity in mesolimbic dopaminergic pathways is suggested to facilitate creativity by driving goal-directed behaviour and by reducing latent inhibition. She suggests that idea generation is distributed along another dimension. At one end of the dimension is rigid, halting thought, driven by abnormal frontal activity. At the other end is facile, loose speech and ideas, driven by abnormal temporal activity. Creative ideation appears to come about in this model when abnormal, though not excessively abnormal, temporal activity is combined with high dopaminergic drive.

Since nearly all of the 'creative' patients described in this paper showed some frontal dysfunction *as well as* temporal dysfunction, we disagree with this model, which essentially regards frontal dysfunction as having a purely negative influence on creativity and temporal dysfunction as having a positive influence. We suggest that frontal and temporal influences are more independent from one another, contributing separately and positively to the genesis of creative activity, at least in the patients described here. As already outlined, temporal dysfunction is modulated in most cases by the hemisphericity of the temporal dysfunction, influencing the modality of artistic output (visual, musical, written). Frontal dysfunction, on the other hand, plays a likely, although less well-defined role in determining the cognitive or behavioural changes that may be necessary for the development of creative activity.

Another compatible interpretation of the phenomenon is that the apparent drive is a practical and inevitable need to communicate the new perceptual (often visual) experiences brought on by brain injury [Miller et al., 2005]. At least two other examples of communicating unusual visual experiences through artistic behaviour can be observed in perceptual neurological phenomena and mental illness. Synaesthesia, a positive neurological phenomenon that occurs from early childhood, affects 4% of the population [Simner et al., 2006]. An otherwise healthy individual has automatic and involuntary experiences in one sensory modality when a different sensory modality is stimulated [Mulvenna and Walsh, 2005]. Different for each synaesthete, examples of these long-term discrete pairings can be simple such as the day Tuesday or the letter F triggering the experience of light pink, or more complex such as the sound of a middle C played on a piano triggering the sensation of a long green solid block moving in space, or the taste of salty burnt chicken. Synaesthesia has frequently been reported among poets, novelists, artists and musicians, such as Rimbaud, Baudelaire, Kandinsky, Nabokov, Scriabin, Messiaen and Heckney. Theories of its neurological basis include hyperconnectivity [Hubbard and Ramachandran, 2005] or disinhibited feedback [Grossenbacher and Lovelace, 2001] between unimodal sensory areas of the cortex and polymodal integration areas in the temporal lobe [Esterman et al., 2006]. fMRI studies and psychophysical tests demonstrate synaesthetes are having perceptual experiences distinctive to non-synaesthetes [e.g. Nunn et al., 2002; Mattingley et al., 2001]. Interestingly, synaesthetes perform better on tests of creativity similar to divergent thinking [Mulvenna et al., 2004] and those who pursue artistic life styles often report needing to communicate these unusual visual experiences through another medium. For example, Oliver Messiaen often composed so his colours triggered by the music 'blended well' together and argued: 'Colors are very important to me because I have a gift – it's not my fault, it's just how I am – whenever I hear music or even if I read music, I see colors' [Cytowic, 2002].

This theme of atypical perceptual experience triggering idea generation for artistic output recurs in reports of patients with dementia with Lewy bodies. Dementia with Lewy bodies is characterized by highly complex visual and auditory hallucinations, often involving animals or people. These are occasionally portrayed in sketches; paranoid delusions are also characteristic of the disease and may be expressed though poetry [Miller et al., 2005; Sahlas, 2003; Chan and Rosser, 2002].

Conclusions

The emergence of de novo artistic behaviours following brain injury is a rare phenomenon and may not even represent the same underlying mechanism throughout the different conditions in which it occurs. There is clearly an important role for hemispheric localization of pathology, which is usually temporal, upon the medium of artistic expression, and a presumed role for mild frontal dysfunction in producing certain behavioural and cognitive characteristics that may be conducive to the production of art. Beyond this, much is speculation; particularly, the nature of the creative drive and the source of idea generation in these patients remain uncertain. Nonetheless it is elucidation of these latter, least-understood aspects that we suspect is required to explain why only a small proportion of patients with the disorders discussed here go on to demonstrate emergence of artistic behaviours.

Further understanding of the aetiology of this behaviour may contribute to the literature on cognitive change after brain injury and on the neurobiological basis of creativity in man. Perhaps most importantly, its increased recognition and responsible nurturing in patients may serve as a source of great comfort to individuals and their families at an otherwise difficult time.

Acknowledgment

The authors would like to thank Michelle de Haan, David Gadian, Bruce Miller, Galit Kleiner-Fisman and Tommy McHugh for their valuable assistance.

References

Carson SH, Peterson JB, Higgins DM: Decreased latent inhibition is associated with increased creative achievement in high-functioning individuals. J Pers Soc Psychol 2003;85:499–506.

Chan D, Rossor MN: '-but who is that on the other side of you?' Extracampine hallucinations revisited. Lancet 2002;360:2064–2066.

Cytowic RE: Synaesthesia: A Union of the Senses, ed 2. New York, Springer, 2002.

Doricchi F, Tomaiuolo F: The anatomy of neglect without hemianopia: a key role for parietal-frontal disconnection? Neuroreport 2003;14:2239–2243.

Esterman M, Verstynen T, Ivry RB, Robertson LC: Coming unbound: disrupting automatic integration of synaesthetic color and graphemes by TMS of right parietal lobe. J Cogn Neurosci 2006;18:1570–1576.

Finkelstein Y, Vardi J, Hod I: Impulsive artistic creativity as a presentation of transient cognitive alterations. Behav Med 1991;17:91–94.

Flaherty AW: Frontotemporal and dopaminergic control of idea generation and creative drive. J Comp Neurol 2005;493:147–153.

Gray JA: Integrating schizophrenia. Schizophr Bull 1998;24:249–266.

Grossenbacher PG, Lovelace CT: Mechanisms of synesthesia: cognitive and physiological constraints. Trends Cogn Sci 2001;5:36–41.

Hubbard EM, Ramachandran VS: Neurocognitive mechanisms of synesthesia. Neuron 2005;48:509–520.

Kapur N: Paradoxical functional facilitation in brain-behaviour research. A critical review. Brain 1996;119:1775–1790.

Lacroix L, Spinelli S, White W, Feldon J: The effects of ibotenic acid lesions of the medial and lateral prefrontal cortex on latent inhibition, prepulse inhibition and amphetamine-induced hyperlocomotion. Neuroscience 2000;97:459–468.

Lubow RE, Moore AU: Latent inhibition: the effect of nonreinforced pre-exposure to the conditional stimulus. J Comp Physiol Psychol 1959;52:415–419.

Lythgoe MF, Pollak TA, Kalmus M, De Haan M, Chong WK: Obsessive, prolific artistic output following subarachnoid hemorrhage. Neurology 2005;64:397–398.

Mattingley JB, Rich AN, Yelland G, Bradshaw JL: Unconscious priming eliminates automatic binding of colour and alphanumeric form in synaesthesia. Nature 2001;410:580–582.

Mell JC, Howard SM, Miller BL: Art and the brain: the influence of frontotemporal dementia on an accomplished artist. Neurology 2003;60:1707–1710.

Mendez MF: Hypergraphia for poetry in an epileptic patient. J Neuropsychiatry Clin Neurosci 2005;17:560–561.

Miller BL, Boone K, Cummings JL, Read SL, Mishkin F: Functional correlates of musical and visual ability in frontotemporal dementia. Br J Psychiatry 2000;176:458–463.

Miller BL, Cummings J, Mishkin F, Boone K, Prince F, Ponton M, Cotman C: Emergence of artistic talent in frontotemporal dementia. Neurology 1998;51:978–982.

Miller BL, Yener G, Akdal G: Artistic patterns in dementia. J Neurol Sci (Turk) 2005;3:245–249.

Mulvenna C, Hubbard EM, Ramachandran VS, Pollick F: The relationship between synaesthesia and creativity. J Cogn Neurosci Suppl 2004;16:188.

Mulvenna C, Walsh V: Synaesthesia. Curr Biol 2005;15:R399–R400.

Nunn JA, Gregory LJ, Brammer M, Williams SC, Parslow DM, Morgan MJ, Morris RG, Bullmore ET, Baron-Cohen S, Gray JA: Functional magnetic resonance imaging of synesthesia: activation of V4/V8 by spoken words. Nat Neurosci 2002;5:371–375.

Sahlas DJ: Dementia with Lewy bodies and the neurobehavioral decline of Mervyn Peake. Arch Neurol 2003;60:889–892.

Schrag A, Trimble M: Poetic talent unmasked by treatment of Parkinson's disease. Mov Disord 2001;16:1175–1176.

Simner J, Mulvenna C, Sagiv N, Tsakanikos E, Witherby SA, Fraser C, Scott K, Ward J: Synaesthesia: the prevalence of atypical cross-modal experiences. Perception 2006;35:1024–1033.

Snyder AW, Bahramali H, Hawker T, Mitchell DJ: Savant-like numerosity skills revealed in normal people by magnetic pulses. Perception 2006;35:837–845.

Snyder AW, Mulcahy E, Taylor JL, Mitchell DJ, Sachdev P, Gandevia SC: Savant-like skills exposed in normal people by suppressing the left fronto-temporal lobe. J Integr Neurosci 2003;2: 149–158.
Thomas Anterion C, Honore-Masson S, Dirson S, Laurent B: Lonely cowboy's thoughts. Neurology 2002;59:1812–1813.
Van Vugt P, Paquier P, Kees L, Cras P: Increased writing activity in neurological conditions: a review and clinical study. J Neurol Neurosurg Psychiatry 1996;61:510–514.
Waxman SG, Geschwind N: Hypergraphia in temporal lobe epilepsy. Neurology 1974;24:629–636.

Mark F. Lythgoe, MSc, PhD
RCS Unit of Biophysics, Institute of Child Health
University College London
London, WC1N 1EH (UK)
Tel. +44 20 7905 2273, Fax +44 20 7905 2358, E-Mail m.lythgoe@ich.ucl.ac.uk

Bogousslavsky J, Hennerici MG (eds): Neurological Disorders in Famous Artists – Part 2.
Front Neurol Neurosci. Basel, Karger, 2007, vol 22, pp 89–104

Marcel Proust's Diseases and Doctors: The Neurological Story of a Life

Julien Bogousslavsky

Department of Neurology, Valmont Clinic, Genolier Swiss Medical Network, Glion-sur-Montreux, Switzerland

Abstract

Marcel Proust (1871–1922), one of the greatest writers of all times, suffered from asthma beginning at age 9, in an era when the illness was considered a 'nervous' disorder belonging to what Beard, in 1870, called 'neurasthenia'. Proust's father, Adrien, was himself a professor of medicine (hygiene) who had met Charcot, and who contributed to neurology with studies on aphasia, stroke, hysteria, and neurasthenia – a condition about which he, along with Gilbert Ballet, published a book in 1897. Through his father, Proust met Edouard Brissaud, the co-founder of the *Revue Neurologique* in 1893, and, in 1896, the author of *The Hygiene of the Asthmatics*, with a foreword by Adrien Proust. Shortly after his mother's death in 1905, Proust contemplated admitting himself to a private hospital to reset his irregular sleep patterns and to improve his asthma. He hesitated in his choice of care between Jules Dejerine in Paris, Henry-Auguste Widmer at Valmont, and Paul Dubois in Bern. Finally, he decided to enter Paul Sollier's clinic, in Boulogne-sur-Seine, on the advice of Brissaud, and stayed there for 6 weeks in semi-isolation. Together with Babinski, Sollier was, at that time, considered the most gifted follower of Charcot. He was a forerunner of studies on emotional memory, which strongly influenced Proust. In Proust's opus magnum work *In Search of Lost Time*, 'involuntary memory' indeed forms the core mechanism of the entire novel, counterbalancing the decaying effects of time. A few years before his death from complicated bronchopneumonia at age 52, Proust became terrified of developing a stroke, like his mother and father, and he consulted with Joseph Babinski, who tried to reassure him. Proust's life followed an unusual neurological itinerary, which has been largely overlooked, but which is in fact critical for an understanding of his literary work.

Marcel Proust (1871–1922) (fig. 1), the greatest French novelist of the 20th century and one of the greatest writers of all times, is well known for a few medical and personal peculiarities that markedly influenced his work: homosexuality, asthma, sleep disturbances, largely self-administered drug therapy, and deep

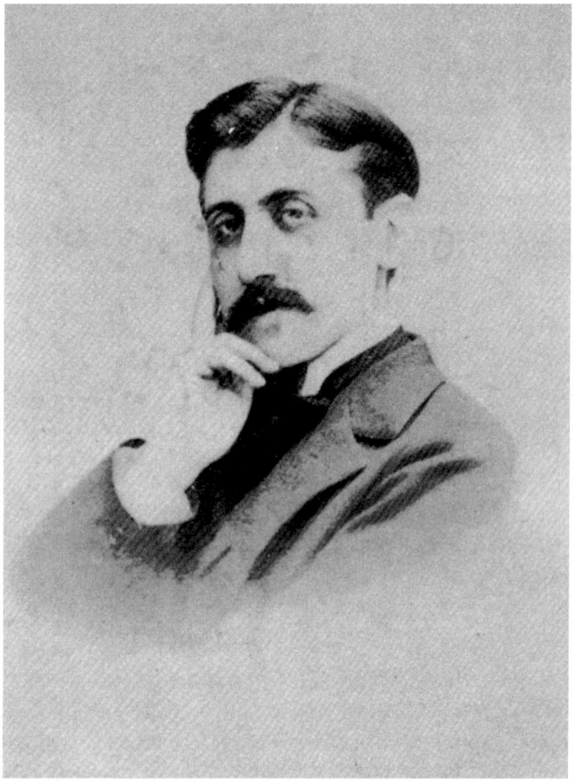

Fig. 1. Marcel Proust. From Abraham P: Proust. Paris, Rieder, 1930.

knowledge of the medical world of his time. Himself both a son and brother of famous doctors, Proust met most of the medical intelligentsia of Paris around 1900 not only as a patient but also privately and at social gatherings, all of which aided in the acquisition of specific information used to introduce several medical characters in his opus magnum, *A la recherche du temps perdu* (poorly translated as 'Remembrance of Things Past'), a 3,500-page novel divided into seven volumes written between 1909 and 1922 [Proust, 1987–1989].

The medical problems of Marcel Proust have already been addressed [Béhar, 1970; Falliers, 1986; Seidmann, 1961; Sharma, 2000; Soupault, 1967; Straus, 1980; Mabin, 1992], but without emphasis on their neurological aspects. Proust suffered recurrent attacks of severe asthma from the age of 9 and developed obstructive pneumopathy before finally dying of infectious pneumonia at age 51. It is striking that most of the famous doctors whom he met were neurologists, probably due to the fact that asthma was largely considered a 'nervous disease' at the time and Proust also categorized himself as being 'a nervous' (i.e. a neurotic). While his father had treated cholera and was subsequently elected to the Chair of Hygiene at the Faculty of Medicine in Paris, he also studied aphasia and wrote on topics of neurasthenia, a group of disorders which today would largely encompass psychosomatic dysfunction, including asthma. All of Proust's biographers have insisted on the importance of his complex relationships with diseases, doctors and medicine but none have highlighted the fact that neurology played a critical role, until recently [Tadié, 1996].

Proust's Father and Other Doctors

Proust's father, Adrien Proust (1834–1903), was an important academic figure in French medicine at the end of the 19th century. By the time he had completed his medical thesis in 1862, Charcot and Potain had recently been appointed to the Medical Faculty in Paris. Before he became famous for his studies on cholera and hygiene, he completed a study on 'Different Forms of Softening of the Brain' to gain his professorship. He also wrote two essays: 'On Aphasia' (1872) and 'Aphasia and Trepanation' (1874), which demonstrated his interest in the brain and its disorders. He became chief of service at La Charité, Lariboisière and Hôtel-Dieu, and was then elected to the Academy of Medicine. Adrien Proust also contributed to the creation of the International Office of Hygiene, the forerunner of the World Health Organization. His most popular book was, *The Hygiene of the Neurasthenic* (1897), which he published together with Gilbert Ballet in the same collection as Brissaud's *The Hygiene of the Asthmatics* (1896). In his book, it seems obvious that the father is making reference to his own son, then aged 26, as he cited the effects of a 'bad education', including too much attention and (maternal) preoccupation, as a source of neurasthenia. However, despite this fact, we know of only three letters from Marcel to his father [Tadié, 1999], while dozens of letters to his mother have been found. Nevertheless, the relationship between father and son was deep and loving. The cliché of Marcel being loved mainly by his mother, while the father only loved Marcel's younger brother, Robert (who became a famous urologist), is inaccurate, and the family seems to have been strong and stable.

Thanks to his father, Marcel Proust heard a great deal about medicine during the family meals at home, where he still lived at age 32 when his father died. He also had the unique opportunity to meet many of his father's colleagues, including Brouardel (Dean of the faculty), Doyen (a famous surgeon), Pozzi (a famous, high-society doctor whose daughter became Paul Valéry's lover), Dieulafoy (famous colleague of his father at the Hôtel-Dieu, whom Proust included by using his name in his novel), Robin (who is said to have mentioned to Marcel that he had better keep his asthma in order to avoid other, more severe diseases), Guyon (a famous urologist who liked jokes, just like professor Cottard in the novel, and who became the teacher of his brother, Robert), Laboulbène, Auguste Broca, and Cotard (who still survives in spirit due to his 'delirium of negation' syndrome, and probably inspired the name of Cottard in the novel), all of whom contributed to some extent to the personalities and features of the doctors who appear in *A la recherche du temps perdu*. Several books that he used as sources of medical information were also at Marcel's disposal at the family home. The main of these was probably, *The New Dictionary of Medicine and Practical Surgery*, which appeared in 40 volumes under the direction of Sigismond Jaccoud, including a 150-page chapter on asthma by Germain Sée.

Through his friend, painter Jacques-Emile Blanche, Marcel Proust also met Blanche's father, Antoine, who cared for Guy de Maupassant when he developed syphilitic general paresis. Antoine was the son of Esprit Blanche, who had treated Gérard de Nerval for several years before he committed suicide. Apart from neurologists who will be mentioned later in this chapter, Marcel Proust consulted many other doctors, mainly in connection with his asthma [Tadié, 1996, pp. 532–536]: Dr. Duplay, who was present when Marcel Proust had his first attack of asthma at age 9 during a walk with his family in the Champs-Elysées (fig. 2), and who more than 10 years later wrote certificates allowing Proust to be discharged from military obligations (he had not been dispended from military service by major Dr. Kopf in 1889–1890); Dr. Merklen, a lung and heart specialist at the Hôpital Laennec; Merklen advised Proust that his asthma had become a 'nervous habit', and recommended that he go to Bern to see Paul Dubois, a psychiatrist who was a colleague and friend of Jules Dejerine; Nicolas Vaschide, a doctor from Rumania who had studied dreams – and about whom Proust made jokes because he could not pronounce the letter 'r', saying 'this is nelvous'; Georges Linossier, who wrote *The Hygiene of the Dyspeptic* (1900); Léon Faisans, whom he asked whether he should see Dejerine for his 'nervous' asthma; Vaquez, who later gave his name to polyglobulia, and whom Proust saw for a 'disturbed pulse'; Dr. Wicart, who was an ENT specialist; Dr. Cottet, a general physician in Evian, and Dr. Henry-Auguste Widmer (1853–1939), a celebrated Swiss physician who owned the well-known Valmont Clinic in Glion-sur-Montreux, where many famous and wealthy Parisians spent a few weeks for medical cures, including Proust's friends Madame Straus and René Blum.

However, the only physician who can be said to have really looked after Proust with his various medical problems during the last 20 years of his life is Dr. Bize, a family doctor recommended by his brother, Robert [Painter, 1979]. From 1904 onward, after Proust was discharged from a 6-week cure at Dr. Sollier's Clinic in Boulogne, Dr. Bize faithfully visited him every Friday until his patient's death. He called him 'Maître' and continued to care for him medically despite

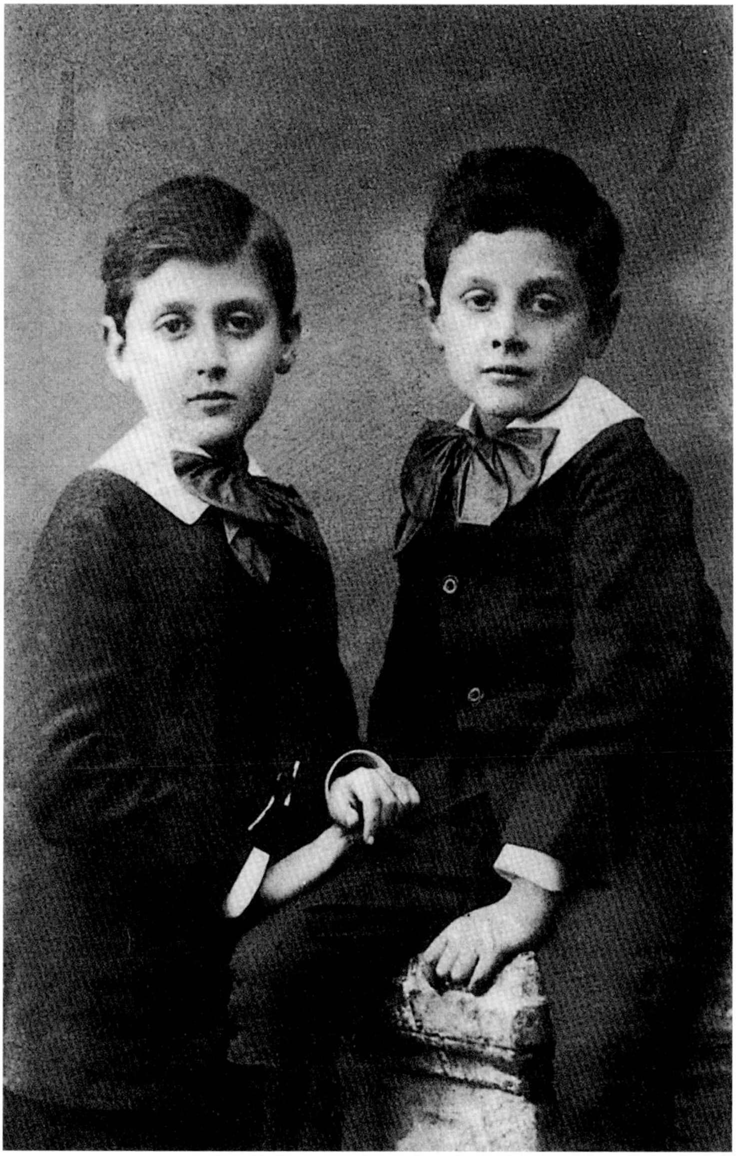

Fig. 2. Marcel Proust shortly after he developed asthma, with his brother Robert. From Abraham P: Proust. Paris, Rieder, 1930.

Proust's attitude disregarding many of his prescriptions, using others to excess and often taking drugs of his own choice. Apart from the very last days when Proust was suffocating with infectious pneumonia, his brother, Robert, never cared for him as a physician, except to advise him regarding other colleagues.

Marcel Proust often exhibited his identification with physicians by advising friends, providing detailed prescriptions and making specific diagnoses, including prognostic features. For instance, letters to the two first readers of his novel, Louis de Robert and Lucien Daudet, include complex discussions of their medical symptoms, with diagnoses and treatments [Proust, 1970–1993]. It is obvious that Proust integrated much of what he heard and read at his family home, so that he could state to his faithful 'gouvernante' Céleste Albaret: 'When one is a doctor's son, one ends up becoming one as well', and 'I am more a doctor than the doctors' [Albaret, 1973]. This is probably why he acquired the habit of selecting and adapting his medications himself, often without following any of the advice of his physicians. In fact, it seems that Proust was probably more interested in consulting the many doctors he met so as to enter into discussions with them, asking them questions with the goal of getting specific medical information for his novel, rather than for personal, medical purposes [Billières, 1961]. In doing so, he was reproducing what he did when he visited so many 'salons' in high Parisian society, where he found the inspiration for and details of the human characters of his future novel, and which gave him the inaccurate qualification of being an upper-class writer [Painter, 1979; Tadié, 1996].

The Diseases of Marcel Proust

In his dedication in the first volume of his novel to Céline Cottin, his housekeeper and cook, Proust signed: 'The sick in perpetuity'. Indeed, sickness was a part of Proust's daily life from childhood to death. It has even been suggested that Proust 'liked' his diseases, and did not do what he should have done to treat himself [Seidmann, 1961]. However, I think that he rather displayed behavior which is common in patients with a fluctuating, chronic disease, in which patients attempt to become familiar with their medical problems and consider disease as a 'partner', because they fear it so much.

After the inaugural attack at age 9, Proust's asthma worsened during adolescence before slightly remitting, to worsen again from age 23 onward. While he had been able to accomplish his military obligations when he was 19, 5 years later he had to be placed on medical leave from his job at the Bibliothèque Mazarine. Proust's asthma has been the subject of detailed discussions [Falliers, 1986; Seidmann, 1961; Sharma, 2000]. While it was associated with allergies and hay fever – and there is no doubt at all that it was a common, severe form of organic bronchial asthma – at that time asthma was largely considered a 'nervous disease', explaining why a famous neurologist like Edouard Brissaud was the author of *The Hygiene of Asthmatics* in 1896, with a preface by Adrien Proust. Asthma was often considered a manifestation of neurasthenia (which mainly covered what we would call psychosomatic disorders today), a topic which was becoming as popular as Charcot's hysteria, and about which Adrien Proust wrote a major book [Proust and Ballet, 1897]. This is also the reason why Proust sought the advice of so many famous neurologists and neuropsychiatrists of his time [Tadié, 1996, p. 663]. It is likely that several nonrespiratory manifestations exhibited by Proust, such as 'cardiac spasms', 'dyspepsia', headache, and back pain belonged to what was then called neurasthenia (and somatization today), and of which no specific organic substrate was ever found.

The treatment of Proust's asthma rapidly became chaotic, with numerous self-prescribed drugs and diets, despite Dr. Bize's good will and faithfulness. Fumigations with antiasthma powders became the mainstay of his management, as emphasized by Albaret [1973]. Antiasthma cigarettes, ether syrup, balsamic substances, opium derivatives, various barbiturates, chloral hydrate, adrenaline, euvalpine, sparteine, aspirin, and other drugs were used by him in various mixtures [Falliers, 1986; Mabin, 1992; Soupault, 1967]. It seems that Proust developed a specific therapy, combining sleep-inducing drugs such as barbiturates (trional, veronal) with stimulants such as adrenaline and coffee. During the few days which preceded his death, his only intake was coffee with cold beer, which Céleste Albaret had to order at the Ritz, Proust's favorite eating place in Paris [Albaret, 1973].

In addition to his attacks of asthma, it is likely that Proust developed what is known as 'chronic asthmatic dyspnea', which corresponds to a chronic obstructive bronchopulmonary disorder with an enlarged anteroposterior chest diameter, as can be seen in the late photographs of Proust (fig. 3). In early October of 1922, Proust developed symptoms of infectious bronchitis, which seriously worsened on October 19 after he went outside, despite being forbidden to do so by Dr. Bize. Dr. Bize isolated pneumococci in the expectorations, and a few days later the picture evolved into infectious bronchopneumonia. Proust rejected his brother's plea that he should be transferred to the Piccini Clinic, and he refused further treatments, claiming that doctors should not prolong 'miserable lives' [Albaret, 1973; Tadié, 1996, p. 907]. According to Albaret [1973], who was present nearly day and night, the last few days were terribly painful and difficult, since the patient suffocated while remaining fully conscious until the end, which supervened on November 18 at 4:30 p.m.

Beside asthma and associated psychosomatic manifestations of neurasthenia, Proust's main medical problem seems to have been iatrogenic, in relation to the many medications which he often took in an erratic way [Mabin, 1992;

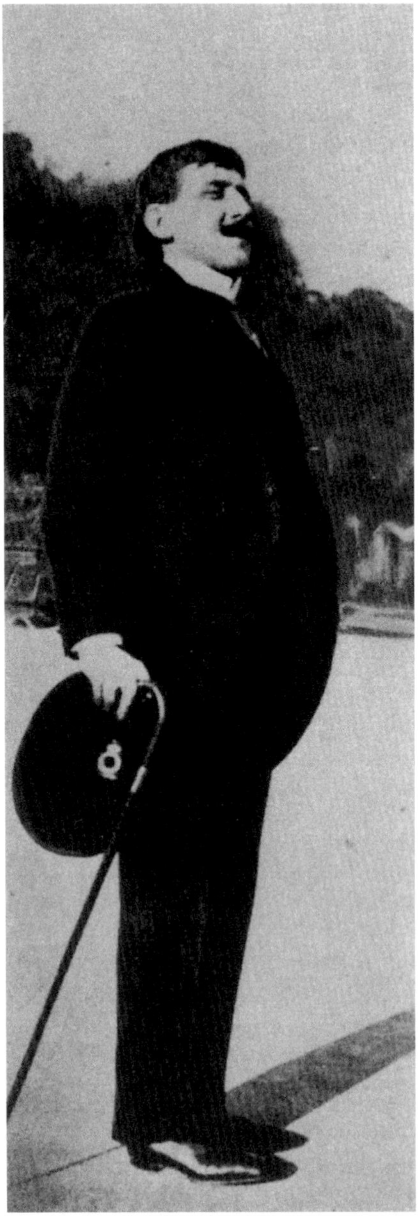

Fig. 3. Marcel Proust a few weeks before his death, showing an enlarged anteroposterior thoracic diameter. From Abraham P: Proust. Paris, Rieder, 1930.

Tadié, 1996]. At least two severe episodes of intoxication accompanied by disturbances of consciousness have been recorded, in 1917 and in 1921 [Albaret, 1973]. Highly likely, these occurred in relation to an excessive intake of sleep inducers such as barbiturates. Interestingly, in 1921 Proust wrote,

'Intoxications are also useful to reassure the patient who learns with pleasure that his paralysis is just a toxic malaise' [Tadié, 1996, p. 870]. Chronic, excessive intake of these drugs alternating with the intake of stimulants may also have resulted in symptoms which alarmed Proust in the last third of his life, including memory dysfunction, slurred speech, dizziness, awkward gestures and falls. It reminded him of the fact that both his father and mother had died of 'apoplexia', and he often expressed a fear of aphasia, which his mother had developed shortly before she died and about which his father had written extensively more than 40 years earlier. He wrote to friends that he forgot to finish writing letters, and that at times he was having problems with 'speech, vision and movement'. Some of these manifestations were introduced by him in his novel, when Bergotte, the famous writer inspired by Anatole France, is afflicted by a series of malaises before he dies of 'apoplexia', although his symptoms today would not be accepted as suggestive of a stroke. Proust was well aware of the problems linked to chronic substance abuse, and he commented to a friend 'chloral is making holes in my brain'.

A last interesting symptom is Proust's modified sense of temperature, since it is well known that, even in summer, he went out wearing furs and scarves. At home, he spent much of his time in bed under a pile of covers, as he wrote on July 14, 1921 – while a patriotic show had been cancelled due to extremely hot weather – that he was writing in bed 'under seven wool covers, a fur, three hot stones and a fire' [Tadié, 1996, p. 858]. The explanation remains unclear, but it may have been related to hypothalamic dysfunction also induced by chronic drug abuse for many years.

Proust, Neurology, and Neurologists

Proust's interest in neurology and neuropsychiatry has been underlined above in connection with his father's studies on aphasia and neurasthenia, while he always considered his diseases as belonging to 'nervous' (in the sense of psychically related) disorders, including asthma. His fear of aphasia was due to episodes of slurred speech and impaired memory, which were probably drug-related, but which reminded him of the death of his parents. Adrien Proust died of 'brain hemorrhage' on November 26, 1903, after 3 days of altered consciousness. His wife died at age 56 on September 26, 1905, of an 'uremic crisis', but with hemiplegia and speech impairment, which is highly suggestive of a stroke. In 1920 Proust wrote that 'a foreigner has taken domicile in my brain' [Tadié, 1996, p. 852], and in his last important article 'About Baudelaire', he identified himself with the poet, who had become aphasic, emphasizing that the disease possibly allowed him to get 'this lucidity of truc suffering' [Tadié, 1996, p. 860].

It is thus not surprising that the most famous physicians whom Proust consulted during his life were indeed neurologists or neuropsychiatrists.

Proust's mother had been a patient of Joseph Babinski (1857–1932), one of the most celebrated clinical neurologists of all times [Haymaker and Schiller, 1970]. Proust first consulted with him during the spring of 1918, when he believed that he might have to undergo brain surgery because he felt that he was developing facial palsy [Tadié, 1996, p. 794]. Proust's friend, Léon Daudet, who completed medical studies before becoming a famous chronicle writer, reported that, along with Sollier, Babinski was the most accurate clinical observer of Charcot's pupils when the master was visiting patients in hospital [Daudet, 1992a]. He also wrote emphatically that Babinski was 'without contest, the premier neurologist in the universe' [Daudet, 1992c]. Proust remembered that Babinski did not know him at all as a writer, and asked him about his job. In March 1919, he again felt the same manifestations that had prompted him to consult with Babinski, and feared a 'grave cerebral cause', although he also suspected that veronal abuse may have been responsible [Tadié, 1996, p. 811]. However, he did not consult with Babinski at that time, and only saw him again in 1921 because of episodes of speech disturbances. Apparently Babinski made him pronounce 'constantinopolitain' and 'artilleur de l'artillerie', and subsequently reassured his patient. On the day of Proust's death, Babinski came to see him at the request of his colleague, Robert Proust, only to confirm that 'it is all over', and suggesting to Robert and Dr. Bize not to perform a last injection, which Proust feared so much and which would not have changed the fatal evolution within the following hours [Albaret, 1973; Painter, 1979; Tadié, 1996]. It is possible that Proust thought of Babinski when working on volume 4 (*Sodome et Gomorrhe*) of his novel in 1921, where he quotes 'a celebrity of nervous diseases'.

Edouard Brissaud (1852–1909) (fig. 4), one of the founders of the *Revue Neurologique*, was probably the neurologist whom Proust knew the best, most likely because he had published a book on *The Hygiene of the Asthmatics* (1896) in the same collection as *The Hygiene of the Neurasthenic* by Adrien Proust, and with a preface by him. Proust liked him, but called him the 'doctor despite himself' in a letter to Anna de Noailles, because he had difficulties getting him to speak about medicine. He also wrote: 'an admirable man, with a vast intelligence, but a poor physician, who thought (I am exaggerating only a bit) that one should live on trional'. However, at the same time Proust was warmly recommending barbiturates to Louis de Robert, mentioning his cousin, the philosopher Henri Bergson, who had been taking trional 'regularly, for years' [Tadié, 1996, p. 812]. In 1904, Proust read for the second time Brissaud's book on asthma, in which the condition is presented as a 'neurosis' occurring in people with a 'morbid, capricious and autocratic personality' [Brissaud, 1896].

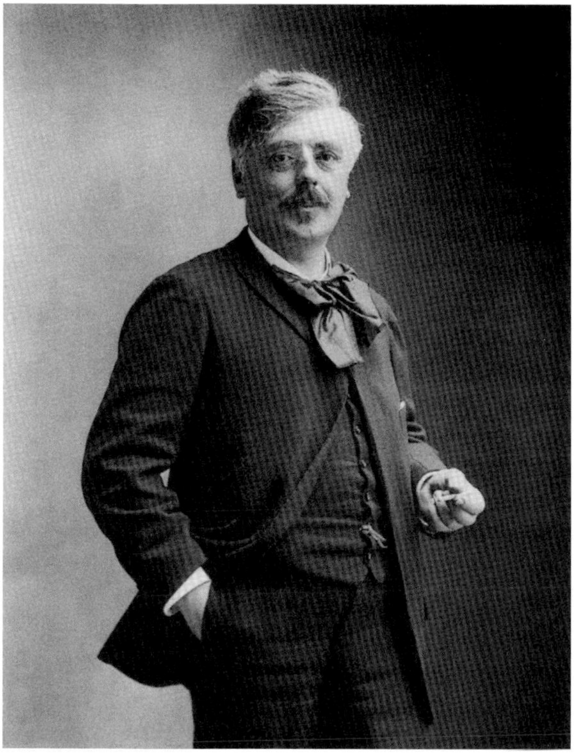

Fig. 4. Edouard Brissaud, founder of the *Revue Neurologique*, who inspired Proust for the character of Dr. du Boulbon in his novel (private collection).

In Proust's novel, Brissaud largely inspired the character of Dr. du Boulbon (and also of Professor E***), who made instinctual diagnoses, while the more scientific and erudite figure of Dr. Cottard was in part inspired by his father. Léon Daudet described Brissaud as 'sentimental and Romanesque', a man who liked to laugh and was as famous for his jokes as his neurology [Daudet, 1992a]. In the second volume (*A l'ombre des jeunes filles en fleurs*) of his novel, Proust describes Dr. du Boulbon: 'A specialist of nervous diseases, the one to whom Charcot, before dying, had said that he would dominate neurology and psychiatry.' However, Brissaud's career was less accomplished than that of other neurologists, such as Dejerine or Marie, a fact that Léon Daudet explained with the fact that he remained unable to emancipate himself from the nihilistic therapeutic attitude of his master, Charcot [Daudet, 1992c].

In 1904, Proust asked Dr. Léon Faisans, a pneumologist, whether he should consult with Jules Dejerine (1849–1917) because his asthma was 'nervous'.

Dejerine was the second successor of Charcot at the Clinique des Maladies du Systèmes Nerveux at La Salpétrière, the world Mecca for neurology, and he was unanimously recognized as the leading neurological figure in France [Haymaker and Schiller, 1970]. Léon Daudet described him as 'precise, and giving the impression of being a misanthrop' [Daudet, 1992c]. Proust however hesitated, because Dejerine's 'cure' was known to include a strict, 3-month isolation in a clinic, which Proust feared very much [Tadié, 1996, p. 552]. Finally, his mother's death caused him, on December 5, 1905, to make an appointment to enter the Clinique des Soeurs de la Sainte-Famille, rue Blomet in Paris, where Dejerine saw and hospitalized his private patients. Apparently he had promised Proust that he would be 'cured' after his famous 3-month isolation stay in the clinic. Nevertheless, Proust became so anxious about the therapy that he cancelled his room the day before admission, and simultaneously made an appointment with Dr. Paul-Auguste Sollier for December 6. Sollier (1861–1938) was another pupil of Charcot, who evolved more in the direction of psychiatry than neurology, and who had been recommended to Proust by Brissaud. Like Cottard in Proust's novel, he became famous for his expertise in 'chronic intoxications'. He worked in a clinic at 145, route de Versailles in Boulogne-sur-Seine, a Parisian suburb, where he admitted patients for a shorter and less strict isolation than Dejerine. This type of cure had been initiated by Camus and Pagniez, with the support of Dejerine. Sollier convinced Proust to follow his therapy and to be admitted to the clinic, where he stayed until January 25, 1906. In fact, for Proust the aim of the stay was to retrain his completely disorganized sleeping schedule [Mabin, 1992] rather than to treat asthma; indeed, his sleep cycle had progressively become totally disturbed by his own habit of working at night, and shortly before his mother died he was waking up at around 8 or 9 p.m., having his mother prepare his breakfast for 11 p.m.! The relationship with Sollier does not seem to have been as good as it should have been, and Proust was upset that the doctor criticized his cousin, Bergson, during one of their first interviews. During his stay in the clinic, where the application of the isolation concept seems to have been quite relative, he wrote: 'I wanted to think that the treatment would have made Mom happy. But my cure is tremendously bad for me.' And shortly after being discharged, early in 1906: 'By the way, I came back here more ill than when I left.'

Proust also had contacts in Switzerland for similar cures in private clinics. Although he never decided to go and see him, he thought several times of consulting with Dr. Paul Dubois (1848–1918), a psychiatrist in Bern who had remained a close friend of Dejerine after they went to school together in Geneva. Dubois had published *The Psychoneuroses and Their Moral Treatment* in 1905, with a preface by Dejerine. He was probably recommended to Proust by his friend, Fernand Gregh, who had been treated by Dubois. In September 1905 Proust and his mother went to Evian, on Lake Geneva, for the purpose of consulting with either Dr. Dubois or Dr. Widmer, who had a well-known clinic at Valmont, in Glion-sur-Montreux, just above Territet, in Switzerland. However, Proust's mother started to develop the serious manifestations which led to her death a few days later, so that she went back immediately to Paris, being followed a few days later by her son. The idea of consulting with Dr. Widmer probably came from Madame Straus, who stayed regularly at the Valmont Clinic from 1904 onward to treat her neurasthenia. When she came back to Paris in 1904, Proust amusingly wrote her about his recent text, 'On Reading': 'Do not read, there are sentences one page long that Dr. Widmer would especially forbid you.'

In 1911, after Proust experienced asthma attacks for the first time by the sea in Cabourg, he again thought of making the trip to Switzerland to see Dr. Widmer [Tadié, 1996, p. 663]. When his friend, René Blum, left Paris for Valmont in February 1913, this reminded Proust that he should also go, 'to change my hours' (he was again living only during the night) in order to be able to make a trip to Florence and see the city in daylight [Painter, 1979, p. 242]. While he did not go at that time because he wanted to keep an eye on his lover-secretary, Alfred Agostinelli, in Paris, records have been kept of Proust's visits to Valmont in 1912–1913.

While he did not consult with him personally, Proust arranged an appointment for Jacques Rivière with Dejerine's famous pupil, Gustave Roussy, Gaston Gallimard's collaborator at the *Nouvelle Revue Française*, even sending him some money in advance for Rivière's consultation. Adrien Proust had met Charcot during the early part of his career, but his son was only 22 years old when the master of La Salpétrière died. However, in 1907 he met his son in Cabourg, Jean-Baptiste Charcot who, after following the footsteps of his famous father in neurology, became even more famous as a polar explorer.

Neurology and Medicine in Proust's Work

Proust's major work *A la recherche du temps perdu* is full of medical references, many of which are neurological. A detailed study of them remains to be done. While Proust's first novel, *Jean Santeuil* (unpublished until the 1950s) [Proust, 1971] contains virtually no medical references, in 1904 – shortly after visiting Brissaud and while working on the first drafts which would lead to his major novel – Proust wrote to Anna de Noailles that he wanted to write a book on doctors. *A la recherche du temps perdu* did not become a book on doctors, but the role of patients, doctors and medicine is significant, and largely based on Proust's personal experiences with his own diseases and doctors, particularly neurologists. Apart from the narrator himself, the eight main patients in the novel include Tante Léonie, the grand-mother, Saniette, Bergotte, Swann, La Berma, and Charlus, who all more or less had the same medical fate leading to their deaths [Béhar, 1970]. Like Proust, the narrator, who also suffers from asthma, stayed (twice) in private clinics. Apart from Cottard (mainly based on Proust's father) the organicist and Du Boulbon (mainly based on Brissaud) the artist, several doctors also appear in the novel, including two real doctors, Dieulafoy and Potain, who were colleagues of his father. None of them gives a very positive and encouraging image of doctors and medicine, corresponding to Proust's own ambivalence, which made him state that medicine mainly prolonged diseases, although not to believe in medicine would still be a greater folly than to believe in it ... Overall, Proust's depiction of doctors is mainly humoristic [Billières, 1961], especially the most famous professors – probably a way for him to accept somehow the failure of medicine to really help him. With this in mind, he came to the conclusion that 'medicine is a compendium of all sequential and contradictory errors of doctors'.

Probably one of the most interesting connections between Proust's life and his novel is how his own memory experiences became a driving force for the intrigue in the book. One of the book's main themes opposes the value of emotional factors in life and artistic creativity of involuntary memory, to the sterile process of voluntary memory which is unable to introduce the reality of the past into the present, because in it 'nothing is left from what one has truly experienced', he stated in *Le temps retrouvé*, the seventh and last volume of his novel which was only published several years after his death. Involuntary memory has nothing to do with conscious associations of ideas, but is triggered by futile, unrelated perceptions which seem to open forgotten, vivid emotions. This theme, which accompanies the reader through all the 3,500 pages of the novel, shed a revolutionary view on the static, mechanistic views on memory, before Freud also came to emphasize the dynamic forces of emotions which lay behind memories and the process of remembering them. Although Proust disliked the comparison, he was close to the concept of 'lived duration' elaborated by his cousin, the philosopher Bergson, at the same time. An interesting background which has not been emphasized adequately is that Proust's father observed that his son's voluntary memory was being altered by his chaotic sleep schedules and his exaggerated drug intake, combining barbiturates with caffeine and other stimulants, together with beer and champagne [Dieguez, 2006]. In *The Hygiene of the Neurasthenic* (1897), Adrien Proust underlines the 'complex play of emotional states', especially in 'awake sleepers', which obviously reminds us of the beginning of his son's novel

(*Combray*), where the narrator describes his emotions during twilight states between wakefulness and sleep. Even more striking in the father's book is the following, which indeed contains no less than what will become the title of his son's novel [Tadié, 1999]: 'L'évocation des souvenirs est défectueuse parce qu'ils (les patients) sont impuissants à soutenir l'effort d'attention nécessité par la recherche du souvenir perdu' (i.e. 'The evocation of memories is impaired, because they (patients) are unable to sustain the effort of attention which is necessary for the search of the lost memory') [Proust and Ballet, 1897, p. 76]. Marcel Proust himself regularly complained of his disturbed, poor memory, referring to difficulties in remembering practical details of his life upon request, i.e. voluntary memory. This disturbance may well have had its counterpart in enhanced bursts of involuntary memories, which could have been facilitated by innocuous stimuli during drug-induced slightly modified states of consciousness. Proust himself acknowledged in his novel that this peculiar process of remembering might be the 'privilege of the nervous'. One could speculate that the frontal mechanisms of voluntary retrieval, the functioning of which is heavily dependent on proper cortical activation, were altered in Proust due to his chronic intake of hypnotics and other drugs, while the emergence of emotional 'involuntary' memories, which are linked to the amygdaloid nuclear complex in the temporal lobe, were not impaired or were even facilitated. The circuitry does not necessitate the high level of cortical activation associated with consciousness, as demonstrated by the common occurrence of such vivid memories during dreams, and the marked difficulties in remembering them after waking up, with consciousness arousal.

Proust used medicine and neurology to analyze, as he did with society in general, the behavior of doctors, whom he knew only too well because of his chronic, debilitating disease. However, his constant comparisons and reference to medicine, diseases and doctors throughout the book go much beyond a mere humoristic description of strange habits and tics of a corporation. It also plunges into the roots of suffering and emotions, as well as the multiple expressions they take in an individual from life to death. As his friend Léon Daudet, whose intervention was critical to Proust for obtaining the Goncourt Prize in 1919 for his novel's second volume (*A l'ombre des jeunes filles en fleurs*), wrote: 'While a part of Marcel Proust's brain admires and tastes, another one criticizes and becomes irritated, and a third one observes, indifferent and as if "spinozied", the interactions of the two other ones' [Daudet, 1992b].

Acknowledgement

I am very grateful to Mark Inglin, MS, for revising the English text.

References

Albaret C: Monsieur Proust. Paris, Robert Laffont, 1973.

Béhar S: L'univers médical de Marcel Proust. Cahiers Marcel Proust, NRF. Paris, Gallimard, 1970.

Billières R: Les médecins et Marcel Proust. Bull Soc Amis Marcel Proust Amis Combray 1961;12: 542–544.

Brissaud E: L'hygiène des asthmatiques. Paris, Masson, 1896.

Daudet L: Devant la douleur; in Daudet L (ed): Souvenirs et polémiques. Bouquins. Paris, Robert Laffont, 1992a.

Daudet L: Salons et journaux; in Daudet L (ed): Souvenirs et polémiques. Bouquins. Paris, Robert Laffont, 1992b.

Daudet L: Rive gauche; in Daudet L (ed): Souvenirs et polémiques. Bouquins. Paris, Robert Laffont, 1992c.

Dieguez S: Proust ou la mémoire involontaire. Cerveau Psycho 2006;14:86–90.

Dubois P: Les psychonévroses et leur traitement moral. Paris, Masson, 1905.

Falliers CJ: The literary genius and the many maladies of Marcel Proust. J Asthma 1986;23:157–164.

Haymaker W, Schiller F: The Founders of Neurology. Springfield, Thomas, 1970.

Linossier G: L'hygiène du dyspeptique. Paris, Masson, 1900.

Mabin D: Le sommeil de Marcel Proust. Paris, PUF 'Ecrivains', 1992.

Painter GD: Marcel Proust. Paris, Mercure de France, 1979.

Proust A, Ballet G: L'hygiène du neurasthénique. Paris, Masson, 1897.

Proust M: Correspondance générale. Paris, Plon, 1970–1993.

Proust M: Jean Santeuil. Paris, Pléiade, Gallimard, 1971.

Proust M: A la recherche du temps perdu. Paris, Pléiade, Gallimard, 1987–1989.

Seidmann E: Marcel Proust et les médecins. Bull Soc Amis Marcel Proust Amis Combray 1961;12: 522–541.

Sharma OP: Marcel Proust (1871–1922): reassessment of his asthma and other maladies. Eur Respir J 2000;15:958–960.

Soupault R: Marcel Proust, du côté de la médecine. Paris, Plon, 1967.

Straus B: The Maladies of Marcel Proust: Doctors and Diseases in His Life and Work. New York, Holmes & Meier, 1980.

Tadié J-Y: Marcel Proust. Biographies NRF. Paris, Gallimard, 1996.

Tadié J-Y: Marcel Proust, l'écriture et les arts. Bibliothèque nationale de France – Réunion des Musées Nationaux. Paris, Gallimard, 1999.

Julien Bogousslavsky, MD
Department of Neurology, Valmont Clinic
Genolier Swiss Medical Network
CH–1823 Glion-sur-Montreux (Switzerland)
Tel. +41 21 962 3701, Fax +41 21 962 3838, E-Mail jb@valmontgenolier.ch

Bogousslavsky J, Hennerici MG (eds): Neurological Disorders in Famous Artists – Part 2.
Front Neurol Neurosci. Basel, Karger, 2007, vol 22, pp 105–120

Heinrich Heine and Syphilis

Christoph auf der Horst

Institute for the History of Medicine, Heinrich Heine University Düsseldorf, Düsseldorf, Germany

Abstract

Though Heinrich Heine died 151 years ago, the underlying illness responsible for his suffering of many years has never been fully clarified. The diagnosis put forward most frequently in retrospect was that of a venereal disease. However, this diagnosis was the result of an interpretation in disregard of the historical context. Only by evaluating and interpreting the entire source material in its historical context (Heine's complete works, his correspondence, records of conversations kept by contemporaries and prescriptions) can this diagnosis be confirmed on a reliable basis. Above all, medical records dated 1848 and their interpretation in the context of contemporary syphilis nosology and therapy show that Heinrich Heine was treated for syphilis from 1848 onward. After 8 years confinement to the proverbial 'mattress grave', Heine's death can ultimately be explained by his long-standing and well-documented abuse of opium.

On February 27, 1856, that is 151 years ago, Heinrich Heine died. Despite intensive research, the cause of Heine's death has not yet been clarified. Pathographers might actually think that they are in a comfortable position, because the sufferings of the poet, critic and feature writer, who had been living in Paris since 1831, are unusually well documented both by Heine himself and also by his visitors.

However good the sources may be, their evaluation is by no means unproblematic. This is because Heine's literary texts as well as the publicistic or literary evidence of his contemporaries do not have an adequate anamnestic quality. Literary texts are fictional texts, and no so-called ego documents (letters, autobiographical texts etc.) can replace any secure medical diagnosis.

As well as the distinction made between text interpretation and anamnesis, a historical interpretation of the disease also has to be distinguished from a retrospective diagnosis. Every attempt at diagnosis may only be undertaken within the contemporary nosology. Every investigation into which disease the historical patient Heinrich Heine suffered from has to be a reconstruction of the disease within the nosology valid at the time. Every other procedural method would be methodologically disputable and historically incorrect, since the definitions of diseases and the explanation of their causes change with time, and in each case are constructs of their cultural environment. In fact, large sections of medical opinion right up to the late 1830s assumed that syphilis and gonorrhea were identical. The Parisian venereologist Philippe Ricord (1800–1889) was the first to make syphilis and gonorrhea generally recognized as being venereal diseases distinct from each other [Dracobly, 2004, p. 538].[1]

Furthermore, the connection between tabes and syphilis as the late stage of a venereal disease (lues IV) was discovered at the earliest in the work of Alfred Fournier (1832–1915) in 1876, i.e. more than that 20 years after Heine's death. Until then, tabes was thought to have been caused in the humoral-pathological sense by excesses of a sexual nature, and was treated by means of evacuative procedures. In contrast, during Heine's lifetime no distinction was made between syphilis and other venereal diseases, such as gonorrhea or ulcus molle. The etiological definition of syphilis valid today was only possible in 1905 after the discovery of its pathogen spirochaete *Treponema pallidum* by Fritz Schaudinn and Erich Hoffmann.

Moreover, a disease is not only a medical phenomenon but also a social one. Certain diseases are stigmatized in society, e.g. AIDS, and not only in modern times, and this stigmatization then has a reactive effect on the subjective perception of the disease. The sick person can suffer as much from the psychosocial consequences of a stigmatized disease as from the disease itself. The patient's understanding of the disease is also historically and culturally influenced. Depending upon the historical and cultural setting, the disease can be considered by the sick person and society to be atonement and punishment, fatal occupational disability, opportunity and challenge, or a benefit obtained through psychological backup by friends or relatives.

The advantage of the historical interpretation when compared with the retrospective diagnosis is to be found in the reconstruction precisely of this interdependent relationship between the patient, the disease and the social environment. In addition to a merely retrospective diagnosis, within the historical interpretation the patient as a person, his disease in contemporary nosology and his perception of and coping with the disease can be reconstructed in each separate case.

[1]I am grateful to Hugh Langridge for the translation of this text.

Anamnesis

What does the source material handed down to us tell us about Heine's symptoms and diseases? Since his early youth Heine had complained about frequently recurring headaches, sensitivity to noise, migraine and just as frequently about pulmonary complaints. At the beginning of the 1830s the first signs of paralysis occurred – only temporarily – in his left hand. After 1837 there are reports about recurrent eye symptoms, but it is not clear how lengthy and serious these were, since, for example, as late as in September 1841 Heine was able to fight a duel with Salomon Strauss. In the mid-1840s he also developed ptosis of the left eyelid. As early as in 1847 Heine's general condition was so poor that the first announcements of his death could be found in German newspapers [Bogner, 1997]. After his physical collapse in May 1848 and until his death, Heine was no longer able to leave his apartment by himself. In the end he had to be carried by a nurse in what had literally become his 'mattress grave'. In addition to the almost complete paralysis of his lower extremities he suffered from painful colics of the gastrointestinal tract and cramps. This agonizing ordeal was made worse by persistent constipation, and in the final months of his life by frequent and exhausting coughing fits.

Heine's Physicians and Applied Therapies

It is unfortunate that none of Heine's numerous physicians left an indisputable diagnosis which would provide clarity for us today about the background of the illness and the immediate cause of death. However, general practitioners in those days were still largely adherents of humoral pathology. They were less concerned about a diagnosis than about a prognosis and therapy. In addition, it is unfortunate that from the point of view of today's differential diagnoses none of the symptoms described would in the end be indicative of a certain illness. Pathographers writing since Heine's death have provided an almost confusing spectrum of different assumptions about his illness, which were collected by Montanus [1995]: venereal infection (syphilis, tabes dorsalis) [Auf der Horst, 2004], multiple sclerosis, amyotrophic lateral sclerosis, acute intermittent porphyria, chronic polioencephalitis, and tuberculosis with subsequent meningoencephalitis. More recently, lead poisoning has been added [Kijewski et al., 2000, 2003; Auf der Horst and Labisch, 1999].

But who treated Heine, and according to which therapeutic schemes? The therapeutic ideas of Karl Friedrich Heinrich Marx (1796–1877), a doctor Heine visited in the early years of his time in Göttingen, are based on the concept of the body and diseases held by the Scottish doctor John Brown (1735–1788). This concept, which became known as 'Brownianism', and was very popular throughout Europe around 1800 due to its simplicity, was based on the irritability concept of Albrecht von Haller. Every disease was due either to excessive irritability (sthenic diseases) or insufficient irritability (asthenic diseases). This resulted in two forms of therapy: the irritability of the diseased organ either had to be increased or reduced, for example by the administration of alcohol or opium.

David Ferdinand Koreff (1783–1851), who treated Heine in 1833, 1836 and in September 1841 after the duel, was also not a supporter of the so-called 'school medicine'. Koreff treated patients according to the principles of animal magnetism, a concept founded by the German doctor and miracle healer Franz Anton Messmer (1734–1815). He claimed that an invisible fluid flows through nature, and that this can be controlled and influenced by particularly gifted people (magnetizers) in order to heal diseases. Magnetic iron rods stroked vertically over the diseased body could, he claimed, act as the bearer of this healing fluid and restore harmony and health to the poorly polarized flows of the human organism.

Another doctor who treated Heine occasionally, but who discontinued the treatment after a physical dispute with Heine's wife Mathilde, was Leopold Wertheim, who propagated hydropathy in Paris.

The recollections of the doctor Heinrich Rohlfs (1827–1898), who was a friend of Heine's, fits very well into this picture of his increased reliance on alternative medical therapies. Rohlfs had visited Heine in Paris in 1851 and published his 'Recollections of Paris in the Summer of 1851' in a multi-part series of articles between June 23 and July 10, 1853 in *Der Bürgerfreund* [Rohlfs, 1853]:

> It is very characteristic of Heine that he is also a free spirit with regard to medicine. In this respect he is an exception to all so-called free spirits whom I had the opportunity to become acquainted with. Regarding their political views they are either Communists or red Republicans, in their religion they are atheists or pantheists; in every matter concerning their physical well-being they are believers, they swear by their doctors and consider every pill prescribed for them to be a sure panacea for their physical weaknesses. They, who reject all beliefs as being absurd, begin to be believers as soon as a part of their body begins to suffer. Almost without exception the atheists are always pietists regarding medicine! Heine is an exception to these.

How little Rohlf's memory here is to be understood as Heine merely paying lip service is revealed by the further course of his admission, which was written down almost word for word.

> 'I do not believe', he said to me one day, 'that hope still exists for me of ever being restored to health again, and in addition I have no trust in the French doctors as healers; they may be excellent surgeons and are well able to diagnose internal diseases, but they do not understand how to heal them' [Rohlfs, 1853, p. 402].

Heine's admission of not having sufficient trust in the healing competence of French doctors clearly indicates his deep skepticism regarding doctors in general. In fact, despite his obvious need for therapy and his great suffering, Heine did not consult the experts of his day nor the specialists in the field of venerology, which was very possibly what he needed. Doctors such as the venerologist Philippe Ricord were not to be found at his sickbed. Ricord who worked at the Hopital du Midi in Paris from 1831 to 1860 as the Chief Surgeon for patients with syphilis confirmed the division of the clinical course of syphilis into three stages, which is still valid today. The fact that as a result of his physical collapse in the Louvre in front of the *Venus de Milo*, which Heine writes about with great mawkishness in the Epilogue to *Romanzero* [Windfuhr, 1975, vol. III, p. 181], King Louis-Philippe's highly respected clinician and personal physician Léon Rostan (1790–1866) and the also highly esteemed clinician Auguste-François Chomel (1788–1858) consulted together is due less to Heine's initiative than to being the achievement of Leopold Wertheim and David Gruby, who were also present at the meeting [Letter from Heine to Maximilian Heine, 3 December 1846; Nationale Forschungs- und Gedenkstätten der Klassischen Deutschen Literatur, 1972]. Dr. David Gruby treated Heine for the first time at the beginning of the 1840s, and from Heine's collapse in May 1848 until his death in 1856 he was responsible for his further treatment.

But who is David Gruby, and why was he not affected by Heine's skepticism of doctors? Four months after his collapse in May 1848 Heine writes to his brother Maximilian that he has 'great hope of recovery thanks to the Hungarian charlatan who, however, robbed me of my last strength through his wonder tincture' [Letter from Heine to Maximilian Heine, 12 September 1848; Nationale Forschungs- und Gedenkstätten der Klassischen Deutschen Literatur, 1972]. David Gruby, who was born in Hungary, is probably meant by this 'Hungarian charlatan'. At this time he dedicated his attention to microscopy, which was still little known (he wrote the first handbook of microscopic pathology). In fact, Gruby only became a registered doctor in 1854 [quoted after Montanus, 1995, p. 358]. Heine's description of him as a charlatan was thus not without foundation in 1848.

In addition, the source material reveals that Heine agreed to the following therapies: he allowed bleeding to be carried out, took laxatives and emetics, and had leeching and blistering plaster applied. He also subjected himself to additional classic humoral-pathological and revulsant methods, such as that of the Seton method or the fontanelle method, two procedures by which wounds are artificially kept open in order to allow serous and purulent fluid to drain off. And finally, Heine was also cauterized – i.e. he was treated by means of red-hot irons or pyrotics. Heine's friend, Alfred Meissner (1822–1885), who had studied medicine, writes later:

> Heine was accustomed to saying that he considered himself to be an experimental animal on which God undertook physiological experiments. It is much rather the case that he

was an experimental animal of his various doctors. These doctors, mostly of German origin, had settled into the French school of medicine. They tested on him the effect of strychnine as a cure for his paralysis, drilled fontanelles in his neck, burnt moxa on him and worked in the area of the lumbar vertebrae with red-hot irons. I had not seen anything like it in all my life. These were the therapeutic methods of which Oppolzer (pathologist in Prague and Leipzig) stated that one should leave them to the slavedrivers, and that their place was in the torture chambers of the Middle Ages [quoted after Montanus, 1995, p. 360].

Tabes Dorsalis

Why, however, did Heine believe that he had to subject himself to these tortures? Heine frequently told friends that he was suffering from tabes dorsalis. The background to this is the expert opinion based on Hippocrates that tabes or locomotor ataxia is the result of a dissipated sex life. The spinal cord as the presumed place where semen is produced was considered to lose substance because of frequent ejaculations [Littré, 1962, p. 471]. The assumption that the spinal cord and sperm are directly connected can be seen, for example, in Leonardo da Vinci's anatomical drawings from the 15th/16th centuries (fig. 1) [O'Malley, 1952, p. 461].[2]

In addition to Heine's own suspicion that he had tabes, as well as the resulting treatment, his work also seemed to speak in favor of tabes. Thus, Arthur Conan Doyle, the literary father of Sherlock Holmes, who is famous for his infallible intuition, mentioned Heine's cycle of poems *Romanzero* in his medical thesis of 1885. The descriptions Heine made in the epilogue were, he claimed, typical of the clinical picture of syphilitic tabes dorsalis:

> Here are the words of Heine, the great German Jewish poet when after seven years of this torture he saw the shades of death gather round his couch. They are interesting as showing the thoughts evolved by a great brain when linked to what was practically a dead body. 'Do I really exist' he writes, 'my body is so shrunken that I am hardly anything but a voice. In my mattress grave in the great city I hear early and late nothing but the noise of vehicles, hammering, quarrelling and piano strumming. A grave without repose, death without the privileges of the dead who at least need not spend any money nor write letters or books – that is indeed a pitiful condition' (fig. 2) [Doyle, 1885].

Thus not only was syphilitic tabes dorsalis introduced as the diagnosis suggested by Heine's pathographics, but, even worse, anamnestic authority was ascribed to literary texts in order to validate a retrospective diagnosis. In fact, the diagnosis of venereal infection with the neurological secondary stage of tabes dorsalis or lues cerebrospinalis still remains the illness from which Heine is most frequently presumed to have suffered.

[2] I am grateful to Prof. Dr. med. Dr. phil. A. Labisch for this reference.

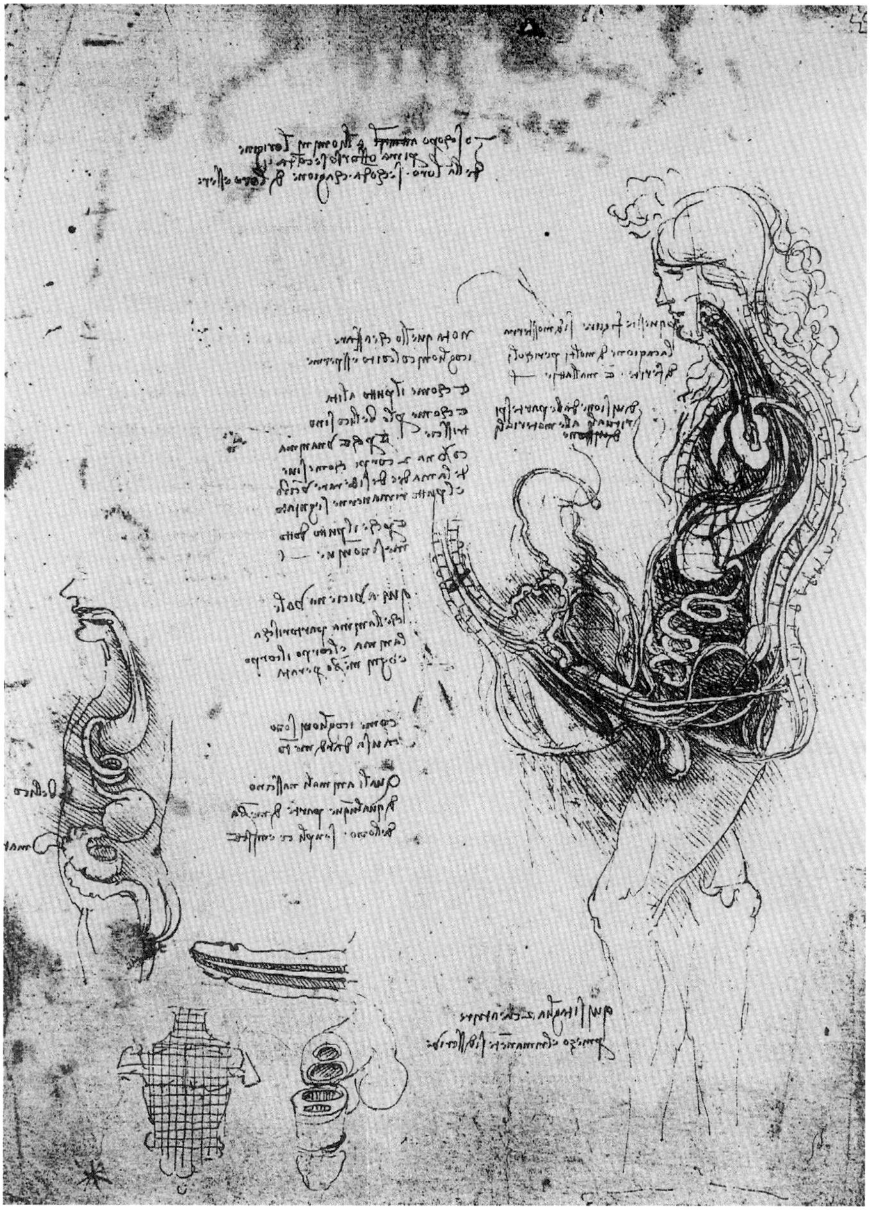

Fig. 1. Sagittal section by Leonardo da Vinci of a coitus, with a direct connection between penis and spinal cord [from O'Malley, 1952].

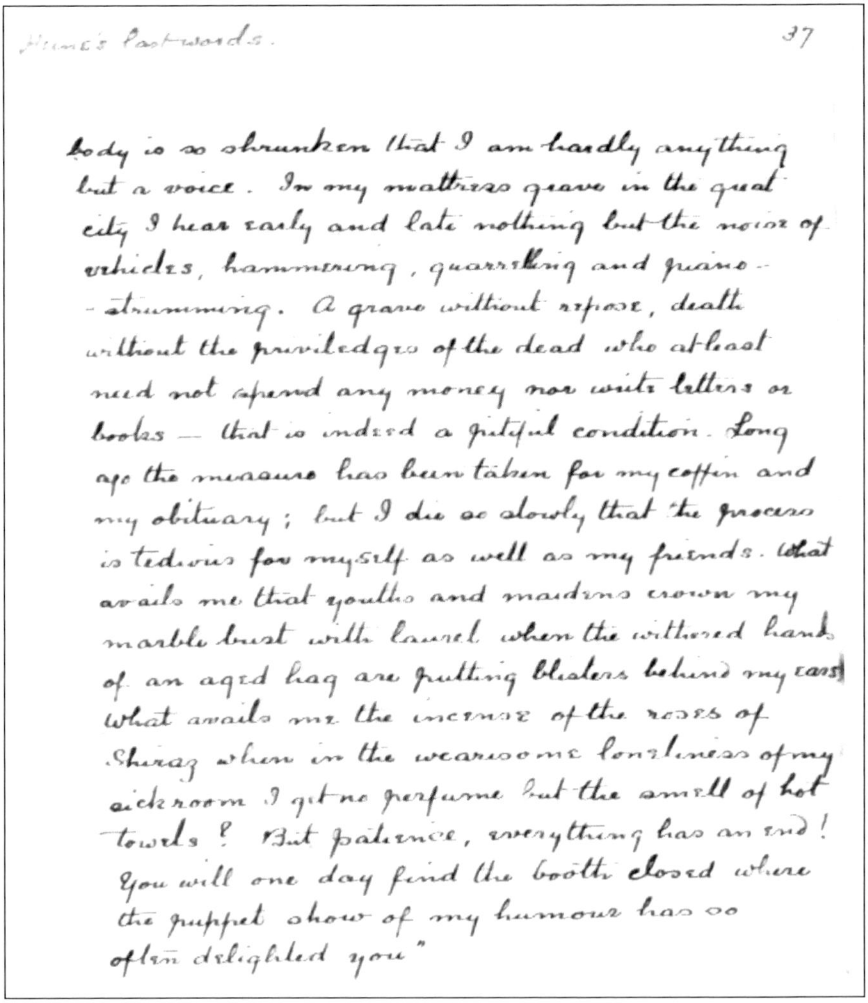

Heine's last words. 37

body is so shrunken that I am hardly anything but a voice. In my mattress grave in the great city I hear early and late nothing but the noise of vehicles, hammering, quarrelling and piano-strumming. A grave without repose, death without the priviledges of the dead who at least need not spend any money nor write letters or books — that is indeed a pitiful condition. Long ago the measure has been taken for my coffin and my obituary; but I die so slowly that the process is tedious for myself as well as my friends. What avails me that youths and maidens crown my marble bust with laurel when the withered hands of an aged hag are putting blisters behind my ears? What avails me the incense of the roses of Shiraz when in the wearisome loneliness of my sickroom I get no perfume but the smell of hot towels? But patience, everything has an end! You will one day find the booth closed where the puppet show of my humour has so often delighted you"

Fig. 2. Excerpt from the part of A.C. Doyle's doctoral thesis [1885] in which he quotes from Heine's *Romanzero*. (The original of the handwritten dissertation is in the Edinburgh University Library.)

Syphilis

A case history that tries to diagnose Heine as suffering from syphilis would initially have to search in the source material for indications of ulcers in the genital region or skin rashes. It is typical that in all the contemporary reports written about Heine's illnesses no diagnostically clearly reliable indication exists concerning skin involvement or ulcus induratum. Knowledge about the dermatological symptoms of syphilis certainly existed during Heine's day and would not have remained unnoticed by a doctor (fig. 3) [Bateman, 1830].

There is, however, also a prescription handed down to us which permits deductions concerning the disease which those issuing the prescription believed they had to treat (fig. 4). At the doctors' meeting of October 9, 1848 which has already been referred to the participating doctors Auguste-François Chomel (1788–1858), David Gruby (1810–1898), Léon Louis Rostan (1790–1866) and Leopold Wertheim (1819–1890) issued the following instructions. Firstly, Heine was to be cauterized along the spine. Secondly, Neapolitan unguent was to be rubbed into the spine. Thirdly, potassium iodide was to be administered internally. Laxatives were to be administered to improve the digestion. As a supportive measure, attention should be paid to appropriate food and nutrition. The doctors who jointly signed the instructions stated that narcotics could also be applied to combat the pain.

What is noticeable about the instructions of this prescription is that a contemporarily current antisyphilitic therapy was described here. This is shown in a comparison between this prescription and a contemporary handbook for practising doctors. The *Nouveau compendium médical à l'usage des médecins practiciens divisés en trois parties*, the first edition of which was published by Antonin Bossu in 1841, the second in 1855 and the fifth in 1874, explicitly agrees with the currently leading venerologist, Philippe Ricord, regarding the lemma syphilis [Bossu, 1855, p. 646]. It was decisive for his successes in the study and therapy of syphilis that Ricord was able to provide a special and successful therapeutic program for the already known division into a primary, secondary and tertiary form of syphilis: mercury for secondary syphilis, but potassium iodide for the treatment of the tertiary form [Dracobly, 2004, p. 546]. In fact, potassium iodide has been successfully employed since the end of the 1840s right up until today for the treatment of symptoms of lues III and the typical syphilitic gummas [Dracobly, 2004, p. 549; Ständers, 1986, p. 194]. In the introductory remarks concerning the syphilis lemma Bossu [1855, p. 647] already points out the advantage of potassium iodide over mercury in antisyphilitic therapy:

> However mercury is not infallible: sometimes it fails or is insufficient, particularly in the already longer existing syphilis of tertiary stage. In this case one has to resort to potassium iodide...

In the section which deals with tertiary syphilis – as prescribed in the third part of the prescription – the internal administration of potassium iodide, thus agreeing with Ricord's recommendations for therapy:

> Mercury is very successful in the therapy of tertiary syphilis. However experience showed that mercury does frequently not affect any more at this tertiary stage and that then the potassium iodide has to be preferred [Bossu, 1855, p. 661].

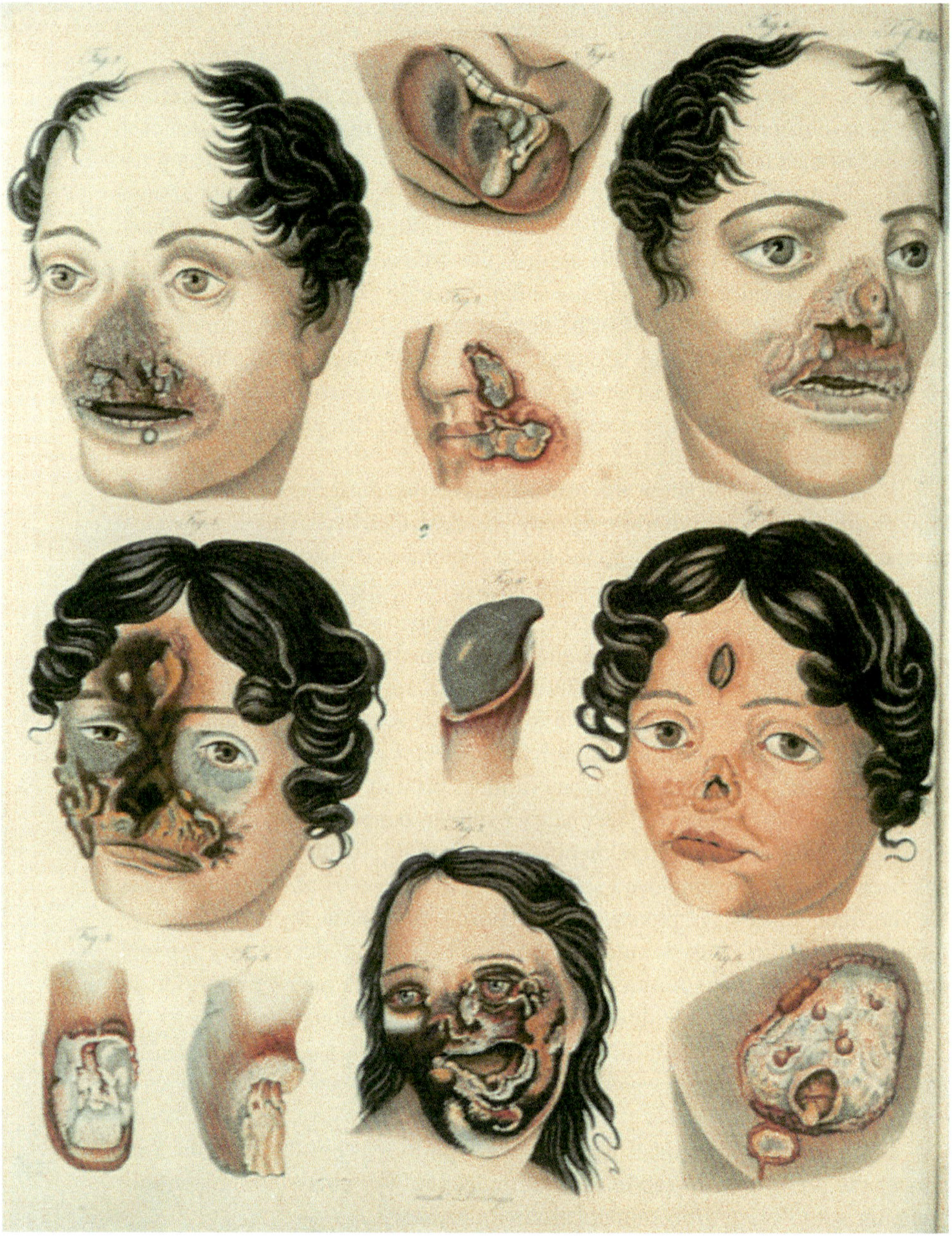

Fig. 3. Illustration taken from the at the time very well-known dermatological atlas of the founder of scientific dermatology, Thomas Bateman (1778–1821).

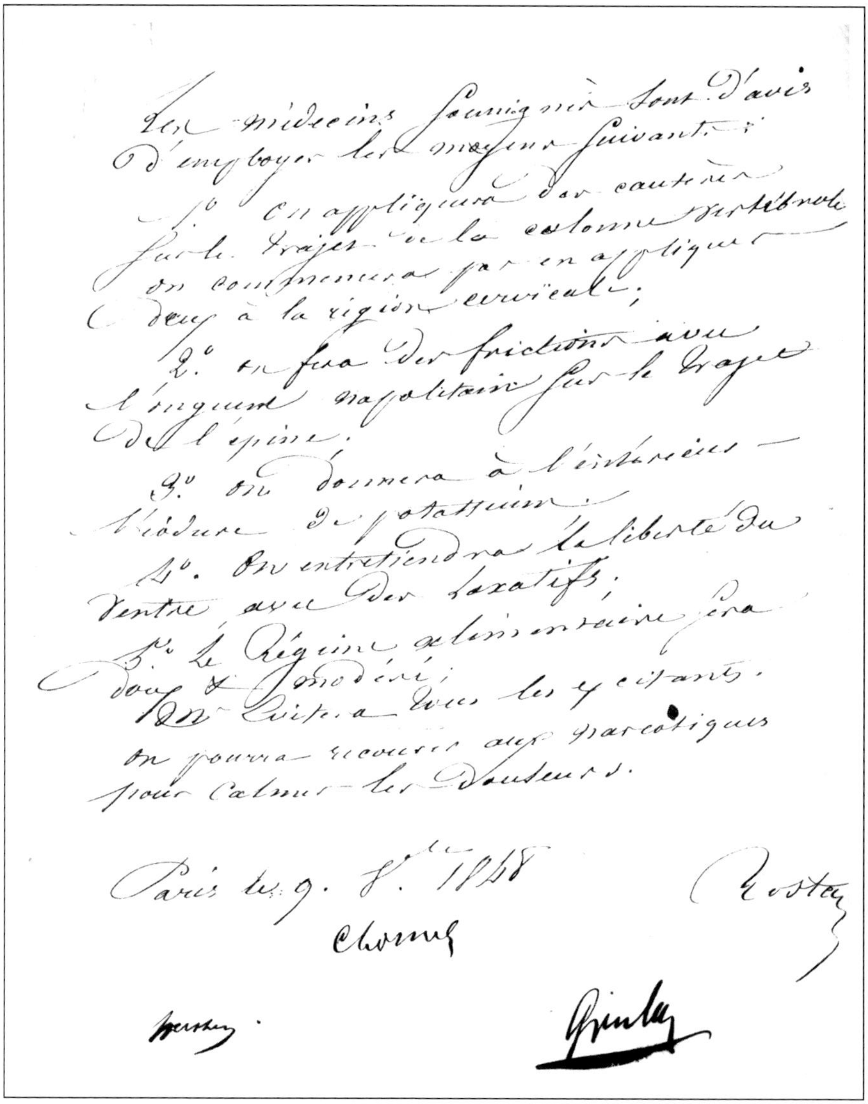

Les médecins soussignés sont d'avis
d'employer les moyens suivants:
1° On appliquera des cautères
sur le trajet de la colonne vertébrale
on commencera par en appliquer
deux à la région cervicale;
2° on fera des frictions avec
l'onguent napolitain sur le trajet
de l'épine;
3° on donnera à l'intérieur
l'iodure de potassium;
4°. On entretiendra la liberté du
ventre avec des laxatifs;
5° Le Régime alimentaire sera
doux & modéré;
On évitera tous les excitants.
on pourra recourir aux narcotiques
pour calmer les douleurs.

Paris le 9. 8bre 1848 Rostan
Chomel
Wertheim Gruby

Fig. 4. The prescription signed in 1848 by the doctors Leopold Wertheim, Auguste-François Chomel, David Gruby and Léon Louis Rostan (with kind permission from the Heinrich Heine Institute Düsseldorf).

As possibilities for internal treatment with potassium iodide the *Compendium* points, among other things, to a general 'tea with iodine' and also to a special tea of Ricord's, in each case giving the ingredients [Bossu, 1855, p. 661]. In addition, the third main section of the *Compendium*, the 'Medical Index', also mentions the tablet form [Bossu, 1855, p. 728].

The second part of the doctor's prescription of 1848, the administration of 'Neapolitan unguent' and the method of its application – 'is to be rubbed in' – is also confirmed in the *Compendium*. Bossu recommends this ointment for the treatment of the syphilitic osteocopic pains of tertiary syphilis [Bossu, 1855, p. 662] and explains the constituents and the method of application of this ointment in the section 'Medical Index':

> Mercurial unguent or mercurial ointment to double portions, Neapolitain unguent. Mercury and balm each to 500 components. 1 to 5 gram are to be rubbed in [Bossu, 1855, p. 742].

It is clear that this ointment, which obviously contains a high level of mercury, is employed against syphilis.

The first part of the prescription, the cauterization of the spine, will have to be interpreted as a reaction to Heine's assumption that he was suffering from tabes dorsalis. The localization of the cauterization directly next to the spinal cord, which was the assumed source of the disease, also supports this, as does the humoral-pathological idea behind it that this evacuative procedure could restore the balance of the fluids. The remaining parts of the prescription can probably be explained by Heine's constipation, which had been known since spring 1847 [Letter from Heine to Caroline Jaubert, 13 April 1847, to Christine de Belgiojoso, 20 September 1847, to Leopold Wertheim, 20 September 1847, to Alexander Weill, 22 September 1847, to Maximilian Heine, 12 September 1848 and to Maximilian Heine, 1 January 1850; Nationale Forschungs- und Gedenkstätten der Klassischen Deutschen Literatur, 1972].

This prescription, in fact, proves that the doctors signing it believed that Heinrich Heine had to be treated for syphilis. The diagnosis itself, syphilis, is not made by them, however. This assumption of the diagnosis of syphilis loses its strength by Heine's remark to the doctor Heinrich Rohlfs, who was a friend of his, a remark which Heine had made to him 3 years after the doctors' meeting in 1848:

> By the way, I am taking no medicine because I do not believe in its effect. The only medication I have taken throughout my illness has been potassium iodide, and I have not perceived that it has brought about any improvement in my condition [Rohlfs, 1853, p. 402].

Rohlfs thus reports that Heine had taken potassium iodide before 1851, but that this medicine had had no therapeutic effect on him. For a diagnosis ex juvantibus it must therefore also be considered that Heine in fact had no late symptoms of syphilis because potassium iodide should otherwise have helped him.

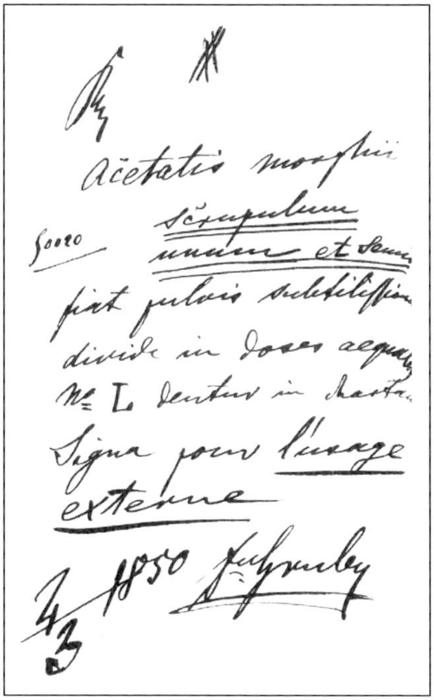
Acetatis morphii
Signa pour l'usage externe
4/3 1850

Fig. 5. Prescription for opium signed by Dr. David Gruby on March 4, 1850 (with kind permission from the Heinrich Heine Institute Düsseldorf).

Heine's Opium Abuse and the Cause of His Death

Heine's underlying illnesses will probably remain a permanent riddle. Until his dying minute Heine had a clear mind. A disease of the peripheral nerves must therefore be assumed. Many of them could be mentioned, all of which have completely different causes. Nevertheless, a distinction has to be made between the underlying illness and the immediate cause of death. What did Heine really die of?

There is, however, one obvious explanation for Heine's death which has not yet been considered. The abdominal cramps can easily be explained by Heine's opium consumption: in fact, in Heine's case history since 1848 nothing has been described in anything like as much detail by himself and by his contemporaries as his opium consumption. Heine's statement that religion is the intellectual opium for suffering mankind [Windfuhr, 1975, vol. XI, p. 103], which, as is known, preceded the more succinct formulation by Karl Marx – religion is the opium of the people – thus assumes a special meaning.

The opium theory can be supported, on the one hand, by the instructions already mentioned for the therapy which were written down and signed on

October 9, 1848. Three additional opium prescriptions also still exist. They were written on July 2, 1849 and on March 4, 1850 (fig. 5). The third prescription, also written by Dr. Gruby, is undated.

Heine's correspondence and the notes taken by others prove that morphine was applied to him by means of percutaneous cones, that every day after June 1854 Heine had morphine sprinkled into a wound kept open in his neck and applied hot poultices to himself to administer morphine [Werner, 1972, vol. II, pp. 99, 123, 132, 195, 269, 345, 373, 375]. The most frequent method of application and also the most convenient was the peroral administration of morphine. Heine frequently took excessively large doses [Werner, 1972, vol. II, pp. 405, 479, 482 and Letter from Heine to Maximilian Heine, 9 January 1850, to Heinrich Laube, 25 January 1850, to Gustav Heine, 15 November 1850 and 21 January 1851, to Julius Campe, 3 August 1854, Nationale Forschungs- und Gedenkstätten der Klassischen Deutschen Literatur, 1972].

In fact, the immediate cause of death could be attributed to morphine abuse. Here it must be remembered that the addictive potential of morphine was noticed for the first time during the American Civil War (1861–1865), and in Europe in the Franco-Prussian War (1870/1871). In August 1854 Heine had moved into new accommodation, which was in fact more comfortable but considered to be damp and cold. After that he suffered from a cold which was resistant to treatment. From a longer sequence of letters about his suffering it is possible to reconstruct a paroxysmal cough which plagued Heine over a period of roughly 1 1/2 years [Letter from Heine to Michael Schloss, 19 February 1855, to Gustav Heine, 3 June 1855, to Elise Krinitz, September 1855, to Betty de Rothschild, autumn 1855 and to Elise Krinitz, 2 January 1856; Nationale Forschungs- und Gedenkstätten der Klassischen Deutschen Literatur, 1972]. This is presumably why Heine valued the cough-relieving effect of morphine. In the case of a painful and unproductive cough the administration of morphine can still be indicated today. In Heine's day the antitussive effect of opium was employed, amongst other things, to counteract 'pains similar to pleuritic stabbing pains, dry, racking, paroxysmal coughing threatening asphyxia'. Morphine was considered to be a 'marvellous palliative, partly against the racking cough' and 'the chest complaint with blocked expectoration' [Sobernheim, 1840, vol. 2, pp. 17, 22, 281].

The attending doctor, Dr. Gruby, writes to Heine's brother on February 17, 1856, in his opinion Heine died 'as a result of weakness caused by violent vomiting'. As he later adds, Heine did not die from the consequences of his long-lasting illness, but of a 'chance indisposition' [Werner, 1972, vol. II, p. 473]. The reports about Heine's final hours by his last female acquaintance, 'Mouche' (Elise Krinitz, 1825–1896), and the nurse also both agree with Dr. Gruby's assumption: Heine died of a vomiting crisis which had got out of control and 'due to the enormous doses of morphine he took during his final days' [Werner, 1972, vol. II, pp. 479, 482]. In addition, Dr. Gruby could not be reached on February 15, 1856. In this emergency an old doctor who lived nearby was called in, and he prescribed a 'tea of orange blossom and water from Vichy with a drop of laudanum' to be taken every half hour [Werner, 1972, vol. II, p. 474]. It is well-known that laudanum is an opium preparation. The doctor, who was unaware of the circumstances, thus possibly treated an overdose of opium with the administration of more opium. The abuse of opium or morphine over too long a period can lead to paralytic intestinal stasis which, for its part, can induce serious vomiting. Alternatively, the vomiting can also be interpreted as the result of acute intoxication after taking an overdose. Nevertheless, this medication is also in very good agreement with contemporary ideas of how serious vomiting is to be treated. According to Bossu's *Compendium*, 'tea of orange blossom' has an antispasmodic effect [Bossu, 1855, p. 738], and the section on 'nervous vomitus' explains that vomiting is to be treated with opium or mineral waters:

> Nowadays it is considered that the anaesthetics should be accounted as main agents of medical treatment. The most applicated substances are Opium and belladonna. Secondly... carbonated beverages, 'la potion de Rivière', magnesium containig water,... [Bossu, 1855, p. 685].

Then, as now, nausea and vomiting are unspecific symptoms. The fact that, nevertheless, mention is made of vomiting due to chronic or acute intoxication is the result of the source material which documents not only the opium abuse in Heine's case history unusually well. The comments by Heine's doctor, his housekeeper and his last female friend also document just as well that these vomiting crises and the previous ones are the result of an overdose of opium. These strongly indicate that Heine died as a result of this last and incorrectly treated overdose.

Medical opinion today states that vomiting lasting 3 days leads to serious alkalosis, and this occurred in the body weakened by year-long colics and serious illness. Alkalosis caused by metabolic processes is due mainly to a lack of potassium. Muscular weakness and a disturbed cardiac function are the results. The body tries to compensate the alkalosis by shallow and slow breathing. This results in irritability, vertigo and also disturbances of consciousness. During Heine's last days, his body, which had been emaciated over a period of years, went into a downward spiral. The administration of laudanum made any escape impossible.

References

Auf der Horst C: Historisch-kritische Pathographien und Historizität. Eine kritische Auswertung der Heine-Pathographien am Beispiel der Syphilisdiagnosen Heinrich Heines; in Labisch A, Paul N (eds): Historizität: Erfahrung und Handeln in Geschichte – Medizin, Naturwissenschaften und Technik. Sudhoffs Arch Z Wissenschaftsgesch Beih 2004;54:121–151.

Auf der Horst C, Labisch A: Heinrich Heine, der Verdacht einer Bleivergiftung und Heines Opium-Abusus. Heine Jahrb 1999;38:105–131.

Bateman T: Abbildungen von Hautkrankheiten, wodurch die characteristischen Erscheinungen der Gattungen und Arten nach der Willan'schen Classification dargestellt werden. Weimar, Verl. d. Grossh. Saechs. pr. Landes-Industrie-Comptoirs, 1830.

Bogner R: Heinrich Heines Höllenfahrt. Nachrufe auf einen streitbaren Schriftsteller. Dokumente 1846–1858. Heidelberg, Manutius Verlag, 1997.

Bossu A: Nouveau Compendium médical à l'usage des médecins praticiens divisé en trois parties. Paris, Ballière, 1855.

Doyle AC: An Essay upon the Vasomomotor Changes in Tabes Dorsalis (handwritten); doctoral thesis, Edinburgh University Library, 1885.

Dracobly A: Theoretical change and therapeutic innovation in the treatment of syphilis in mid-nineteenth-century France. J Hist Med Allied Sci 2004;4:522–554.

Ewald CA: Handbuch der allgemeinen und speziellen Arzneiverordnungslehre, ed 11 (newly revised and enlarged edition). Berlin, Hirschwald, 1887.

Kijewski H, Huckenbeck W, Reus U: Krankheit und Tod des Dichters Heinrich Heine aus der Sicht spurenkundlicher Untersuchungen an Haaren. 1. Haarmorphologische Untersuchungen. Rechtsmedizin 2000;10:201–211.

Kijewski H, Huckenbeck W, Reus U: Krankheit und Tod des Dichters Heinrich Heine aus der Sicht spurenkundlicher Untersuchungen an Haaren. 2. Mineralstoffbestimmung und Symptomatik. Rechtsmedizin 2003;13:131–136.

Littré E, Œuvres Compleins d'Hippocrate. Traduction nouvelle avec le texte en grec. Amsterdam, Hakkert, 1962.

Montanus H: Der kranke Heine. Stuttgart, Metzler, 1995.

Nationale Forschungs- und Gedenkstätten der Klassischen Deutschen Literatur: Heinrich Heine. Werke, Briefwechsel, Lebenszeugnisse. Weimar-Berlin, Akademieverlag, 1979.

O'Malley CD: Leonardo da Vinci. On the human body. The anatomical, physiological, and embryological drawings of Leonardo da Vinci. New York, Henry Schuman, 1952.

Rohlfs H: Recollections of Paris in the summer of 1851. Der Bürgerfreund, June 26, 1853, vol 51, p 402.

Sobernheim JF: Handbuch der praktischen Arzneimittellehre für angehende, praktische und Physikats-Ärzte, so wie als Leitfaden für den akademischen Unterricht. Berlin, Förstner, 1840.

Ständers C; Praxis der Haut- und Geschlechtskrankheiten. München, Wien, Baltimore, Urban & Schwarzenberg, 1986.

Werner M: Begegnungen mit Heine. Berichte der Zeitgenossen; in Fortführung von H.H. Houbens 'Gespräche mit Heine'. Hamburg, Hoffmann & Campe, 1972.

Windfuhr M: Heinrich Heine. Historisch-kritische Gesamtausgabe der Werke. Hamburg, Hoffmann & Campe, 1975.

Dr. phil. Christoph auf der Horst
Institute for the History of Medicine, Heinrich Heine University Düsseldorf
Universitätsstrasse 1
DE–40225 Düsseldorf (Germany)
Tel. +49 211 81 15 8 20, Fax +49 211 81 15 8 16, E-Mail chorst@uni-duesseldorf.de

Bogousslavsky J, Hennerici MG (eds): Neurological Disorders in Famous Artists – Part 2.
Front Neurol Neurosci. Basel, Karger, 2007, vol 22, pp 121–149

Baudelaire's Aphasia: From Poetry to Cursing

Sebastian Dieguez[a], *Julien Bogousslavsky*[b]

[a]Brain Mind Institute, Laboratory of Cognitive Neuroscience, Lausanne, and [b]Department of Neurology, Valmont Clinic, Genolier Swiss Medical Network, Glion-sur-Montreux, Switzerland

Abstract

At 45 years of age, Charles Baudelaire suffered a left hemispheric stroke that left him with a right hemiplegia and severe aphasia. In this chapter, we investigate the nature of his symptoms, drawing mostly on his own and his contemporaries' correspondence. Before specifically examining his aphasia, we put the poet's life, work, and health in context, notably his tormented mind, his probable syphilitic infection and the intellectual milieu of 19th century France. The time when Baudelaire was struck with aphasia coincides with early discoveries and debates that centered on the nature and implications of this neurological disorder. Many of the questions raised at that time still await definitive answers. Here, we compare Baudelaire's language disorder with recent research that has shed new light on the poet's disease. Most interestingly, we explore the nature of his dramatic use of the expletive *Cré nom!*, which was the only word he was able to express. Finally, we discuss the links between disease and creativity and dismiss the frequent notion that Baudelaire, in the end, paid the price of his genius.

Plains-moi! . . . Sinon, je te maudis!

(Epigraphe pour un livre condamné, *Les Fleurs du Mal*, added in the third edition, 1868 – excerpt)

Mon cerveau est un palimpseste et le vôtre aussi, lecteur.

(*Les Paradis Artificiels*, chap. VIII)

Charles Baudelaire is perhaps the quintessential poète maudit (cursed poet), with all the genius, misery, mental derangement, dissolute lifestyle, provocation and dandyism that the concept entails. Arguably, he is also one of the most talented and creative writers of the modern era. Victor Hugo himself saw a 'new thrill' (un frisson nouveau) in his work. Paul Valery spoke of a 'continual charm'.

However, 'maudit' can also be understood as 'incompris' (misunderstood), for it is well known that Baudelaire's personality and the contents of his works did not make it easy for his contemporaries to accept his art. In his piece *L'Albatros*, he vividly captured the image of the sublime celestial abstraction of the poet confronting its degrading and grotesque presence down on earth:

> The Poet bears a likeness to that prince of the air,
> who mocks at slingshots, and haunts the winds:
> on earth, an exile among the scornful, where
> he is hampered, in walking, by his giant wings.

Hampered he was, as this chapter will show, and not only by his 'giant wings'. Baudelaire was not a vigorous man and had a very sad end. He was struck by hemiplegia with aphasia before his 50s and died after having survived 18 months with this terrible condition, without being able, of course, to work again. As with many artists, we can only say of their lives and diseases what they themselves and their relatives wrote about them, and what scholars have discovered.

His subversive writings, dissolute lifestyle and frightening demise are all excellent ingredients to spark a debate as to the links between disease and creativity, personality and art, life and work, aphasia and intelligence. What is more, what we know of his symptoms is interesting in its own right to introduce peculiar and still poorly understood features of motor aphasia, namely automatisms, stereotypes, cursing and catastrophic reactions. In this chapter, we will focus on these aspects of Baudelaire's aphasia, but we will also say a few words about his other symptoms – as he was very likely a victim of syphilis since early adulthood – and of the relationship of some of his creative powers to disease and death. But first, we start with a brief introduction to Baudelaire's life and works.

Life and Works

Short Biography

Baudelaire was born in Paris on the April 9, 1821, to a 61-year-old father and a mother of 26. His father died when he was 5. Only later would he learn that his father was a defrocked priest. The next year, his mother, Caroline, would marry Jacques Aupick, a high-ranking army officer, with whom Baudelaire would always have a conflicting relationship. The young man chose to study philosophy at high school, from which he was dismissed for protecting a comrade by swallowing a contentious paper note. As it may be of some interest to neurologists, it is worth mentioning that Charles Lasègue then became his private tutor in 1839 (Baudelaire was 18) to nevertheless help him pass his baccalauréat. He then intended to study law but obviously preferred enjoying the bohemian opportunities provided by Paris, such as meeting writers, friends and prostitutes. By this time, he had no job, a lot of debt, and was about to suffer from his first health problems, likely resulting from syphilitic infection (see below). As his family was understandably worried not only about him but also about his stepfather's reputation – he was a general by then – in June 1841 they decided to send him to India on the *Paquebot des Mers du Sud*. However, the ship encountered a tempest and the voyage was cut short at Mauritius Island. Baudelaire embarked in November and by February 1842 he was back in France. Of these few exotic months Baudelaire kept vivid images that would forever fuel his works.

By then a young adult, he was allowed to receive the inheritance of his deceased father. However, the money was soon squandered and again he got himself into serious pecuniary trouble. He was even placed under a restraining order by his mother. For the rest of his life he would be running after money, or rather eluding his creditors. In the meantime, he met Jeanne Duval, a young mulatto actress and prostitute, with whom he would have a relationship with ups and downs for about 14 years. He began at this time to have some of his writings published, mostly critical studies of painters, and some poems. By 1846 he had discovered hashish and the works of Edgar Poe. In February 1847, he became involved in political riots and was heard screaming along with others that: 'General Aupick must be killed.' He became less interested, or at least less physically involved, in political matters after 1850 and, instead, focused on writing his poems and translating Poe. In 1855, a collection of his poems was published under the title *Les Fleurs du Mal* (Flowers of Evil). He also issued a few *Poèmes en prose* and an essay on laughter in the arts the same year. In 1856 his tumultuous relationship with Jeanne Duval came to an end. Baudelaire would never marry or have children. Many have written that he was impotent, or even a virgin, though it is hard to say whether there might have been psychological or physical reasons for this.

His *Fleurs du Mal* – arguably one of the treasures of mankind – quickly came under attack, mainly from the conservative journal *Le Figaro* that qualified its author as a 'dry fruit' and the book a compendium of 'monstrosities'. Influenced by this libel, the public prosecutor decided to seize the book and to sue its author and publisher (Auguste Poulet-Malassis, who would remain one of Baudelaire's closest friends). They were convicted and fined, and six poems were suppressed. In 1860, *Les Paradis Artificiels* – a study of hashish and opium – and many poems added to *Les Fleurs du Mal* were published.

In the spring of 1864, apparently fed up with the Parisian cultural atmosphere, he decided to go to Brussels, in Belgium. He planned to give some conferences there, and to look for a publisher. Obviously, he also left Paris to elude his creditors. All of this would be a striking failure. He was left there on his own, wandering aimlessly, sick, melancholic and more and more misanthropic.

He decided to express his disgust in a book on Belgium titled *Pauvre Belgique* (Poor Belgium). But, as his dreadful fate took over, this project would remain at a sketchy stage.[1]

Overview of Works

We will certainly not dare add anything here to the thousands of pages devoted to the analysis of Baudelaire's works and the 19th century zeitgeist. More than enough has already been said about this by the greatest minds of literature. However, it seems important, in a book such as this, to say a few words about the content and context of Baudelaire's work, as the reader will not necessarily be acquainted with them. After all, a discussion of Baudelaire's disease would only be relevant in light of some understanding of who he was, what he did, and when and where he lived.

Baudelaire's work takes place in what Léon Daudet called the 'stupid 19th century'. This is a period of dazzling change in society, politics, religion, philosophy, art and science. Thinkers and laymen were forced to deal with what has been seen as the advent of 'modernity'. No wonder some minds were confused by these exceedingly rapid transformations. Baudelaire was at the same time a representative and a critic of that era. Some of his writings read like quasi-philosophical preoccupations with esthetics, the switch to 'modern life', the threat of 'progress' and the clash between religion, occultism and secularism. It is, of course, impossible to capture the essence of his style in a few lines, but suffice it to say that Baudelaire had a fondness for opposites and contradictions. He could convey the sense of the purest beauty from revolting scenes, and conversely savage the pleasurable to the point of evoking disgust. Though the topics of death, evil, sexuality and disease are omnipresent in his works, one can often find a sense of love, perfection and the infinite hidden behind their appearances.[2] His fascination with the work of Edgar Poe should come as no surprise, as both were representative of the same kind of post-romantic decadence. Indeed, some have said that Baudelaire did more for Poe's glory than for his own. What is clear is that few have written as well of the tortures of the modern mind, the inescapability of boredom and melancholy (what he called spleen), the corruptibility of the body and the quest for a new meaning after official religion was declared bankrupt. It is safe to say that, on

[1]This short biographical summary is liberally inspired by the chronologies available in Baudelaire [1980] and Jackson [2001]. There are innumerable books on Baudelaire's life; in French, we warmly recommend Pichois and Ziegler [2005].

[2]Favourite examples include *The Clock*, *The Voyage*, *Mademoiselle Bistouri*, *The Death of Lovers*, *A Carcass*, *The Hard-Working Skeletons*, or *Danse Macabre*.

these grounds, Baudelaire's masterful poetry was revolutionary. The psychological properties of time, space, perception, emotion and the self were all scrutinized and intermixed under his pen, at such a level that many see in him a good example of the synesthete (see Appendix). Contradictions and form shifting were not only to be found in his work, but also in his life. Courbet, who made a famous portrait of the poet, was struck by the constant changes in Baudelaire's appearance. This was not only evident in the dandy's perpetual quest for stylish elegance and originality; apparently even his face could seem surprisingly different from day to day. Indeed, he himself wrote: larvatus prodeo ('I move forward like one possessed', or less literally, 'I am a man of many masks'). In *Fusées, Hygiène* and *Mon coeur mis à nu* – autobiographical works where he dissects his tormented mind – we can further see his constant changes of habits, goals and beliefs. This was, in part, voluntarily sought through the use of drugs and alcohol to explore altered states of consciousness and new creative pathways, a dangerous exploration to which we owe *Les Paradis Artificiels*. There are really many Baudelaires, which is why there are so many contrasting comments and essays on his works and psychology.

Health before Aphasia

Baudelaire's life and works, however, were accompanied by many health problems. We will focus here on the medical facts that we know mostly through the correspondence of Baudelaire and his relatives. Accordingly, we will only briefly mention that some authors have insisted on psychoanalytical and literary approaches, apparently implying that, in the end, Baudelaire's brain and body have little involvement with the ultimate cause of his demise. Sartre [1947] is notorious in his analysis of Baudelaire's psyche for having rather exclusively focused on the poet's *will* (or rather the lack of it). 'This long and painful dissolution had been chosen; Baudelaire made the choice to experience time backwards' (p. 152). He concludes his essay with these lines: 'Thus he was at twenty, thus we find him on the eve of his death: he is merely gloomier, more nervous and less sharp... The free choice that man makes with himself matches absolutely what we call his destiny' (pp. 178–179). Of course, the extent to which one *chooses* to have half one's brain destroyed is a matter that Sartre and fellow existentialists should take some time to explain to our patients in the neurological ward [for heartfelt replies to Sartre's opinion of Baudelaire, see Bataille, 1957; Angles, 1948].

The French writer Lévy [1988] offers a fictional account of Baudelaire's last days. This would seem like an interesting source for our topic, but we must be careful with that kind of work which is, after all, largely fictional. Though this book has been incredibly publicized in France, it is hard to find something useful either in it or in the stupendous number of press articles generated by it, at least as far as Baudelaire's life is concerned. Pichois [2005] perhaps offers the best analysis of what we actually know, without further embellishment or excessive speculation [Lebrun et al., 1971, also wrote a fine article on Baudelaire's aphasia]. According to Pichois, it was the progressive overlapping of different disorders that led to the 1866 stroke. Thus, the cause was a polymorphous ailment of infectious, toxic, and 'nervous' origins, which we will describe in the next sections.

Venereal Infection and Dermatologic Disorders

From 1839 on, Baudelaire started to complain in his letters of various problems that seem to hint at venereal disease. In November 1839, he writes to his stepbrother: 'I have no more pains. Almost no more headaches, I sleep much better; but I have ghastly digestion, and a continuously small stream, with no pain at all; all of this with such a wonderful complexion that nobody suspects anything' [Pichois, 2005, p. 111]. This 'anything' is often taken to be indicative of syphilis, although a more careful interpretation of the fragment would merely indicate gonorrhea. What is clear, nevertheless, is that Baudelaire at this time had many encounters with prostitutes and, considering the era and the place in which these took place, it would be quite astonishing if he managed to dodge the pox. As he wrote: 'We all have the republican spirit in our veins, just as we have the pox in our bones. We are democratized and syphilised' and 'On the day that the writer corrects his first proof, he is as proud as a schoolboy who has just caught his first pox' [in Hayden, 2004, pp. 112–113]. It is usually to Sara 'la Louchette' that the infection is attributed, but he had other favorites that could just as well have been the culprit.[3] In a letter to his mother dated 1860, Baudelaire complains of what he had to endure for the previous 19 years, but this is ambiguous and, in any case, does not take us back to 1839, as has sometimes been wrongly calculated. Nevertheless, it is widely accepted that, by 1841, Baudelaire *has* the pox and his stepfather decided to send him to the islands for a few months. Syphilis then assumes its other mask and begins to attack his skin and mucous membranes, his arteries and his visceral organs. Despite treatment with potassium, diverse baths and perhaps mercury, by 1848 he has pain in the joints, spots on his skin, fatigue is exacerbated and he starts losing his hair. The symptoms will show up intermittently in association with tremendous breakdowns of mood. In May 1861 he writes to his mother:

[3]For Sartre, of course, Baudelaire is the only one to blame: 'He was the architect up to and including his very syphilis... That syphilis which tortured him all through his life, which led him to senility and to death: is it an exaggeration to say that he asked for it?' [Sartre, 1947, pp. 82–83].

> You know that when very young I caught a venereal infection, which I had later supposed had been totally cured. In Dijon, after 1848, it erupted again. It was made to subside once more. Now it has returned in a novel form, with markings on the skin, and causing extraordinary stiffness in all the joints... Perhaps in the state of sadness in which I am plunged, my terror makes it worse [in Hayden, 2004, p. 113].

Visceral and Gastrointestinal Disorders

Other symptoms of secondary syphilis did not spare Baudelaire either. From 1847 on, he complained of throat and laryngeal ulcers, and of a 'perpetual idleness commanded by a perpetual discomfort'. At this time, the 26-year-old Baudelaire has deep financial worries and indulges excessively in wine and laudanum. He is also an opium and ether enthusiast, not only for poetic purposes, but presumably to calm his gastric pains. Indeed, his stomach will be a recurrent topic of complaint in his letters. In March 1853 he writes about his stomach being wasted by 'this abominable existence and brandy'. Until his stroke, he will suffer from ingestion disorders, colic, vomiting, feelings of chocking, palpitations, fevers, insomnia, neuralgias, fatigue, and constipation.

'Nervous' Disorders

On the June 30, 1845 Baudelaire writes to Ancelle about suicide: 'The fatigue of going to sleep and the fatigue of waking up have become insupportable. I kill myself, because I am useless to others – and *dangerous to myself.* I *kill* myself because I believe in my immortality, and because I have *hope*' [in Hayden, 2004, p. 115, emphasis in original]. He failed to do so, however, after having written a testament. Whether this was a serious alert or mere simulacrum, we can backdate his 'nervous' disease more accurately to 1854. These 'nervous' complaints are most likely linked to his use of alcohol and opium and also to secondary manifestations of his syphilis. Pichois lists an impressive catalogue from 1854 to 1866: feeling stupid, body and mind illness, dark veil before the eyes, eternal racket in the ears, weakness of will, sadness, difficult gait, clumsiness of the hand, insomnia, migraine, neuralgia above the right eye, and stupor [Pichois, 2005, pp. 113–115]. In a letter to his mother, in 1855, he confides his worry at seeing his 'admirable poetic skill, the sharpness of ideas and the power of hope, which all really constitute my stock, wear out and collapse' [Jackson, 2001, p. 258]. And in December 1856: 'What I feel is an immense sense of discouragement, an insupportable feeling of isolation, a constant fear of some vague calamity, a complete distrust in my strength, a total lack of desires.' Though these lines are indicative of a depressive illness, one must not take at face value the many complaints of Baudelaire. Sartre, continuing with his theory that Baudelaire 'has chosen to suffer' [Sartre, 1947, p. 89], insists on the fact that the poet could radically change his position depending on whom he was writing to. When he writes to his mother, Sartre thinks that 'his display of suffering clearly has two goals. The first one is to satisfy his grudges, he wants his mother to be smitten by remorse. The second one is more complex: Ms. Aupick represents the judge, the Good. He humiliates before her, he seeks condemnation and absolution at the same time' (p. 86). In his letters to other persons, Baudelaire often does not appear depressed or ill. Nevertheless, in 1860, the year *Les Paradis Artificiels* is published, he experiences 'a singular crisis': 'I believe I have had something like a cerebral congestion'.

We do not know what this 'congestion' was about, perhaps it was a transient ischemic attack or perhaps a side effect of drugs and alcohol. In any case, it is the idea of hysteria that soon becomes omnipresent. Inspired by the reading of Flaubert's *Madame Bovary*, he wrote:

> Hysteria! Why wouldn't this physiological mystery be the basis… for a literary work? This mystery, which the Academy of Medicine has yet to solve, and which, expressing itself in women by the sensation of an ascending and asphyxiating sphere (I am only talking about the main symptom), translates into all kinds of impotencies in nervous men and also into a propensity for all excesses [in Pichois, 2005, p. 128].

Apparently, this was an appropriate diagnosis for doctors who could not make sense of all his complaints, and who were unaware of his syphilitic history. He had no problem endorsing the diagnosis of hysteria in himself, as these two oft-quoted and intriguing passages make clear: 'The sickness persists. And the doctor has pronounced the big word: hysteria. In plain French: I throw my tongue to the dogs [I give up],' 'Morally and physically, I've always had the feeling of being on the brink of the abyss, not only the abyss of sleep, but also the abyss of action, of memory, of desire, of regret, of remorse, of beauty, of numbers, etc. I have cultivated my *hysteria* with enjoyment and terror. I always have vertigo now, and today, January 23, 1862 I have experienced an unusual warning: I felt pass over me *the winds of the wing of foolishness.*' Vallery-Radot [1956] read these last quotes as 'signs announcing the paralysis with aphasia which, 4 years later, would shatter his 'giant wings' (p. 518). During these years, Baudelaire would often be seen on the streets with a bandaged head, presumably to quiet his neuralgias and migraines. We will never know if these were hysterical or neurological in nature, and, in any case, neurologists are already hard pressed to make the distinction nowadays.

By this time, Baudelaire is in his 40s. It is hard to say to what extent all of his symptoms were causally linked or to some extent independent of each other. It is even harder to say in what way his complaints and his 'hysteria', together with the all-too-real venereal infection, were related to the cerebrovascular problems that would follow. In any case, it is disturbing that, in his letters, Baudelaire somehow foretold the upcoming events. On February 12, 1866, he wrote: 'all too often, in these unending days spent in my bed, I would say to myself: all right now, let's think! If it is apoplexy or paralysis that is coming, what would I do and how would I put some order in my things?' [in Pichois and Ziegler, 2005, p. 714]. Alas, he was right on target.

Stroke

Before he became aphasic, Baudelaire had an ictal prodrome essentially of the motor type. This happened during his stay in Belgium. On the March 15, 1866 he fell down in St. Loup Church – 'merveille sinistre et galante' – in Namur. He wanted to see this Baroque church one last time before he left Belgium. About this episode, Eugène Crépet wrote:

> While he was admiring and showing to Poulet-Malassis and Rops, who accompanied him, the richly sculpted confessionals, he tottered, struck by a sudden dizziness, and fell on a march. His friends picked him up; he didn't look frightened and claimed that his foot slipped. They pretended to believe him; but on the following morning, upon waking up, he showed signs of mental confusion [apparently he was found immobile near the washbasin, absent-minded with a toothbrush in his hand, which he suddenly slipped into his pocket when he realised he was being observed]. He was promptly brought back to Brussels: but as soon as he was on the rail car he asked his friends to open the window, when in fact it was already open[4] [in Pichois and Ziegler, 2005, p. 717].

A few days later, around March 20, he made another mistake: 'at eleven in the evening, as he was parting company with his friend, the photographer Neyt, he said, 'see you tonight!'' [Lebrun et al., 1971, p. 310]. Neyt went home, but worried about his friend's bizarre behavior, so he decided to check whether Baudelaire got back safely to the Hôtel du Miroir. As he was not there, Neyt went looking for the poet in Brussels' cafés. He finally found him at the Taverne Royale, at one in the morning. There he was, Neyt wrote, alone in a corner, 'looking prostrate... I urged him to go home, telling him it was unwise for him to stay up this late. Finally he stood up; I accompanied him... to his hotel, with many difficulties. But when we had to climb up the stairs, I was forced to haul him up... I installed him in his room... but I had to leave; he refused obstinately my help and shouted his head off: Go away! Go away! I tell you! The following day... he was lying on his bed, all dressed up... It was nine in the morning. I woke him up; he opened his eyes, but he kept still and was unable to say a word' [in Lebrun et al., 1971]. Doctor Léon Marcq [or, unlikely, Dr. Oscar Max, appointed to the Hôtel du Miroir, see Lebrun et al., 1971] diagnosed 'an hemiplegia with subsequent aphasia. The muscles of one half of the body were paralyzed.' This narration is based on the testimonial of Neyt to Kunel, long after the

[4]This has been interpreted as a semantic paraphasia.

events. So one should be cautious about this early diagnosis, as it appears that actually Baudelaire was not aphasic at this time. Besides, it seems unusual for an aphasia to have the kind of paraphasic prodrome that was described. Baudelaire, hence, must have suffered one or more subsequent strokes.

Indeed, back at the Hôtel du Grand Miroir, we know he was still able to move and write. His last letter in his own hand dates from March 20 (to his mother): 'I'm neither well nor bad. I work and I write with difficulty. I'll explain why later.' This is rather indicative of mild paresis, though the handwriting is actually better than in some previous letters, and in that letter he even manages to discuss an orthographic matter. In the following days, around the 22nd and 23rd, there must have been a worsening – perhaps another stroke – as he can no longer write, but he is nevertheless well enough to dictate a few letters and to correct some proofs. His friends and doctors seem quite optimistic, provided he takes some rest and changes his lifestyle. Sadly, his state worsens irremediably on March 31, likely the result of a more severe stroke. Unaware of the situation, his mother – ironically – on that same day received a letter from Dr. Marcq, which stated, 'I announce to you with assurance that B's disease will have a favourable end.' But unfortunately, that very day the doctor wrote to Poulet-Malassis: 'I just saw Baudelaire, I find his state to be notably worse.' And Poulet-Malassis, then, to a friend: 'Baudelaire's situation is very serious', followed by a postscript, 'I reopen my letter to say that the state of B. has become, in a few hours, of the most extreme gravity.' Indeed, Baudelaire is now severely hemiplegic on the right side and completely aphasic. That day, Ms. Hugo writes: 'Baudelaire is finished... The illness has almost entirely invaded his brain. They despair of the invalid and it is mostly feared that he will survive his own intelligence' [in Pichois and Ziegler, 2005, p. 722]. On April 1, Poulet-Malassis writes to Asselineau: 'Yesterday the paralysis was visible on the right side and the softening of the brain is obvious... There is, so to speak, no hope to save our friend. I just left him, he barely recognized me' [in Pichois and Ziegler, 2005, p. 723].

Baudelaire can no longer be kept at the Hôtel du Miroir. On April 3 he is taken to the Institut Saint-Jean et Sainte-Elisabeth, the only clinic in the area, which is run by Augustinian nuns. According to the registry, the cause of hospitalization was 'apoplexia'. Baudelaire was placed in a common room. He stayed there for about 2 weeks. He is soon deemed 'condemned' by doctors and friends, even his brilliant biographers Pichois and Ziegler [2005] call him, at this stage, the 'living dead' and they state that there is nothing to say for a biography of Baudelaire from these months of 'vegetative life' (p. 725). These are harsh words, not only for Baudelaire, but for all aphasics. It is in that religious institute that Baudelaire began to display his famous *Cré nom* (see below). Barral writes: 'He shouted Pas! Pas! Sacré Nom!... Sacré Nom de Dieu!... Nothing is more harrowing than the spectacle of aphasia's ravages on a superior mind' [in Lebrun et al., 1971, p. 311]. And Starkie: 'The only two words he could remember were "sacré nom" which were always interpreted as an oath. With these two words, he who had loved and practised the art of conversation was obliged to express the whole gamut of his feelings and thoughts – joy, sorrow, anger and impatience – and he sometimes flew into a rage at his inability to make his meaning clear, and to answer those who spoke to him… Thought still lived in him, as could be divined from the expression in his eyes, but it was imprisoned in its dungeon of flesh, and without means of communication with the outside world' [in Lebrun et al., 1971, p. 311].

After some hesitation, Baudelaire's mother decided to go to Brussels to care for her son. She was convinced when she realized – after some exchange of letters with the Sister Superior – that the religious institute was not a good place for her son: 'she [the Sister Superior] told me, after explaining the state of health of my poor son, that he's got no religion and that it is very hard for her to have in her house an unreligious man and she asked me to help her. This gives me reason to fear that she does not wish to keep him…And another fear, no less important, is that the sisters, doubtless animated by good intentions, will torment him; and by talking him too soon into God things, will harm him' [in Crépet, 1932]. Indeed, they had some unreasonable demands for a man who was probably apraxic: 'The sisters impose some observances on him; when he is about to eat, they want him to cross himself; and so he reacts sweetly, with admirable patience, closes his eyes and turns his head away without getting angry. He pretends to be asleep when they torment him, but they could as well provoke a scene that would kill him' [in Crépet, 1932]. Though not mentioned explicitly, the reason for the Religious Superior's complaints was probably Baudelaire's involuntary (?) blasphemous cursing *Cré nom*. However, there was no other place for patients like him in Brussels. As the Sisters complained more and more about their frightening patient, Ms. Aupick decided to take him back to the Hôtel du Miroir. At this time, the hemiplegia had substantially reverted – he could move by himself with a cane – but not the aphasia. His mother, interestingly, seemed to misunderstand Baudelaire's expletive, either voluntary or unconsciously: '*Non, quie, quie*, the only words he can articulate, he shouts his head off with them' [in Pichois and Ziegler, 2005, p. 729].

As soon as the hapless patient was gone, the Sisters proceeded to do some purifying ceremonials. In a dramatic account, it was said that, 'as soon as the door of the institute closed on Baudelaire, the Sisters fell on their knees, shed abundant tears, sprayed the spaces previously occupied by their terrifying patient with holy water and only calmed down when they saw the stole of the hastily queried exorcist priest' [in Lebrun et al., 1971, p. 311]. He was then brought back to Paris with his mother (July 2, 1866), stayed a few days in a hotel near the Gare du Nord, and was taken to the Maison de Santé' of Doctor

Duval. Soon, he was unable to leave his bed and began to cease all efforts to communicate. On August 31, 1867, he died.

In his last moments he is said to have exclaimed, 'Beau' while showing the *Dôme des Invalides* through the window and then 'Dieu!'. But this story is usually replaced by a more likely one. He became calmer in the last days and died in the arms of his mother, who wrote: 'He looked asleep, with his eyes open; he passed away very gently, with no agony, no suffering. I was holding him for an hour, waiting for his last breath. I was saying tokens of tenderness to him, persuaded that despite his state of prostration and muteness, he must understand me and could answer me' [in Crépet, 1932, p. 663] and 'He died without agony, very gently, and *smiling*' (p. 667).

Baudelaire's mother was very pious; she asked the Sisters and his friends to watch out for her son's spiritual well-being: 'Think of his soul, I beg you', she wrote to Ancelle. 'Despite appearances, despite his writings, he believes, there is something religious deep down in him' [in Crépet, 1932, p. 647, footnote 1]. The first offer made by a priest only resulted in more furious 'Cré nom!'. However, a few weeks before he died, he ended up receiving the last sacraments. 'My poor child received all his sacraments, well aware of what he was doing, and with much fervour. I had the chance to catch him in a good moment' [in Crépet, 1932, p. 647, footnote 1]. Though it is not our duty to judge the sincerity of both Baudelaire and his mother, the matter of ultimate conversion in neurologically impaired patients seems to us, at best, somewhat dubious. But why not? In a way he *was* a religious man. Catholic Belgian newspapers surely adopted this point of view when they published the following necrology: 'Before dying, Mr. Charles Baudelaire, who had recovered all his senses, asked to receive Church sacraments and he confessed to the priest. The author of *Flowers of Evil* died as a Christian' [in Lebrun et al., 1971, p. 314]. Pichois and Ziegler [2005] also acknowledge that Baudelaire received the last sacraments by his own demand (see pp. 759–761). However, exactly how he made himself clearly understood and managed to confess is not explained.

Aphasia

In the remainder of this paper we shall describe in more detail specific aspects of Baudelaire's aphasia, namely its relationship with intelligence, its typology, the peculiar use of the expletive *Cré nom*, violent emotional reactions, the question of awareness of impairment, the evolution of symptoms, and we will go back to the question of etiology and discuss possible lesion sites.

Thought and Language

Aphasia was a fairly well-known disorder in Baudelaire's time, albeit poorly understood. Many of Baudelaire's relatives and contemporaries had something to say about his condition. These comments reflect how aphasia was appraised in those early times, so we will quote some of them. On April 26, 1866 Poulet-Malassis encourages Asselineau to read Trousseau's work on that matter, as both are worried about their friend's condition. These pages are not optimistic, however:

> As for aphasia with paralysis... I believe we must confess our almost total powerlessness. We can no more cure the aphasia than the accompanying paralysis; nature alone can be mostly accountable for any improvement, which in any case is always incomplete. The aphasic patient remains forever as struck with regard to his understanding as with the immobility of one side of his body. He will always limp with his intelligence [in Pichois and Ziegler, 2005, p. 731].

That last sentence has remained notorious in subsequent discussions of the aphasic mind. To decide whether Baudelaire limped or not with his intelligence, we first have to figure out as much as we can about the nature of his aphasia. Asselineau [1869/1990], in his biography of Baudelaire, writes an interesting account of his encounter with the aphasic poet:

> Contradictory rumours began to spread on Baudelaire's disease. There had been talk of insanity because of certain violent behaviour that was all too explainable by his inability to make himself understood.... Upon seeing me, he greeted me with a long, loud and persistent burst of laughter, which made my blood run cold.[5] Was he actually crazy? I had been with him for a mere quarter of an hour, and alas! was completely reassured on that matter. I became convinced that Baudelaire had never been more lucid and subtle. Seeing him lending his ear, while having a wash, to the hushed conversations near him and not missing a word of it, which I could observe through the signs of approbation or impatience he manifested, exchanging smiles with me, shrugging his shoulders, nodding, displaying, in a word, the marks of the most sustained attention and the clearest intelligence, I had no doubt that the part that illness had spared in him was completely sane and active and that his mind was as free and nimble as I saw it the previous year. Moreover, this fact had been acknowledged by the doctors who saw him the following days, Piogey, Lassègue and Blanche. When at Brussels, despite claims to the contrary made by people who barely knew him or only for a short time, the integrity of his intelligence had already been acknowledged by the man who was observing and caring for him the more assiduously, namely Poulet-Malassis. He wrote to me, 'The gravity of his disease, it seems to me, appears to be entirely in his inability to express himself. And it is clear that he is aware of this inability; but still he acts like a quasi-mute, who would articulate one single word and try to make himself understood by varying intonations. I understand him quite often, as far as I'm concerned; but it's hard...' (pp. 91–93).

[5]Baudelaire was known to have a frightening laugh, often compared to the devil's laughter itself [Benjamin, 1955/2002, p. 239].

Many ideas are to be found in this fragment, the main one being at the center of all discussions on aphasia of that era: what is it exactly that the aphasic patient lacks? The doctors in Paris told Baudelaire's mother: 'Without having his tongue paralysed, he lost the *memory of sound*...' [Pichois and Ziegler, 2005, p. 728]. And Emile Crépet: 'As for complete insensibility [i.e. dementia], it seems that Baudelaire never slipped into it; he would only exhibit an extreme despondency in the last few weeks. As for reading, this became impossible for him from the day after his second stroke' [Crépet, 1932, p. 643]. So, according to some doctors, his friend Asselineau, and many others, it seems that Baudelaire had only lost the ability to express himself. Crépet mentions that he was also unable to read, but curiously this is seldom mentioned by other authors. Cognitive psychology, of course, did not exist at that time, and the concept of modularity had just been resuscitated from the ashes of phrenology, thanks, in part, to the work of Broca. So language and intelligence were somehow nonfractionated concepts and it was hard to make sense of a disorder such as Baudelaire's without confronting these ideas. It would seem that an inability to read was irreconcilable with an entirely spared inner mental life, which would explain why the problem was not addressed by his friends. A purely motor disorder would be fairly acceptable, but an impairment of *thought* would entail no less than a disruption of the soul [see, e.g. Daudet, 1922].

Back in 1862, Baudelaire famously wrote: 'I felt pass over me *the winds of the wing of foolishness*.' Though it is hard to make sense of the exact meaning of this 'foolishness', some have interpreted this as a prodromic sign of mental deterioration. Lévy [1988], through the voice of a mysterious narrator, captures the issue quite rightly: 'The big question which, generally, agitated our circles, was whether only speech was affected – leaving intact, so to speak, the resources of an intelligence that would find other paths to express itself – or whether, if one goes together with the other, ideas with their words, the wreck was a total one' (p. 308). The narrator of this novel offers his own 'theory of aphasia', which, in his naiveté, may not be uninteresting for our understanding of 'folk neurology'[6]:

> On the one hand, there are the simple aphasias... These are integral muteness, in which speech is lost without allowing another kind of language to take over... On the other hand, there are more complex aphasias, with a strong substitutive coefficient, in which the patient continues to express himself through thousands of gestures and pantomimes... In the meanwhile, all of the difficulty resides in learning to see in these gestures more than gestures and

[6]'Folk neurology' is an analogy to the epistemological fields of folk psychology and folk physics that cognitive philosophers deal with, and might be described as the people's naïve understanding of brain functions and disorders [see, e.g., Croquelois et al., 2005].

to decrypt the hidden meaning which has anatomically withdrawn into it. Baudelaire's aphasia, of course, was of the second kind (p. 309).

There are indeed many kinds of aphasias; what is lost and what is spared in each patient involves not only the functions of language, but more widely the capacity for communicating, abstracting, symbolizing, conceptualizing, and judging, all of which are usually encompassed in the overreaching notion of 'intelligence'.

Sometimes it takes someone less familiar, less *concerned* with the patient to detect signs of mental deterioration. Speech pathologists are well aware that often persons closely related to an aphasic patient overestimate his capacities, as wishful thinking is inevitable when a loved one is struck by disease. Less involved observers may thus offer a more realistic account, albeit a rather blunt one sometimes.

A newspaper published the following notice on September 2, 1867: 'Mr. Charles Baudelaire has just passed away, after long days of suffering. For more than one year, the poet had lost speech and his mind, and death had already taken half of him. Today, it takes him entirely, and his friends dare not lament a long awaited death, which puts to an end an agony much too long' [in Lebrun et al., 1971, p. 314].

Dr. Lasègue, who had not seen the ill poet, sent a note to Ms. Aupick:

> It will be a long and, unfortunately, uncertain treatment... With an aphasia that serious, it is impossible to quantify feelings and intelligence, as expression is lacking even for the simplest ideas... [If] irritability is violent, unruly and almost unmanageable, there is no choice. Coercion is always worse for patients at home than in an institution. At home, they don't accept taking orders, and they refuse to suffer the authority of parents, whereas they resign, almost effortlessly, to the injunctions of strangers [in Crépet, 1932, p. 671].

Maxime Du Camp, in his *Souvenirs littéraires*, writes a rather negative account of Baudelaire's state: 'seated in a big armchair, hands white, face with the grubby palor which is the make-up of dementia, eyelids swollen, eyes vacant and inquiring. No trace of emotion on his thinned face; sometimes he seemed to lift himself in an incomparable effort to answer what was being said; he shouted: "Non, non, cré nom, nom!" These were the only two words – the only two notes – he was able to articulate' [in Lebrun et al., 1971, p. 313]. Jules Vallès is another example of a rather negative opinion of Baudelaire's intelligence:

> He could only articulate one word, like a child, but that word, he groaned it, he sniggered it, and, with gulps of anger or joy, he translated his supreme impressions! He was shown a flower: he gave it a little smile, like a lunatic's smile. – Cré nom! Cré nom! He cooed, swaying his head, like he was moved by the perfume and the radiance. Cré nom! It was now a greeting, now a curse, depending on whether he was shown a thing or a name he used to love or hate! Cré nom! Maybe it was also the groan of despair! Who knows? Perhaps it might mean: 'Ah! Why have I played the comedian all my life? I drove myself crazy, I know

it but I cannot say it, and could I, proud as I am, I wouldn't!' [in Bandy and Pichois, 1957, p. 322].

Well, one could indeed go on speculating about the meaning and intentions of Baudelaire's stereotyped utterances and about what remained of his inner mental life. It is very easy to put in those patients' mouths and minds exactly what we would like.

What thought is without language is one of the oldest questions of philosophy, and it has received enormous input through the study of aphasic patients [Laplane, 1997]. However, as far as the specific case of Baudelaire is concerned, the question will forever remain unanswered.

What Kind of Aphasia?

All in all, we are left with two different pictures: that of Broca's aphasia with relatively well-spared comprehension, and that of global aphasia, which seems more likely given the presence of the aspects which are described in the following sections.

The lack of information and formal testing of Baudelaire does not allow much room to discuss the specific cognitive nature of his deficits. We have hinted at what his relatives believed was or was not spared, but this, of course, is largely unreliable. What can be done is to compare Baudelaire's case to more recent data on the architecture of linguistic functions. As we have just seen, the general question of intelligence will remain a moot point as far as the poet is concerned. If we try to be more specific, can we safely assume that his comprehension was spared, or at least relatively spared? Would Baudelaire score honorably on a routine bedside assessment, notwithstanding specific scales or standardized tests used by aphasiologists?

It is now widely agreed that Broca's aphasia usually entails important comprehension deficits and the patient Leborgne, Broca's princeps case, himself is now considered – ironically – *not* to be a good example of Broca's aphasia but of *global* aphasia, on the grounds that there exists 'a robust relationship between stereotypical utterances and global aphasia' [Selnes and Hillis, 2000, see below for more on Leborgne]. Lebrun [1986, 1987] also states that most patients with monophasia have comprehension difficulties. It is worth recalling an important fact that all practitioners with aphasic patients should be aware of: comprehension in patients with global aphasia may appear surprisingly well preserved if they are contextually involved in a situation of immediate relevance, that is, if the meaning of the question or statement they are told is unambiguously derivable from the overall context. So facial expressions, anger or goal-directed movements are by no means evidence that verbal comprehension is spared in a patient if these reactions are immersed in a socially familiar and meaningful context. There is much more involved in communication than phonological assemblies alone.

As we have seen, Baudelaire certainly lost the ability to speak, while reading and writing were most likely totally impaired as well. Now if, as the previous considerations suggest, comprehension was also considerably compromised, it would seem that the whole of his language system was initially entirely reduced to the ability to curse *Cré nom* (though he was later able to express other, very short formulas), pointing to a rather severe instance of global aphasia.

Cré Nom!

The most striking feature of Baudelaire's aphasia is, of course, his recurrent and almost singular use of the expletive *Cré nom*.[7] As we have seen, this caused some stir at the religious pension where he was put, in Brussels, and the utterance did not remain unnoticed by virtually anyone in literary circles. Indeed, one can only imagine the effect of Baudelaire's blasphemous utterances in that era of pioneering aphasiology, considering the provocative content of his works. Even nowadays, neurobehavioral clinicians are required to devote a great deal of time informing patients' relatives of the mechanical side of their symptoms, just to dissipate some misconceptions regarding the patients' presumed lack of will, possession by the devil, sinful personality or plain simulation, all of which we have heard in our ward. Interestingly, Lévy [1988] fabricates the narration of Père Dejoncker at the St. Elisabeth Institute, which deals with just that:

> I felt in his screams, his movements, I perceived in this burst of vehemence that exploded to my ears, a hell of a vitality which was not from the dying. I say 'hell', but don't assume that I'm speaking like these simple minds who see your friend [Baudelaire] like a creature of the devil. Nevertheless, it is true that, in such an insurrection, something frightening was compelling... I quickly became convinced that I was dealing with a pain that looked so striking only because it affected the soul as much as, or even more than, the body. This pain of the soul, nothing could soothe it (pp. 320–321).

Indeed, language has often been seen as the highest of human faculties, God's gift. Its disruption must be due to a defect of the soul, especially when the patient is blasphemous, a plain localized disorder of the brain just does not seem like a satisfying explanation [Daudet, 1922].

The French writer, Philippe Muray, also has his own explanation: 'Now, he has insulted everything' [Muray, 1984, p. 658]. Hence, Baudelaire's use of a

[7]We would like to say a few words about this *Cré nom*. It is short for *Sacré nom de Dieu*, literally: 'Holy name of God'. In French, the expletive is now really outmoded, be it in its complete or short form, and would only count as 'blasphemous' to extremely pious ears. Its closest counterpart in English would be 'Goddamn' or even 'Damned'.

curse as his ultimate verbal contribution is merely the logical conclusion to a whole life devoted to the destruction of everything sacred. That being said, if we want to have a sound neurological explanation of the use of single utterances by aphasic patients [also called 'recurrent utterances', 'stereotyped aphasia', and even 'monophasia', see Lebrun, 1986], be they expletives, trivial catch phrases or nonsensical syllables, we have to admit that this largely remains a mystery. What could be the origin of such peculiar behaviour[8]? Why would these patients use certain words rather than others? What is the diagnostic and localization value of this intriguing symptom? There are no definite answers to these questions, though we have some clues about the likely mechanisms involved.

To demystify the cursing of Baudelaire, the first thing to do is to acknowledge that he was not, by far, the only patient to display such a disorder. It is rarely acknowledged that Broca himself wrote about these kinds of singular utterances:

> ...the perfectly sensible answer they [the aphasic patients] would like to make is reduced to a very small number of articulated sounds, always the same and always arranged in the same way; their vocabulary, so to speak, is made of a short series of syllables, sometimes a monosyllable which expresses everything, or rather nothing, as this unique word is more often than not alien to all vocabularies... In ordinary circumstances, they invariably pronounce their favourite word; however, when they feel angry, they become able to articulate a second word, most likely a gross curse; which they were presumably previously acquainted with, before their disease... Mr Auburtin has observed a patient... who requires no excitation to pronounce this stereotyped curse. All his answers begin with a bizarre six-syllable word and end invariably with this supreme invocation: Sacré nom de D... [Broca, 1861, pp. 113–114].

It is not well-known that patient Leborgne – arguably the princeps case in the modern history of aphasiology – actually said other things than 'tan'. Indeed, later in the same paper, Broca writes: 'If one did not understand his [Leborgne's] gestures, he easily became irate, and added to his vocabulary a gross swear word, only one, and precisely the same one that I mentioned previously while discussing the patient observed by Mr. Auburtin. That is, *Sacré nom de Dieu!*' [Broca, 1861, pp. 123–124]. So this specific blasphemy hardly seems an original symptom of motor aphasia, since it was described almost from the beginning. In another early observation, a patient of Trousseau, when angry, would shout *sacon!*, probably a contraction of *sacré nom!* [Lebrun, 1986]. Other examples of recurrent utterances include Valery Larbaud's poetic 'Bonsoir les choses d'ici-bas' or short phrases like 'better, better', 'I can try', 'factory', serial numbers, yes or no, and proper names [Code, 1982; Lebrun, 1986]. There are also patients who utter meaningless syllables, like Leborgne's 'tan' and a personal patient who was only able to say 'ipou'.

[8]Stand-up comedian Billy Connolly offers a funny theory – which we cannot detail here – regarding his own father, a victim of a stroke who was only able to utter with great difficulty the expletive: 'Fffffuuuck' [see Connolly, 2005].

If recurrent utterances are not infrequent in aphasic patients, what mechanisms could be involved? Clearly, language is not entirely confined to the left hemisphere (nor is language the sole function thereof, by the way). In many experimental and clinical studies, the right hemisphere has been shown to participate in various aspects of language processing. However, it remains a widely shared opinion that the two hemispheres take over different roles in language subcategories (motor planning, grammaticality, emotional expression, meaning appreciation, etc.). Hughling Jackson was the most vocal defender of this thesis. In fact, he followed the writings of the French clinician Baillarger to develop this idea. What Baillarger conceptualized as two different kinds of speech – voluntary and involuntary – Jackson proposed to implement in the brain. Loosely defined, Jackson's notion of 'propositional speech' corresponds to 'voluntary speech' and is located in the left hemisphere, whereas nonpropositional speech (involuntary or automatic) involves the participation of both hemispheres. Further, 'Jackson saw aphasic speech automatisms as primitive and automatic behaviour and the expression of levels lower down the ontogenic and phylogenic neural hierarchy which have been released from higher level inhibition' [Code, 1997, p. 42]. What is meant by 'primitive' speech are utterances which do not entail much conscious thought and include formulaic speech made of overlearned, familiar, holistic, conventional, invariant and context-bound sentences (also called 'sealed units' or 'packages'). They are clichés and stereotypes, motorically easy to formulate, which are produced quite automatically in social and emotional aspects of communication. Examples are: slang, idioms, polite exchanges, catchy pop lyrics, proverbs, verbal 'tics' and, of course, cursing [Code, 1997]. Arguably, these involve pretty much all our daily use of language. Whether they should be labelled 'nonpropositional' is, of course, a debatable issue, as most of the time they have some pragmatic meaning and actually refer to something. However, what is proposed is that they somehow bypass higher cognitive units, rather like the practiced car driver or tennis player who does not spend a great deal of time thinking when executing complex behavioral sequences.

Cursing in aphasia was discussed in detail by Jackson in terms of a disinhibition of this emotional-automatic speech. Gowers also thought that cursing followed aphasia because 'the will is needed not to cause, but to restrain emotional speech' [in Brown and Kushner, 2001, p. 542]. Anatomically, this could be analyzed in two different ways: what is disinhibited are either 'lower centers', for example subcortical structures, or the right hemisphere (the latter being seen as more 'primitive' than the left in early neuroscience). As an aside, this discussion influenced Freud's idea of repression. In his 1891 book on aphasia, Freud saw cursing by aphasics as emerging from the destruction of more highly organized and repressive articulate speech. Uncontrolled swearing by aphasics results, Freud wrote, from 'functional retrogression (dis-involution) of a highly organized apparatus and therefore corresponds to earlier states of its functional development. This means that under all circumstances, an arrangement of associations, which having been acquired later, belong to a higher level of functioning, will be lost, while an earlier and simpler one will be preserved' [in Brown and Kushner, 2001, pp. 542–543]. Apparently, even mute persons with aphasia of sign speech will sometimes display automatic eruptive cursing via signs [Brown and Kushner, 2001, p. 543]. Drawing on coprolalia in Tourette's syndrome [Singer, 1997], one might postulate the involvement of dysfunctional basal ganglia, limbic and frontal circuits in cursing in aphasia, which would not be totally at odds with the above explanation in terms of a release of 'lower-centers' [Code, 1997]. This would also be compatible with an account in terms of right hemispheric disinhibition. We know that Baudelaire was able to recognize his friends' names [Crépet, 1932, p. 655] and became very emotional when hearing words such as Paris or the mention of his mother [Crépet, 1932, p. 644]. He was also able to enjoy music: two young musicians were brought to him to play *Tannhäuser*, as he had a fondness for Wagner, and he showed clear signs of appreciation. Thus, it would seem that a link between sound input and emotion was spared, presumably involving right hemispheric functions – as the latter is dominant for the processing of emotionally self-relevant stimuli [Keenan, 2003] and emotionally significant music [Alfredson et al., 2004]. In the same vein, the production of recurrent utterances must tap into spared pathways that are normally involved in the execution of automatic speech, and this may well be mediated by the basal ganglia or the limbic system via the right hemisphere [as discussed by Code, 1997]. Furthermore, the recognition that Baudelaire could modulate the prosody of his monophasia is certainly indicative of an involvement of the right hemisphere [Gorelick and Ross, 1987]. In any case, a 'spared' pathway is obviously necessary if one wants to account for so-called Baillarger-Jackson's '*dissociation automatico-volontaire*', which is precisely what is at issue with recurrent utterances (though it is not clear whether Baudelaire could or could not utter *Cré nom* on purpose or in a repetition task).

As for the specific 'choice' of the expletive *Cré nom*, this is even harder to account for. A quite intuitive solution is the 'last word before stroke theory', which was held, more or less in that form, by Jackson, Gowers, Alajouanine and Critchley [see Lebrun, 1986; Code, 1982, 1997]. In this account, the patient was saying or was about to say something when his brain suffered the stroke. Somehow, the system then remained 'stuck' with that particular utterance. However, in the case of Baudelaire, we simply do not know what his last words were before aphasia and, as far as we know, there is no evidence that he was particularly fond of the expletive *Cré nom* or even the complete *Sacré nom de Dieu* for that matter (remember, he was a poet, after all). Another similar approach is that the *first* word said in aphasia becomes the recurrent utterance, and this might indeed be the case for Baudelaire. The idea that aphasic nonpropositional speech is somehow 'primitive', a regression in the scale of language acquisition is, of course, also seductive and was captured by Baudelaire's mother, who really saw and cared for her 'poor child' like – well – a child.

Catastrophic Reactions

A frequent observation of Baudelaire's aphasia is a tendency to displays of anger. Presumably, these unpredictable reactions and the blasphemous *Cré nom* were the reasons why the Augustinian Sisters had such a hard time with him (notwithstanding the fact – which would seem perfectly excusable to any rational person – that he was just not *able* to recite the obligatory prayers). It is not clear whether Baudelaire became angry in all circumstances and with everybody. For example, he seemed quite docile with Asselineau: 'We are taking a walk in the greenery... I am making the most cheering conversation I can with him. When I bring him back he has expressed but the pleasure of living and contentment, gazing from time to time heavenwards with an expression of resignation, after a vain attempt at speaking' [Asselineau, 1869/1990, pp. 91–93]. As with many aphasic patients, he mostly became very upset with people who did not understand him. However, it was with his mother that he most easily lost his temper (giving weight to Sartre's account that Baudelaire did everything to make the old lady feel bad). In a letter to Poulet-Malassis, she wrote:

His book of poetry (*Les Epaves* [the prohibited poems of *Les Fleurs du Mal*]) has often been the cause of terrible fits of anger: he has something to say about this strange book that I cannot figure out. Recently, while taking a look at that unfortunate book, he stuck it in my face to the point of making me back away and threw a furious tantrum because I could not understand..., he ended up, exhausted, throwing himself to his armchair, where a few minutes later he resumed shouting loudly, wiggling his legs in the air... like some ferocious beast [in Lebrun, 1971, p. 12].

Ms. Aupick, for sure, was not unaware of her son's selectivity: 'He has always been sweet and polite with everybody. Me, alone, I have to suffer his great tantrums, surely because he has things to tell me that he doesn't tell to the others, or else, because he doesn't put himself out much with me, as he knows my weakness.' She was told by Dr. Duval: 'For a long time I wanted to tell you to cease your visits, as he gets excited and angry only with you' [Crépet, 1932, pp. 656–657].

Pichois and Ziegler [2005], following Asselineau, seem to interpret the *Cré nom* as a form of frustration: 'The sisters and their superior concluded that he had no religion, whereas... Baudelaire's cursing – the notorious *Cré nom* – resulted from his suffering and his impatience with not being understood' (p. 730).

Of course, catastrophic reactions and recurrent utterances are not independent explanations for the use of *Cré nom!* by Baudelaire. Both could arguably be the consequence of the other, although, to our knowledge, the links between these two manifestations of severe aphasia have not been thoroughly studied. Nevertheless, common mechanisms might be at play, especially the aforementioned limbic and right-hemispheric release [Carota et al., 2005].

Anosognosia?

To what extent can we say that Baudelaire was aware of his condition? Recall that Poulet-Malassis wrote: 'The gravity of his disease, it seems to me, appears to be entirely in his inability to express himself. And it is clear that he is aware of this inability' [Asselineau, 1869/1990]. It is indeed common wisdom among neurologists to ascribe awareness of impairment to motor aphasia and anosognosia to Wernicke's aphasia. However, the picture may not be as clear-cut. In a review of anosognosia in aphasics, Lebrun [1987] states that aphasic patients who recover from their condition often are quite surprised to learn that they repeatedly used a specific word. It appears that motor aphasics are aware of their incapacity to speak, but often unaware of the specific kind of errors or speech they produce. Among other explanations, an impaired auditory feedback might prevent these patients from hearing their own stereotypy as they produce it. So it is far from certain that Baudelaire actually *knew* he was cursing when he attempted to speak [Lebrun, 1987].

Course of and Attempts at Rehabilitation

Did Baudelaire's aphasia show any progress during his year and a half of survival after his stroke? Here is a realistic account: 'The illness would show many ups-and-downs during the eighteen months that it lasted. Many times, the hemiplegia showed a significant improvement, allowing the patient to take strolls and even to take part in a small dinner organized in his honour. The aphasia, however, resisted all treatment' [Crépet, 1932, p. 643]. Notwithstanding, it seems that Dr. Duval made some efforts towards speech therapy. Ms. Aupick wrote: 'I am told he can now say: *bonjour monsieur*. I would like to know whether he says it spontaneously, by himself... or whether he merely repeats it when Mr. Duval exercises him in pronouncing a few words. What a distressing thing, the state of my poor son, forced to learn to speak like a child!' [in Lebrun et al., 1971, p. 312]. She tried to make him write with the left hand, but only managed to stir his anger [Crépet, 1932, p. 652], which would indicate a complete agraphia or apraxia. All along, his mother showed pathetic expectations of her son's progress. She constantly asked his friends and doctors about signs of improvement in his speech. Asselineau seemed to be more realistic: 'He says four new words: bonjour monsieur, bonsoir monsieur, adieu and the name of his doctor. The latter is triumphant about this result, which to me does not seem so glorious. The problem will not have achieved much progress merely because Baudelaire can say a few more words... Everything he will say in his illness is mere parrot talk. Doctor Duval... triumphs stupidly in my opinion' [in Lebrun et al., 1971, p. 313]. Another example of the hopeless optimism of his mother is when she cheered at these new words: '*Passez-moi la moutarde* [pass me the mustard]. This gives me hope his speech could come back, maybe all at once.' And 'Charles has gained a few words: he says *oui* always opportunely now; *très bien*; he was once heard saying *Piogey* when we were trying to find this doctor's name; but he couldn't repeat it. May that improvement... continue!' [Crépet, 1932, p. 657]. Instead, his state kept worsening. It is now acknowledged that no total recovery, be it progressive or sudden, is to be expected from global aphasics, and to our knowledge, there has not been a single case of 'miraculous' return to normality in a patient with global aphasia.

Etiology

What caused Baudelaire's stroke? This is hard to say, because we have no official medical documents on him. We must search for clues in his correspondence and anamnesis. First, one has to look at his burdened family history. Baudelaire was born to a 61-year-old man and a mother of 26. While this would not necessary be a risk factor, one has to admit that even for the 19th century it is somehow unusual. His biological father died at 65 of a stroke. His mother died hemiplegic and aphasic, 4 years after Baudelaire. She was said to suffer from the same kind of ailment as her son, with good abilities to understanding but poor word finding, semantic paraphasias and automatisms [these being quite different from the blasphemous *Cré nom*; she apparently said 'cinquante centimes' or 'quatre-vingts centimes', see Pichois, 2005, p. 110, footnote 1]. Alphonse, Baudelaire's stepbrother, had diabetes and neurosyphilis. He died of a right-sided brain hemorrhage. Many have thus seen a hereditary factor in Charles Baudelaire's destiny, perhaps some genetic proneness to cerebrovascular disease. But this also fits quite well with contemporary 'degeneracy' theories. According to Muray [1984, p. 659], the poet himself seemed to agree with that idea in these quite prophetic verses:

My father dead hemiplegic
My brother Alphonse dead hemiplegic
My mother will die hemiplegic
Me, son of a 'priest', will die hemiplegic
My ancestors insane or maniacs
All victims of terrible passions
In solemn apartments
All dead of syphilis
All had the pox... all had the pox

However, we could not locate this excerpt in any work of Baudelaire, so it may be hagiographic (however, like the Italians say: *se non e vero, e ben trovato*). Be that as it may, it appears that even Jeanne Duval became hemiplegic, some time after they ended their relationship.

The concept of 'degeneration', of course, is closely interlinked with the question of syphilis, the plague of the 19th century. Charcot himself overlooked the evidence available at his time of the infectious origins of tabes dorsalis and preferred an account based on family history. Certainly, an early infection by *Treponema* could be a plausible cause of arteritis leading to cerebrovascular disease, but in the case of Baudelaire, a 'meningo-encephalitis', such as Doctor Oscar Max diagnosed, is unlikely. Indeed, there was no progressive mental deterioration in the months preceding Baudelaire's stroke, so general paresis of the insane is not a plausible diagnosis. Furthermore, even after the stroke, many had the feeling that he was not frankly demented or intellectually diminished. However, this idea is still mentioned, probably due to the writings of Cesare Lombroso in his notorious book *The Man of Genius* [1891], which presented Baudelaire as a case study of 'progressive paresis of the insane'. More recently, Hayden [2004] promoted the idea that Baudelaire died at an early stage of general paresis, the 'paretic stage', thus leaving him no time to develop signs of insanity (though, of course, in tertiary encephalitic neurosyphilis mental deterioration usually comes first and 'general paresis' later, if ever).

Baudelaire's drug use must also be mentioned (mostly opiates and alcohol). Although there were no severe episodes of withdrawal, dependency, amnesia or hallucinations, many of his ailments were surely to be explained by his bad habits, and he knew it. Indeed, before it was too late, he had sometimes been resolute in changing things in his life: 'Obey to the strictest principles of sobriety, the first one of which is the suppression of all excitants... Work entails necessarily good habits, sobriety and... consequently health', 'to be cured of everything, of misery, of disease and of melancholy, there lacks only the taste for work... Hygiene. Too late, perhaps!' [in Vallery-Radot, 1956, p. 517]. However, these excesses are to be considered as the consequence of various ailments and pains, rather than their cause. The question of personality proneness may also be addressed: he was emotional, unstable, impulsive, hypochondriacal, depressive and somewhat phobic and paranoid. Recall that he wrote of his own 'hysteria'. Some of his complaints might then have a *functional* origin, due to a tendency to somatize his inner struggles. Sartre even implied that he simply made up most of them. Indeed, the poet was well aware of timely scientific discussions of hysteria, malingering and neurosis. He wrote: 'How to heal oneself? How to make hope out of despair; will out of cowardice? This disease, is it imaginary or real? Did it become real after having been imaginary? Is it the result of a physical weakening, of an incurable melancholy after so many years full of shock, spent without solace in solitude and uneasiness?' [in Murphy, 2003, pp. 511–512]. Could his peculiar personality have somehow led to the stroke? This would not be altogether a preposterous hypothesis, as there are many things that remain to be understood in the relationship between cerebrovascular disease, mood and personality [see Dieguez et al., 2004].

Lesions

Notwithstanding the obvious lack of radiological information and the scarcity of clinical evidence, can we pinpoint the precise location of the brain damage that Baudelaire suffered from? In the light of what we have discussed about the course of events and his symptoms, we can offer some speculative insights. First, as we have said, Baudelaire very likely suffered various strokes from March 15 to 31, 1866 [see also Asselineau, 1869/1990, p. 91]. These were likely ischemic in nature, perhaps transitory for the first (March 15) and second attack (March 22). The stroke leading to aphasia must have been quite a severe infarct, involving the softening of extensive regions of the perisylvian area of the left hemisphere, though it is unclear if the origin was the left carotid artery or the middle cerebral artery [Lebrun et al., 1971]. As we know that his hemiplegia recovered better than his aphasia, at least for the lower limb, we might say that the stroke was accompanied initially by a penumbra that involved large territories of the sensorimotor areas and underlying subcortical structures and which was then slowly resorbed. However, the basal ganglia likely remained largely damaged, as this is usually the case in patients with recurrent utterances [Lebrun, 1986; Code, 1997]. Catastrophic reactions seem to occur mostly after lesions in the superficial territory of the superior division of the left middle cerebral artery, involving the insula, the frontal operculum or the angular gyrus [Carota et al., 2001]. Stereotypes and automatisms have poor localization value, as they occur mostly in extended lesions leading to global aphasia. These involve large portions of the left frontotemporal lobes and underlying subcortical structures.

Conclusion: Disease and Creativity

The question one is bound to ask is that of the relationship between Baudelaire's health and his art. Léon Daudet, son of the writer Alphonse Daudet, sees a link between obstacles to health and genius, meaning that the former allow the artist to sharpen and improve his creativity: 'The road of his existence, which was that of a sick man, a sexual impotent, a bohemian and also a very unhappy man... helped him to polish his sensitivity and the exaltation of his thought' [Daudet, 1929, p. 204]. Baudelaire himself wrote: 'I claim that inspiration is somehow linked to stroke and that every sublime thought comes with a nervous shock... which rings up to the cerebellum' [in Vallery-Radot, 1956, p. 518]. But can we say that his disease had a more direct impact on his work? As we have seen, his stroke entirely prevented him from writing again. There is also no evidence of deterioration in his writings a few weeks before his stroke [notwithstanding the graphological analysis defended by Pichois, 2005]. Of course, his conferences in Brussels were a disaster and his notes on Belgium were sparse and poorly organized. But we also know that his last letters were quite well written and did not have more mistakes or any changes in style compared to the older ones. Throughout his life, his changes in creative ability seem better explained by psychological and physical disturbances than by symptoms of brain dysfunction.

To some, however, aphasia – especially seen from the perspective of literary critics poorly acquainted with facts of neurology – is not a disease like any other. In these circles Baudelaire's aphasia seems to almost *make sense*, in a way. This implies that Baudelaire's life be examined retrospectively so that one can fully see the ironies of fate at work. Indeed, the poet himself was fond of predicting his own demise. It is almost as if Baudelaire's ending as an aphasic was some sort of retribution for his dissolute lifestyle. 'He asked for it', some authors seem to imply, 'genius has a price', others might say. From this perspective, we have seen that Sartre described the poet as a self-made victim. It is up to the individual to decide whether or not to become a *poète maudit*, and the individual is consequently responsible – guilty – for the condition in which he finds himself. Creativity seems to be inextricably linked to a willingness to remain in a state of suffering. But does one have to lead a horrible life to write about the darkest corners of the human mind? Pichois [2005] seems to think so, as rather surprisingly he has a benevolent stance towards Sartre's essay: 'I have cultivated my *hysteria* with enjoyment and terror.' One can even think, as Sartre [1947, p. 128], that Baudelaire asked for it and found it, in order to feel himself exist, to be another person. Thus, according to Pichois, Baudelaire used hysteria as a mask to convey his legend, of which the works are but a sprouting. Then, disease and health complaints, in the guise of 'hysteria', were mostly an *excuse* for the poet's impotence and excesses, so he knew perfectly that he had to give his 'tongue to the dogs' and was prepared for it. Somehow, he also knew he was condemned, not to die, but to lose something sacred. Pichois, like many others, seems convinced that, indeed, poetry and genius have a price. Getting rid of his own self and all possibilities to actually *lead* his life (not to mention the possibility of salvation), the poet is left with the sole purpose of creating. 'L'art pour l'art' would thus demand an empty and already condemned self. Once his immortal verses were written, aphasia made sure in the surest possible way that he added nothing else.

Could Baudelaire have written works other than the ones we know? Could someone else, for that matter someone positive, responsible and healthy, have written the same poems? These are questions impossible to answer and such an attempt would be futile. In the end, one might wonder if there really is some 'logic' in an artist such as Baudelaire to become aphasic. Many commentators surely would like it to be so, but we opine that some things might best be explained by plain, unfortunate mechanisms operating in an indifferent universe. And we are quite sure that nobody *demands* or even *deserves* to become aphasic. Here, of course, we have taken a neutral stance, and merely sought to understand his symptoms and etiology from the point of view of neurobehavioral science, *pace* Sartre, Pichois and all literary and psychoanalytical critics engulfed in their 'malediction' belief.

A Short Appendix on Synesthesia

Some authors have implied that Baudelaire may have had synesthesia [e.g. Harrison and Baron-Cohen, 1994] and some even find the hypothesis 'undoubtedly genuine' [Critchley, 1994]. Synesthesia can be defined as the mixing of sensations which are normally experienced separately. In oft-quoted verses from the poem *Correspondances*, Baudelaire powerfully conveyed this idea:

Like prolonged echoes mingling in the distance
In a deep and tenebrous unity,
Vast as the dark of night and as the light of day,
Perfumes, sounds, and colours correspond.

He wrote to Alphonse Toussenel: 'I have been saying for a long time that the poet is supremely intelligent, he is the quintessence of *intelligence*, that *imagination* is the more *scientific* of all faculties, because it encompasses the *universal analogy*, or that which a mystical religion would call a *correspondence*' [in Jackson, 2001, p. 258].

Arguably, this is best described as 'literary synesthesia' rather than 'psychological synesthesia', though the frontier between both might not always be clear-cut. From a neuroscientific standpoint, synesthesia has been associated with a modularity breakdown, aberrant connectivity, anomalous hemispheric dominance and genetic factors. Is any of this relevant to Baudelaire's disease and aphasia? We leave this question open, but we would like to stress the fact that, although Baudelaire is always cited in discussions of synesthesia, the truth is that we simply do not know if he was a 'clinical' synesthete or not. For that matter, all poets might be synesthetes. Synesthesia, after all, is what metaphor is all about and certainly Baudelaire intuitively thought that the general concept of 'correspondances' might be the ticket to understand the origins of language and creativity, as has recently been proposed by neuroscientists [Ramachandran and Hubbard, 2001].

References

Alfredson BB, Risberg J, Hagberg B, Gustafson L: Right temporal lobe activation when listening to emotionally significant music. Appl Neuropsychol 2004;11:161–166.
Angles A: Sartre versus Baudelaire. Yale French Stud 1948;2:119–124.
Asselineau C: Charles Baudelaire. Paris, Le Temps qu'il Fait, 1869/1990.
Bandy WT, Pichois C: Baudelaire devant ses contemporains. Monaco, Editions du Rocher, 1957.
Bataille G: La littérature et le Mal. Paris, Gallimard, 1957.
Baudelaire C: Œuvres complètes. Paris, Robert Laffont (Bouquins), 1980.
Benjamin W: Charles Baudelaire. Paris, Payot, 1955/2002.
Broca P: Remarques sur le siege de la faculté du langage articulé, suivies d'une observation d'aphémie (perte de la parole). Bull Soc Anat Paris 1861;6(36ème année, 2e série): 330–357. Reprinted in Broca P: Ecrits sur l'aphasie (1861–1869). Paris, L'Harmattan, 2004.
Brown KE, Kushner HI: Eruptive voices: coprolalia, malediction, and the poetics of cursing. New Lit Hist 2001;32:537–562.
Carota A, Dieguez S, Bogousslavsky J: Psychopathologie des accidents vasculaires cérébraux. Psychol Neuropsychiatr Vieillissement 2005;3:235–249.
Carota A, Rossetti AO, Karapanayiotides T, Bogousslavsky J: Catastrophic reaction in acute stroke: a reflex behavior in aphasic patients. Neurology 2001;57:1902–1905.
Code C: On the origins of recurrent utterances in aphasia. Cortex 1982;18:161–164.
Code C: Can the right hemisphere speak? Brain Lang 1997;57:38–59.
Connolly B: Live in New York. Universal (DVD), 2005.
Crépet J: Les derniers jours de Charles Baudelaire. Nouv Rev Fr 1932;21:641–671.
Critchley EMR: Synaesthesia; in Critchley EMR (ed): The Neurological Boundaries of Reality. Northvale, Aronson, 1994, p 116.
Croquelois A, Assal G, Annoni JM, Staub F, Gronchi A, Bruggimann L, Dieguez S, Bogousslavsky J: Diseases of the nervous system: patients' aetiological beliefs. J Neurol Neurosurg Psychiatry 2005;76:582–584.
Daudet L: La fin d'un dogme scientifique. Action Française, March 10, 1922.
Daudet L: Flambeaux. Paris, Grasset, 1929.
Dieguez S, Staub F, Bruggimann L, Bogousslavsky J: Is poststroke depression a vascular depression? J Neurol Sci 2004;226:53–58.
Gorelick PB, Ross ED: The aprosodias: further functional-anatomical evidence for the organization of affective language in the right hemisphere. J Neurol Neurosurg Psychiatr 1987;50:553–560.
Harrison J, Baron-Cohen S: Synaesthesia: an account of coloured hearing. Leonardo 1994;27:343–346.
Hayden D: Pox: Genius, Madness, and the Mysteries of Syphilis. New York, Basic Books, 2004.
Jackson JE: Baudelaire. Paris, LGF, 2001.
Keenan J: The Face in the Mirror. London, Harper Collins, 2003.
Laplane D: La Pensée d'outre-mots. Le Plessis-Robinson, Les empêcheurs de penser en rond, 1997.
Lebrun Y, Hasquin-Deleval J, Brihaye J, Flament J: L'aphasie de Charles Baudelaire. Rev Neurol 1971;125:310–316.
Lebrun Y: Aphasia with recurrent utterances: a review. Br J Disord Commun 1986;21:3–10.
Lebrun Y: Anosognosia in aphasics. Cortex 1987;23:251–263.
Lévy B-H: Les derniers jours de Charles Baudelaire. Paris, Grasset, 1988.
Lombroso C: The Man of Genius. London, W. Scott, 1891.
Muray P: Le XIXe siècle à travers les âges. Paris, Gallimard, 1984.
Murphy S: Logiques du dernier Baudelaire. Paris, Honoré Champion, 2003.
Pichois C: La maladie de Baudelaire; in Pichois C (ed): Retour à Baudelaire. Geneva, Slatkine Erudition, 2005.
Pichois C, Ziegler J: Baudelaire. Paris, Fayard, 2005.
Ramachandran VS, Hubbard EM: Synaesthesia: a window into perception, thought and language. J Consciousness Stud 2001;8:3–34.
Sartre J-P: Baudelaire. Paris, Gallimard, 1947.

Selnes OA, Hillis A: Patient Tan revisited: a case of atypical global aphasia? J Hist Neurosci 2000;9:233–237.
Singer C: Tourette syndrome. Coprolalia and other coprophenomena. Neurol Clin 1997;15:299–308.
Vallery-Radot P: Baudelaire: médecine et médecins. La Presse Médicale 1956;64:517–518.

Sebastian Dieguez
Brain Mind Institute, Laboratory of Cognitive Neuroscience
EPFL, Dorigny, Station 15
CH–1015 Lausanne (Switzerland)
Tel. +41 21 693 1681, Fax +41 21 693 1770, E-Mail sebastian.dieguez@epfl.ch

Bogousslavsky J, Hennerici MG (eds): Neurological Disorders in Famous Artists – Part 2.
Front Neurol Neurosci. Basel, Karger, 2007, vol 22, pp 150–168

Memory and the Creation of Art: The Syndrome, as in de Kooning, of 'Creating in the Midst of Dementia'

An 'ArtScience' Study of Creation, Its 'Brain Methods' and Results

Carlos Hugo Espinel

The Blood Pressure Center and Georgetown University School of Medicine, Washington, D.C., USA

Abstract

The creation of abstract art demands high intellectual capacities. Willem de Kooning, nonetheless, accomplished his last paintings while crippled by impairments diagnosed as Alzheimer's disease. Until my research neither art nor science offered an explanation, or a thinking method, for identifying this phenomenon, for solving a mystery that pertains to human discovery and creation. In this 'ArtScience' study of the de Kooning phenomenon I use 'Thinking Methods' which I devised by a systematic application of information on the workings of the brain, the 'Brain Methods'. With my 'Method of Observation' I examined de Kooning's paintings, created both before and during dementia, and found them comparable in technique and expression. This demonstrates the authenticity of art created in dementia. With my 'Cognitive Analysis' I identified in de Kooning the syndrome herein called 'Creating in the Midst of Dementia'. This Syndrome, unique in mechanisms and presentation, is characterized by (1) a specific combination of brain functions and malfunctions, in this case, preservation of three memory systems – working, procedural, and episodic – and deficit of the semantic memory system, and by (2) a response to precise stimuli, one that triggers brain reactivation, and as a consequence enables creating in the midst of dementia. My work offers: (1) The identification of the 'Syndrome of Creating in the Midst of Dementia'. It (a) presents its definition, the criteria of diagnosis, mechanism, rationale, and possibility of 'cognitive repair' and (b) solves the mystery of de Kooning creating art while crippled by dementia. (2) New Thinking Methods, the 'Brain Methods', that based on information on the workings of the brain, open a new path in the pursuit of truth. The 'Method of Observation' serves to define stimuli, and the 'Cognitive Analysis' to assess cognitive faculties. (3) The integration of art and science into a new discipline of study, 'ArtScience'.

The Creation

The Phenomenon

It would be a mystery, a cognitive wonder, indeed a phenomenon meriting scientific attention, if masterpieces of abstract art can be created in dementia. Abstract art is not just the mechanical copy of an image, not even the rendition of the seen, but the invention of an image that is both nonrecognizable and yet capable of stimulating thoughts and emotions [Chilvers et al., 1994]. This creation is therefore an achievement that demands high intellectual capacities. Dementia, on the other hand, is an acquired, sustained deterioration of memory and other cognitive abilities that impairs even performance of activities of daily living [Bird and Miller, 2005; Neugroschl et al., 2005].

With my 'Thinking Methods', by observing the art and by investigating the cognition of the creation, I had found how Willem de Kooning (1904–1997) created his last abstract masterpieces while crippled by dementia (figs. 1, 2) [Espinel, 1996a]. In this 'ArtScience' study I present my Thinking Methods; with it I show that, and why, the de Kooning phenomenon meets the criteria of what I have identified as a unique neurocognitive Syndrome, that of 'Creating in the Midst of Dementia'.

Art, the Mystery

In February of 1995, an extraordinary conference of art experts took place in New York City. The gathering, its secluded and exclusive nature, and the participants, their preeminence in the art world, hint at the sensitive nature of the matter to be discussed. They included the directors of the San Francisco Museum of Modern Art, SFMOMA, of the Walter Art Center in Minneapolis, the curator of modern art at the New York MOMA, a Professor of Art at the University of Texas, and the distinguished artist, Jasper Johns [Garrels, 1995; Storr, 1995]. The conference sought an informed opinion for an upcoming exhibition of de Kooning's paintings.

De Kooning's paintings, coveted by collectors, bringing high prices in the art market, being exhibited in museums worldwide, leading the 'abstract expressionist' movement, contributed to the historical beginnings of American modern art. Starting in the 1930s with figurative works, evolving every few years, inventing new forms, many extracted from his representation of womanly curves, experimenting all the way from black and white to multiple dissonant color combinations, de Kooning advanced to the creation of the pure abstract image (figs. 3, 4). It was as if de Kooning had the capacity to renew his art, and perhaps himself. Until in the late 1970s, now in his 70s, de Kooning began to slow down. He had

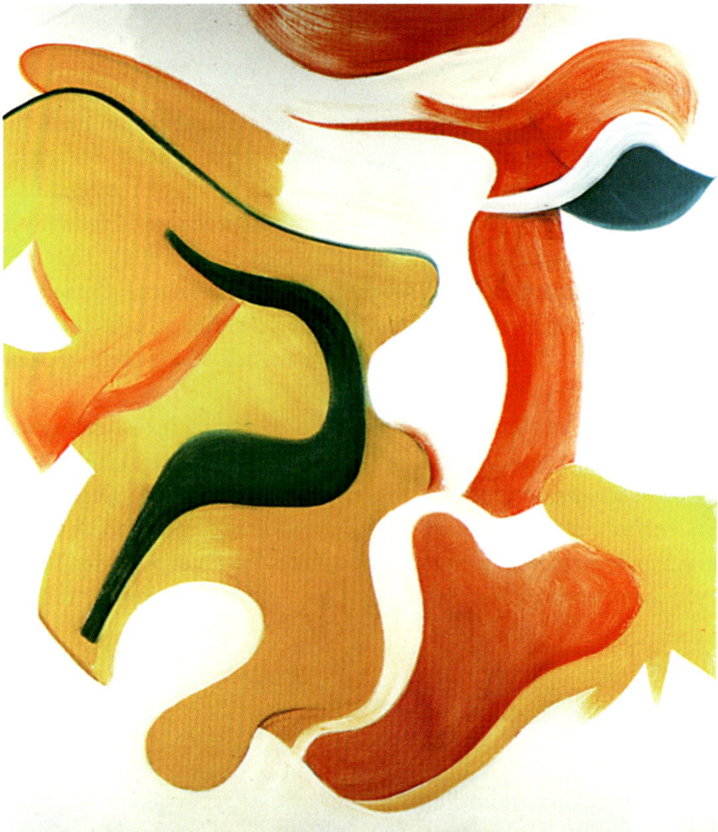

Fig. 1. Willem de Kooning, *Untitled XIII*, 1985, oil on canvas, 203.2 × 177.8 cm. Collection of the Cleveland Museum of Art. Leonard C. Hanna, Jr., Fund (copyright 2007, The Willem De Kooning Foundation/ProLitteris, Zurich).

become forgetful, confused, disoriented. He withdrew from the art scene. In fact, de Kooning stopped painting [Garrels, 1995; Storr, 1995; Larson, 1994].

Then in 1980, de Kooning began to paint again, and went on to do so for years. This resurgence stunned the art world. Its results, though, these last paintings, had to be assessed, their quality judged, and that is why the experts met in New York (fig. 1) [Garrels, 1995; Storr, 1995]. The conference was recorded, and I, in the course of investigating the neurocognition of discovery and creation, examined the tapes.

No one in the history of art had seen anything like this. These were not just 1 or 2 mindless scribbles a demented old man might have scrawled on a piece of paper. These were works of abstract art, many masterpieces. They were rendered

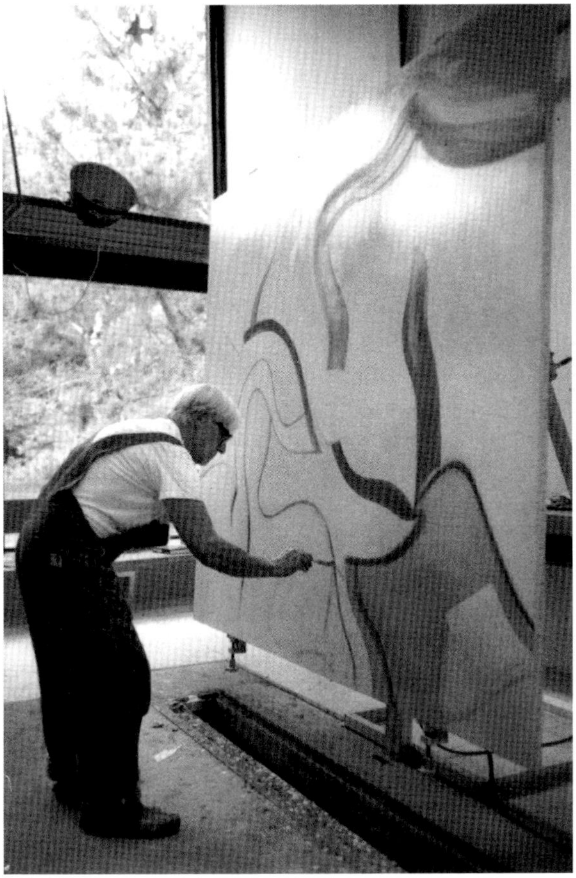

Fig. 2. Adelaide de Menil: Willem de Kooning at work, photo, 1983 (copyright A. de Menil, with kind permission).

on massive canvas, each different, each in distinct phases of compositional development. The images defied depth, came to the surface of the paintings, the forms intermingled in harmonious combinations, the colors surged in stunning ever-changing shapes (fig. 1). The disease, though, introduced controversy to the conference. In the same paintings some experts found 'signs of faltering control' while others deemed them 'highly controlled and sophisticated'. They had learned that the art was produced while de Kooning had lost control of his life; while his mental condition had deteriorated to such degree that he could not perform activities of daily living; that the courts of New York had declared him legally incompetent to handle his own affairs [Garrels, 1995; Storr, 1995]. For art, then, the creation was a mystery.

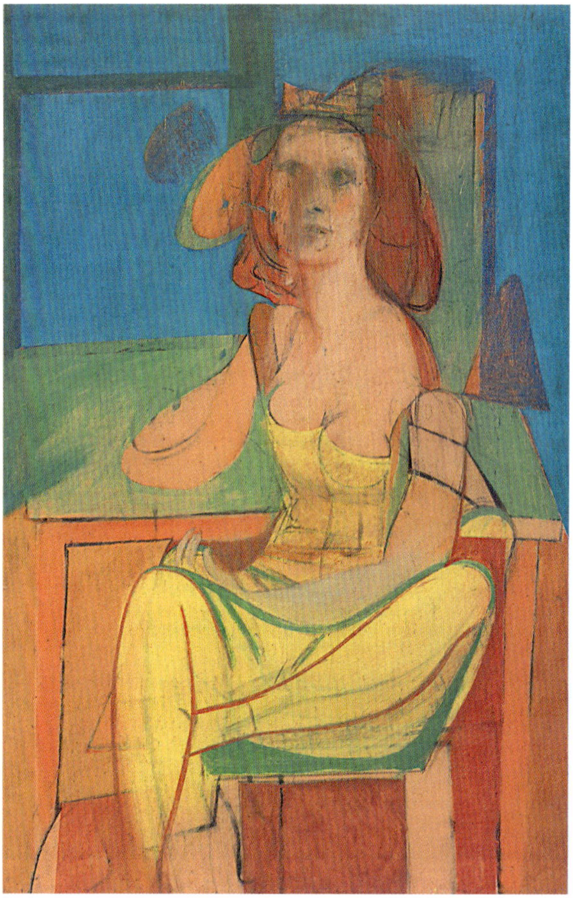

Fig. 3. Willem de Kooning, *Seated Woman*, ca. 1940, oil and charcoal on masonite, 137.2 × 91.4 cm. Philadelphia Museum of Art. The Albert M. Greenfield and Elizabeth M. Greenfield Collection (copyright 2007, The Willem De Kooning Foundation/ProLitteris, Zurich).

De Kooning's last paintings were shown to the public at the San Francisco MOMA (where I examined them), and at the Walter Art Center in Minneapolis. The catalogue at the end summarizes the experts' overall appraisal. With no evidence provided, for example in visual features that any viewer could verify, the consensus was that: 'these paintings of the 1980s are among the most beautiful, sensual, and exuberant abstract works by any modern painter' [Storr, 1995].

De Kooning's clinical diagnosis was that of Alzheimer's disease. This diagnosis compounded the mystery, as the creation of his art challenged not only art, but science itself.

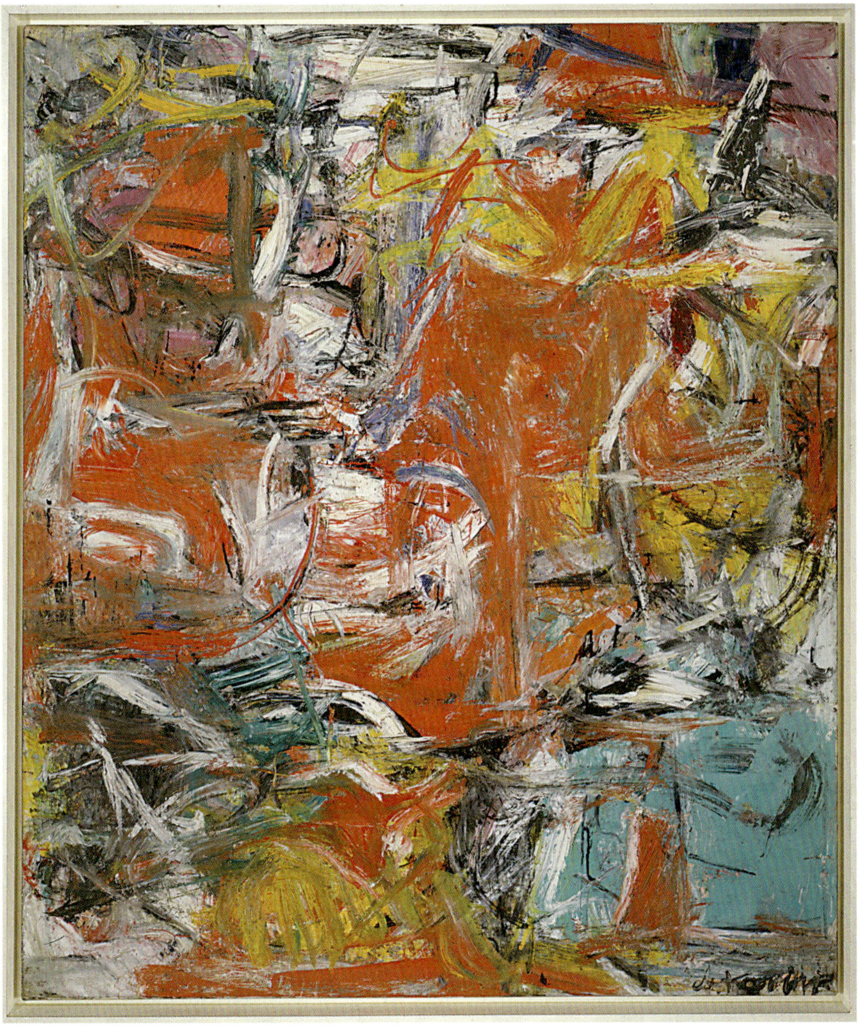

Fig. 4. Willem de Kooning, *Composition 1955*, oil, enamel, and charcoal on canvas, 79 1/8 × 69 1/8 inches (201 × 175.6 cm). Solomon R. Guggenheim Museum, New York, 55.1419 (with kind permission).

'ArtScience', My Investigation

Investigating the phenomenon of de Kooning's creation, I thought, concerned not only art. It extended to the very frontiers of neurocognitive science, to the complex issue of how we think, discover, of how we create.

Its study demanded, as I saw it in the discipline of ArtScience, the fulfillment of new and rigorous investigative criteria. It had to satisfy stipulations of art and of science. It had to demonstrate certainty of four conditions: (1) the creation; whether the paintings, produced in dementia, met the challenge of being abstract, were true to art, and whether they belonged to de Kooning, not just his hand, but his intellect, were true to the artist himself, (2) the dementia; whether de Kooning was indeed demented, showed evidence for the sustained loss of memory and mental capacities, (3) the creative process; whether de Kooning had created while demented, and whether during the process he did or did not receive assistance fundamental to the creation, either intellectual or physical, from anyone, or from therapy, or pharmacological agents, and (4) the neurocognitive coherence; whether the fact of the creation fell into the realm of the possible in neurocognition; that is, whether the phenomenon, if previously unexplored and complex, still fit information on the workings of the brain.

Only evidence that satisfied the criteria I set would have lent validity to the study.

To investigate the de Kooning phenomenon I applied Thinking Methods I had developed for the study of problems in science and art, procedures based on neurocognitive information on the workings of the brain [Espinel, 1994, 1995, 1998a, 2003a]. I proceeded systematically. I studied the paintings with the 'Method of Observation' I devised to examine the science image [Espinel, 1994, 1995, 1998a, 2003a], and studied the creation process with the 'Cognitive Analysis', devised to investigate the brain's faculties and their operation [Espinel, 2002a, 2003b]. For more than 15 years I have applied these Methods to investigate creation and invention, and have made discoveries that impact art and science, and integrate both into a new discipline of study that I call 'ArtMedicine' or 'ArtScience' [Espinel, 1994, 1995, 1996b, 1997, 1998a, b, 1999, 2002a, b, 2003a, b].

I examined de Kooning's paintings created both before and during his dementia, and exhibited in museums in the US and abroad, and found in private collections. I consulted curators and art experts. And I located and interviewed his attorney and those persons involved with de Kooning's care while incapacitated [Espinel, 1996a, unpubl. interviews, 1995–1996].

The 'Method of Observation'

My 'Method of Observation' has two steps: the 'Gathering of Information' and the 'Recognizing the Observed' [Espinel, 1994, 1995, 1998a, 2003a].

Step 1: Gathering of Information

The Method begins with the Gathering of Information on the lines, surfaces and colors of the observed. Specifics that I call 'Visual Features', since they, as visual stimuli, make the observed visible [Espinel, 1994, 1995, 1998a, 2003a].

Lines

In de Kooning's paintings one can observe two types of lines (figs. 1, 3, 4). One type is drawn on the canvas with brush, charcoal, or scratched with spatulas, knives, and paint tube tips. This line is not original to de Kooning. Ancient cave and Chinese art shows that for millennia human beings have drawn lines with all kinds of utensils [Espinel, 1996b]. The other line is created by juxtaposing surfaces of different colors. One can observe this type of line in the Giotto frescos of the early 14th century. And, for example, in the depiction of the earliest evidence of a neurological syndrome I discovered in Masaccio's portrayal of an invalid (1427–1428); it is an intricate juxtaposing of colors that delineates the complex muscular malformations that are diagnostic of poliomyelitis [Espinel, 1995]. It is the type of line I observed in Caravaggio's *Sleeping Cupid* (1608) outlining forms that had eluded art experts for centuries, and that I discovered are signs of a fatal type of rheumatism in a boy [Espinel, 1994]. The invention of this line is then part of an awesome intellectual achievement, the creating of images that appear real. Images that, as I showed in my analysis of the depiction of a pregnant woman by Vermeer (ca. 1664), a neurocognitive study of 'How the Brain Sees', impact the viewer's brain as do images of the real world [Espinel, 1998a].

Throughout his career de Kooning combined the various types of lines to define space and form in both realistic and abstract images. Pertinent to this investigation is that one observes the same types and use of lines in his last paintings (figs. 1, 3, 4).

Surfaces

De Kooning's surfaces are of two types (figs. 1, 3, 4). One is the result of applying paint, the other is the priming of the canvas being left exposed. He primed the canvas by sand papering either a previous painting or a new canvas covered with paint [Sylvester, 1994; Prather, 1994]. De Kooning's surfaces are not his invention. Applied pigments as a surface can be traced all the way back to millennia-old cave paintings. Areas of exposed priming, on the other hand, are observed representing space in Michelangelo's frescos in the Sistine Chapel (1508–1512). And in Rembrandt's 1654 self-portrait I discovered that a spot of exposed priming depicts a dark wound (most likely temporal arteritis) on the master's forehead [Espinel, 1997].

In de Kooning's paintings, in both his previous and the last, the two types of surfaces serve to represent space and vivify abstract forms.

Colors

Except for his 1940s black abstracts, de Kooning's paintings show a gamut of colors [Sylvester, 1994]. By applying the brush to the canvas with varying pressures, de Kooning changes color tone and saturation. An effect I observed in Raphael's *La Fornarina* (ca. 1520), with which I found the master had depicted a mass, a skin retraction, and discoloration in the left breast, and that I discovered are signs of breast cancer [Espinel, 2002b]. De Kooning, also, by smearing paint, by rubbing the canvas with fabrics, paper, or spatula, invents new color variations to create unrecognizable images [Espinel, 1996a] (figs. 1, 3, 4).

Critical to this research is that one observes that except for favoring primary colors, de Kooning's last paintings compare in color – in technique, tone, and intensity – to his previous works (figs. 1, 3, 4).

The first step of my Method of Observation provides evidence, therefore, that de Kooning's last paintings preserve, in lines, surfaces, and colors, in concrete Visual Features, the pictorial expressions that had characterized his work while he enjoyed full possession of mental capacities.

Step 2: Recognizing the Observed

In this step of the Method I observe the 'Patterns' in which the Visual Features of the observed configurate, and I notice whether the Patterns are recognizable, or not [Espinel, 1994, 1995, 1998a, 2003a].

In de Kooning's abstract paintings (figs. 1, 4), the Visual Features arrange in nonrecognizable Patterns. No matter from what perspective the paintings are looked at, even upside down, one cannot find a Pattern that matches any familiar image, nor do the Features superimpose, change in size, or arrange in linear perspective to show depth. This is why the art experts, and any viewer for that matter, see de Kooning's images as if close to the painting's surface. I must note that the creation of these visual effects is a complex intellectual undertaking. It requires first the mastering of techniques used to represent the real, and then being able to avoid, or obliterate, any semblance, even accidental, of recognizable form or space. It was Picasso who (in the summer of 1910, in the village of Cadaques, Spain) first achieved the complexity of the nonrecognizable image, and opened the possibility of abstract art [Richardson, 1991]. Picasso derived his Patterns from straight, 'cubic' configurations; many of de Kooning's Patterns derive from the curvilinear female body.

The Method's Recognizing step shows, therefore, that de Kooning's last paintings satisfy the complex nonrecognizability requirements of abstract art.

The Method's results – that de Kooning's last paintings adhere in technique and pictorial expression to the artist's previous work and meet the stipulations of the abstract image – fulfill my investigation's first condition. They demonstrate the authenticity, the truth of the art created in the midst of dementia.

It was, therefore, the integration of art and science, ArtScience, that permitted a cogent assessment of the complex creation.

Creating in the Midst of Dementia

Symptoms

From the mid-1970s de Kooning's forgetting of recent facts became obvious to himself and others. In conversations he filled memory gaps with gags, in private (his assistants told me) he vented his frustration throwing brushes, thrashing around his messy studio. Curiously, though, he could remember his remote past. He suffered anxiety and panic attacks, increased alcohol consumption, disregarded his sleep, nutrition, and personal hygiene. At times he did not know where he was, and with whom. He required several hospitalizations. He stopped painting. He was taken for dead, the art world spoke of de Kooning in the past [Garrels, 1995; Storr, 1995; Espinel, 1996a, unpubl. interviews, 1995–1996].

Care

In 1978, his estranged wife, Elaine, returned to him and organized care that included alcohol abstinence, scheduled sleep, balanced nutrition, and exercise. She assembled a team of assistants (2 were painters) to attend de Kooning's needs. His studio was cleaned and organized. A canvas was placed on his easel. Oil paints, brushes, spatulas, and other painting utensils were laid out by the canvas. His own previous sketches and paintings were placed around the studio [Storr, 1995; Sylvester, 1994; Espinel, 1996a, unpubl. interviews, 1995–1996].

From then on de Kooning was on his own.

Everyone I interviewed corroborated to me that de Kooning received no advice or assistance, nor drugs, psychotherapy, or any other kind of treatment while he created his last paintings [Espinel, 1996a, unpubl. interviews, 1995–1996].

Confirmation

An assistant reassured me that from what she heard (silences of brush work broken now and then by the 'shuh-shuh-shuh' of his rubbing of the canvas) and what she saw, his unfaltering brush activity, his engrossed, his quiet examining of the images, at times his distant smile, de Kooning 'functioned pretty well' (fig. 2). Only when I pressed further, when I enquired, specifically, about his performance of activities of daily living, did she reveal key information to me. That de Kooning, yes, still: (1) became disoriented, 'alone in the street, he'd get lost'; and (2) did not recall facts, addresses, names, words, even faces. He, for instance, 'did not recognize a famous movie actor (his name not disclosed here) who came to the studio for a filming session', and 'he confused his wife with his sister' [Espinel, 1996a, unpubl. interviews, 1995–1996].

Painting (figs. 1, 2)

De Kooning started a new painting with a sketch of one of his own previous images, as he had done before becoming incapacitated. From the mid-1980s he sketched from images projected on the canvas with a machine (an assistant informed me) he had acquired before his dementia. De Kooning then colored the sketch, and adding lines he devised new forms, and with spatulas and cloth spreading the paint over the canvas, he created new spaces. He would rotate the canvas and make changes. Some paintings went through up to 16 stages. One day he would stop painting on a canvas, and leaving it on the easel signaled his assistants he had finished the work [Storr, 1995; Sylvester, 1994; Prather, 1994; Espinel, 1996a, unpubl. interviews, 1995–1996].

Photos of the painting's stages show [Storr, 1995] and his assistants confirmed it (told me of noticing it when taking the work from the easel) that de Kooning's final images do not resemble, whatsoever, the initial sketch [Espinel, 1996a, unpubl. interviews, 1995–1996]. The new painting is a creation, original in form, color, and expression.

The evidence, therefore, meets the second and third conditions of the investigation. It shows that de Kooning was demented, and the creation took place in the midst of dementia.

Science, The Mystery

Unable to understand de Kooning's creation in terms of art, the art experts turned to science – to neurology – for an explanation. The exhibit catalogue summarizes their efforts [Storr, 1995].

The catalogue first cites a neurology professor's assertion that Alzheimer's disease is a global mental deterioration that spares no faculty [Storr, 1995; Larson, 1994], which would make creating impossible. Then it cites an Alzheimer's specialist's affirmation that the disease strikes mental functions differently, 'affecting conscious while sparing procedural memory' [Storr, 1995; Larson, 1994]. This, the experts note, would allow tracing on a surface, some level of drawing. But then a memory specialist consulted on de Kooning contradicts the above, saying that 'if color perception endures, the faculties associated with drawing weaken early in Alzheimer's disease' [Larson, 1994]. Faced with these contradictions about the disease, the art experts tried yet one more neurologist. One who had reported 'Clinical Tales' of unexplainable behaviors happening in some demented patients, the catalogue quotes, 'that even in cases of wide-spread brain damage, and in dementia, there can be sudden, remarkable, if transient restitutions of function, that hold integrity for hours or minutes' [Sacks, 1990].

The above opinions, though provided by eminent scientists, do not, however, address the cognitive phenomenon of de Kooning's creation. His images are not just mechanical tracings, they are complete paintings, more than 300 of them, many masterpieces. His was not a transient restitution of function. De Kooning worked (I found out from his assistants) for up to 8 straight hours a day, day after day; the creative feat lasting, the paintings show it, more than 8 consecutive years [Espinel, 1996a, unpubl. interviews, 1995–1996].

For science, then, as for art, the de Kooning phenomenon was also a mystery.

Until my research, until ArtScience, neither art nor science, that I found, could explain or indeed offer thinking methods for exploring, much less for identifying a cognitive phenomenon that concerns not just some paintings, or disease, or, for that matter not even the great de Kooning, but the very marvel of human creativity [Espinel, 1994, 1995, 1996a, b, 1997, 1998a, b, 1999, 2002a, b, 2003a, b].

The 'Cognitive Analysis'

In the Cognitive Analysis I do not examine the intellect in isolation [Espinel, 2002a, 2003b]. Such wonders as creation and discovery are investigated integral to the workings of the brain. I have assessed de Kooning's paintings in relation to his memory. Systematically, and separately, I have analyzed each of the four memory systems – working, procedural, episodic, and semantic – as they might have worked in his creation. The *integration* of art and science, ArtScience, I devised to open new ways in the pursuit of truth [Espinel, 1994, 1995, 1996a, b, 1997, 1998a, b, 1999, 2002a, b, 2003a, b].

Short-Term or Working Memory

De Kooning's last paintings, purely abstract and capable of stimulating thoughts and emotions, suggest reasoning and planning behind their creation. The paintings have, furthermore, a vast number of bits of information expressed in multiple combinations of Visual Features and Patterns (fig. 1). This suggests that in the creation de Kooning must have held in his consciousness a small number of information bits (say, the curve and thickness of a brush stroke) as he, second by second, rendered each detail of line, surface, and of color, and as he, simultaneously, to achieve the abstract ideal, went on avoiding, or obliterating, recognizable Patterns. This type of recall was also indispensable for his sketching of his previous images. In my cognitive investigation of creation I have likened this achievement in art to the operation of working memory in language [Espinel, 2002a, 2003b], in which a few words are held second by second to grasp the meaning of a sentence, towards understanding the idea [Squire et al., 1993; Baddeley and Hitch, 1974].

This short-term memory faculty, processed in the prefrontal areas of the brain, is critical to planning and reasoning [Squire et al., 1993; Baddeley and Hitch, 1974]. His last paintings, then, suggest the operation of working memory in de Kooning's brain.

Long-Term Nondeclarative ('Procedural') Memory

The lines' precision, the surfaces' smoothness, and the colors' scrupulous separation observed in his last paintings indicate in de Kooning the mastering of drawing skill (figs. 1, 2). The many changes (shown in photos), and the production of a painting a week, suggest speed, automaticity: years of skeletal muscle conditioning to the procedure of painting. Skill and automaticity have previously been lumped into 'procedural memory'; but recent neurocognitive studies show that they operate separately, and in separate brain organizations. Skill depends on the workings of the dorsal striatum; and conditioning of skeletal musculature, that facilitates automaticity, on the operation of the cerebellar and brain stem pathways [Squire et al., 1993; Schacter, 1987].

Not only the vast variety but the quality of Visual Features in the last paintings suggest in de Kooning's brain, therefore, the workings of the long-term nondeclarative, 'procedural' memory systems.

Long-Term Declarative Episodic Memory

De Kooning, unable to retrieve recent facts, could remember remote events. I found that he recalled with much pain his childhood in Rotterdam, and remembered with excitement his immigrating to the US (in his 20s, illegally, through Norfolk, Va.), and his beginnings as a house painter in Connecticut. Once he did not recognize an old friend, an artist, but as in the course of the conversation his style was brought up, de Kooning then described their first meeting. He remembered the studio, its old walls, its colors, and his friend's features, his gestures, and de Kooning spoke animatedly of the joy, of the feelings of the encounter [Espinel, 1996a, unpubl. interviews, 1995–1996]. It was as if de Kooning, I think, was seeing the scene, was reliving the event.

This conscious, autonoetic, recalling of previous life episodes as experienced, this reliving them with a wealth of facts, thoughts and emotions, is intrinsic to the workings of episodic memory. A faculty that is a privilege solely of the human. A system served by a network of cortical and subcortical brain regions that overlap with and extend beyond the hippocampus and those of other memory systems [Tulving, 2002].

I have previously shown how episodic memory might have been crucial to the process of creation in Pollock's masterpiece, *Lavender Mist* (1950), and in Picasso's monumental *Guernica* (1937), works that led me to suggest the 'Autonoetic Hypothesis on Creativity' [Espinel, 2002a, 2003b]. For de Kooning, demented, confined to his studio, his brain receiving no *outside* stimuli, episodic memory had to be the faculty that permitted him to *autonoetically* go back to the past and relive his experiences [Espinel, 2002a]. Remembering that must have provided information and emotions, I think, that de Kooning rendered in his last paintings in vivid forms and colors [Espinel, 1996a].

Long-Term Declarative Semantic Memory

What then might have happened to de Kooning?

His inability to recall recent facts, his failure to retain and use new knowledge, indicates in de Kooning a deficit of the memory of facts, semantic memory. A system that depends on the workings of neurons in the temporal and frontal lobes [Squire et al., 1993; Schacter, 1987, 1998; Tulving, 2002]. Unable to retrieve facts of New York, of his address, he was disoriented to place, and of names and faces, disoriented him socially. De Kooning must have appeared distant, lost, gone.

Semantic memory deficit must have also, of course, limited de Kooning's art.

The Syndrome of 'Creating in the Midst of Dementia'

My observations identify in the de Kooning phenomenon what I suggest is a distinct neurocognitive Syndrome, one that I call 'Creating in the Midst of Dementia'. Identifying the Syndrome in the artist solves the mystery of de Kooning's last paintings.

The Syndrome is characterized by (1) a specific combination of brain functions and malfunctions, in this case, preservation of three memory systems – working, procedural, and episodic – and deficit of semantic memory; and (2) a response to precise stimuli, one that triggers brain reactivation, and as a consequence, creating in the midst of dementia.

Neurocognitive Coherence

Specificity of Diagnosing Memory Systems

The Cognitive Analysis showed that de Kooning's dementia was not a global jumbled mental deterioration. My Thinking Methods permitted a precise diagnosis of memory systems. They revealed the uniqueness of a specific combination of brain functions and malfunctions: the preservation of working, procedural, and episodic memory and the deficit of semantic memory.

Neurocognitive research has shown that memory is not just one global function. Rather the data demonstrate that the faculty of recall involves at least the four memory systems listed above operating integratedly. Each system resides in separate brain structures, possesses a distinct capacity, operates at a different recall speed, relates to consciousness in a distinct manner, and each participates, differently, in the process of thought and emotion [Squire et al., 1993; Baddeley and Hitch, 1974; Schacter, 1987, 1998; Tulving, 1995, 2002].

The unique combination of functions and malfunctions that characterizes the Syndrome of Creating in the Midst of Dementia falls, therefore, within the realm of the possible in the workings of the brain. The Syndrome, therefore, has neurocognitive coherence.

Rationale of the Syndrome

If demented, how then did de Kooning create?

Specificity of Response

My investigation suggests that it was the response to sensory stimuli, visual and precise, that reactivated de Kooning's brain. That solved the mystery. Three sets of evidence – in the care, an event that may be considered an experiment, and information on the workings of the brain – lend support to my proposal.

(1) The Care. During the creation de Kooning received neither artistic assistance nor drugs, psychotherapy, or any kind of known treatment. He stayed in his studio, he remained in isolation, and what he saw was not random images but his own art, in other words, his *external* stimuli were visual, and specific.

(2) The 'Experiment'. Ideally de Kooning's creation should have been examined experimentally. A fortuitous event that occurred during these years of creation serves, as I see it, the function of such an experiment.

De Kooning started a painting, both before and after becoming incapacitated, by sketching one of his previous images. From the mid-1980s he carried out the procedure by projecting the image on the canvas. In 1989, a relative of his, perhaps concerned over the validity of the art, ordered the projecting stopped. De

Kooning's response to the removal of the images I confirmed in all my interviews. Suddenly faced with the empty canvas, de Kooning looked at it, drew a few swirls, stared at them, and sat. In the next days he added a few lines here and there but weeks passed, and he never completed a painting. It did not matter that the rest of the care continued the same, de Kooning remained sitting in one place, inert, lost. Subsequently, however, the order was reversed. And as he saw his own images, de Kooning stood up, and sketched them, and was able, once again, to complete paintings, to create [Espinel, unpubl. interviews, 1995–1996].

The previous exposure to, and now the removal of and the re-exposure to the images show, like an experiment, albeit fortuitous, the specificity of de Kooning's response, and the precision of the effecting stimuli that mediated the creating.

(3) The Workings of the Brain. Neurocognitive experimentation has shown that the two declarative long-term memory systems – semantic and episodic – operate in series and in parallel [Tulving, 1995, 2002; Schacter, 1998]. Remembering a fact, an image, a sound, a scent, establishes the connection, stimulates reliving an entire event. The fact, semantic memory, triggers the reliving, the operation of the episodic memory. We all have experienced this wonder. As we have experienced, in our daily living, and in our attempts at creation, how remembering an event moves us to new thoughts and emotions, and to action, that is served by the function of the entire brain.

A Mechanism, 'Surrogate Memory'

I have shown that the de Kooning phenomenon met the criteria for the Syndrome of Creating in the Midst of Dementia. That the artist's brain, if in possession of working, procedural and episodic memory, suffered a deficit of semantic. The brain then lacked the facts, what it had built through a life dedicated to art, what served it as *internal* stimuli. Without these pieces the brain could not establish the connection, it was paralyzed.

It is possible, then, that the exposure to his previous images reintroduced the facts, the missing pieces, in other words, that the paintings, the *external* stimuli, served as the brain's *surrogate* semantic memory. This is why, I think, that seeing and sketching his images worked. Because the pieces being specific, 'fit in', precisely, into already existing mechanisms. A fit that triggered the operation of the episodic and other memory systems. And the brain, its function reactivating, began the cognitive repair that permitted creating masterpieces of abstract art, the cognitive wonder, while crippled by dementia (fig. 5).

All factors, the function and malfunction of memory systems, the response to specific stimuli, and the possible mechanism and repair, fall within the capacities of the workings of the brain. The study thus meets the fourth and final condition, that of having neurocognitive coherence. And this in turn provides rationale for the Syndrome of 'Creating in the Midst of Dementia'.

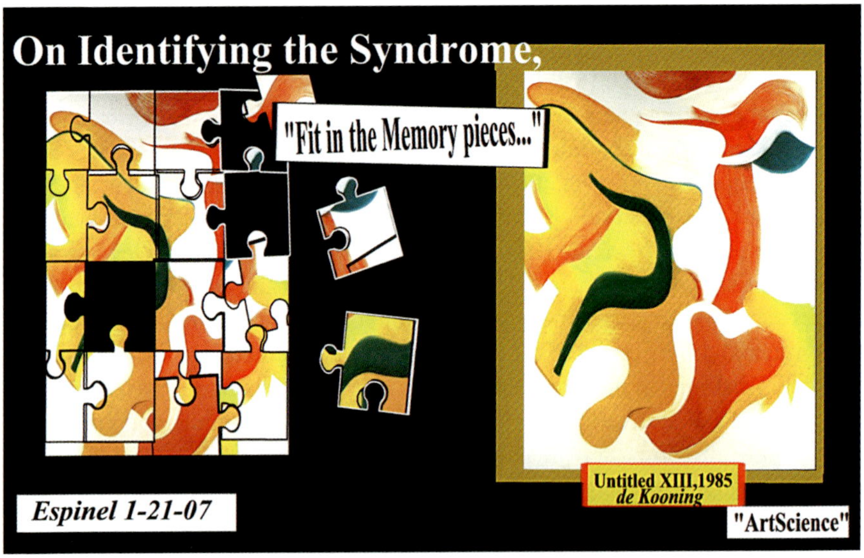

Fig. 5. C.H. Espinel. *On Identifying the Syndrome*, 2007. Digital ArtScience image. This digital composition illustrates the brain's response to specific stimuli and possibility of 'cognitive repair' in the Syndrome of Creating in the Midst of Dementia (copyright C.H. Espinel).

ArtScience, as I introduce the discipline herein, opens a path for the exploration of brain and creation.

Brain, Memory, and Creation

My work offers:

(1) The identification of the 'Syndrome of Creating in the Midst of Dementia'. This ArtScience study: (a) presents its definition, its criteria of diagnosis, mechanism, rationale, and possibility of cognitive repair, and (b) by identifying the Syndrome in Willem de Kooning, solves the mystery of his creating art while crippled by dementia.

(2) New Thinking Methods, the 'Brain Methods', that based on information on the 'workings of the brain' open a new path in the pursuit of truth. The 'Method of Observation' serves to define stimuli, and the 'Cognitive Analysis' to assess cognitive faculties.

(3) An integration of art and science into a new discipline of study, 'ArtScience'.

References

Baddeley AD, Hitch G: Working memory; in Bower GA (ed): The Psychology of Learning and Motivation. New York, Academic Press, 1974, pp 47–89.

Bird TD, Miller BL: Alzheimer's disease and other dementias; in Kasper DL, et al (eds): Harrison's Principles of Internal Medicine, ed 16. New York, McGraw-Hill, 2005, pp 2393–2406.

Chilvers I, Osborne H, Farr D: Abstract art; in The Oxford Dictionary of Art. New York, Oxford University Press, 1994, p 2.

Espinel CH: Caravaggio's 'Il Amore Dormiente': a sleeping cupid with juvenile rheumatoid arthritis. Lancet 1994;344:1750–1752.

Espinel CH: Masaccio's cripple: a neurological syndrome. Its art, medicine and values. Lancet 1995;346:1684–1686.

Espinel CH: De Kooning's late colours and forms: dementia, creativity and the healing power of art. Lancet 1996a;347:1096–1098.

Espinel CH: Chou Ch'en's street character: deformity in the art of the Ming dynasty. Lancet 1996b;348:1714–1716.

Espinel CH: A medical evaluation of Rembrandt. His self-portrait: ageing, disease, and the language of the skin. Lancet 1997;350:1835–1837.

Espinel CH: Art and neuroscience: how the brain sees Vermeer's *Woman Holding a Balance*. Lancet 1998a;352:2007–2009.

Espinel CH: Art and mind: book review of Adolf Wolfli: draftsman, writer, poet, composer. JAMA 1998b;279:1405–1406.

Espinel CH: Michelangelo's gout and renal disease in a fresco by Raphael. Lancet 1999;354:2149–2152.

Espinel CH: The 'Autonoetic Hypothesis on Creativity': memory and cognition in Pollock's abstract work; in Gray WD, Schunn CD (eds): Proceedings of the Cognitive Science Society. London, Laurence Erlbaum, 2002a, vol 1, p 1002.

Espinel CH: The portrait of breast cancer and Raphael's *La Fornarina*. Lancet 2002b;360:2061–2063.

Espinel CH: The portrait of breast cancer and the Espinel 'Observation Method'. Lancet 2003a; 361:1130.

Espinel CH: The 'Autonoetic Hypothesis on Creativity': memory and cognition in Picasso's *Guernica*; in Gray WD, Schunn CD (eds): Proceedings of the Cognitive Science Society. London, Laurence Erlbaum, 2003b, vol 2 (on CD).

Garrels G: Three toads in the garden: line, color and form; in Jenkins J, Engberg S (eds): Willem de Kooning: the Late Paintings, the 1980s. Minneapolis, Wallace Carlson, 1995, pp 9–37.

Larson K: Alzheimer's expressionism; in Village Voice, May 31, 1994, vol 39, pp 41–44.

Neugroschl JA, Kolevzon A, Samuels SC, et al: Dementia; in Sadock BJ, Sadock VA (eds): Kaplan and Sadock's Comprehensive Textbook of Psychiatry, ed 8. Philadelphia, Lippincott, Williams & Wilkins, 2005, pp 1068–1077.

Prather M: Catalogue; in Smyth FP, Curry T (eds): Willem de Kooning Paintings. Washington, National Gallery of Art, 1994, pp 75–223.

Richardson J: A Life of Picasso. London, Jonathan Cape, 1991, vol 1, pp 1881–1906.

Sacks O: The Man Who Mistook His Wife for a Hat and Other Clinical Tales. New York, Harper Perennial, 1990, p 6.

Schacter DL: Implicit memory: history and current status. J Exp Psychol Learn Mem Cogn 1987;13: 501–518.

Schacter DL: Memory; in Posner MI (ed): Foundations of Cognitive Science. Cambridge, MIT Press, 1998, pp 683–725.

Squire LR, Knowlton BJ, Musen G: The structure and organization of memory. Annu Rev Psychol 1993;44:453–495.

Storr R: At last light; in Jenkins J, Engberg S (eds): Willem de Kooning: the Late Paintings, the 1980s. Minneapolis, Wallace Carlson, 1995, pp 39–80.

Sylvester D: Flesh was the reason; in Smyth FP, Curry T (eds): Willem de Kooning Paintings. Washington, National Gallery of Art, 1994, pp 15–31.

Tulving E: Organization of memory: quo vadis? in Gazzaniga MS (ed): The Cognitive Neurosciences. Cambridge, MIT Press, 1995, pp 839–847.
Tulving E: Episodic memory: from mind to brain; in Fiske ST, Schacter DL, Zahn-Waxler C (eds): Annual Review of Psychology. Palo Alto, Annual Reviews, 2002, vol 53, pp 1–25.

Carlos H. Espinel, MD, FACP
1715 North George Mason Drive, Suite 401
Arlington, VA 22205 (USA)
Tel. +1 703 522 6908, Fax +1 703 522 6918, E-Mail espinelmd@aol.com

Bogousslavsky J, Hennerici MG (eds): Neurological Disorders in Famous Artists – Part 2.
Front Neurol Neurosci. Basel, Karger, 2007, vol 22, pp 169–183

Persisting Aphasia, Cerebral Dominance, and Painting in the Famous Artist Carl Fredrik Reuterswärd

F. Colombo-Thuillard[a], *G. Assal*[b]

[a]Department of Neuropsychology, Hôpital Cantonal, Fribourg,
[b]Chauderon 38, Lausanne, Switzerland

Abstract

What about artistic creativity following a cerebral lesion? We studied the case of a prominent right-handed Swedish painter and sculptor who suffered a cerebral hemorrhage at the age of 55 years. The patient displayed a lesion of the left capsular lenticular region, which resulted in a right hemiplegia and sensory loss, with aphasia of the subcortical type. The linguistic impairments recovered well but at 1 year postonset, the right hand was still completely paralyzed. After a period of a few weeks, during which the patient refused to use his nondominant hand, he produced his first left-handed drawing, and by 1 year postonset, he had once again resumed an intensive artistic activity using his nondominant hand. The pictorial works were reviewed by several renowned art specialists: changes of style and even of contents were judged without loss of artistic quality. The result was described as a gain in emotional and artistic intensity. We discuss our observation in the context of the literature and focus on the crucial role of cerebral dominance and hand preference. We conclude that pictorial creativity and language are distinct forms of expressions.

What about artistic creativity and consciousness following a cerebral lesion, leading to aphasia? According to Chatterjee [2004], the work produced by artists following a cerebral lesion can help to understand a possible change in their world representation. Artistic production in aphasics may contribute to answering this question, in the field of literature, music and painting [Alajouanine, 1948; Gardner et al., 1991]. We studied pictorial activity after onset of aphasia in a prominent Swedish artist, who had a stroke at the height of his artistic career.

Table 1. Aphasia in an artist: case studies in the literature

Authors	Patient	Hemiplegia	Change of hand	Change of style
Bonvincini, 1926	Vierge	+	+	'more impressionist, magical work of an artist'
Engerth and Urban, 1933	academic sculptor	+	–	'more anxious, loss of symbols'
Alajouanine, 1948	painter	–	–	'gained a more intense and acute expression'
Gourevitch, 1967	M	–	+	'new kind of expression, like hieroglyphs'
Zaimov et al., 1969	ZB	+	+	'birth of a new painter, fusion of reality and dream'
Reinvang, 1987	OJH	+	–	'naïve and concrete'
Kaczmarek, 1991	RL	+	–	'no more abstract, symbolic pictures, but concrete art'
Gardner et al., 1991	GM	+	+	'less sophisticated amorphous forms'

– = Absent; + = present.

Painting in Aphasics: Literature Overview

The chronological list of scientific case studies concerning aphasic artists (table 1) starts with Bonvincini [1926] who described Vierge, a Castilian painter, suffering a heavy stroke at the age of 31, resulting in a high-grade Broca's aphasia and right hemiplegia. The paralysis of the dominant right side forced Vierge to change his working hand. Two years postonset the talented artist was able to take up his regular work again and accomplished this with the same productive imagination as before his illness. However, contemporary art critics spoke about a change of style with more impressionist components. They reviewed the postmorbid paintings as the magical work of an artist. The quality of the poststroke creations was in no way judged as less valuable in spite of the evident chronic aphasia. In 1933, two Austrian pupils of Pötzl, Engerth and Urban [1933], published the case of what they called an 'academic sculptor' who at the age of 57 underwent a stroke with a severe persisting Wernicke's aphasia, discrete hemiplegia and neuropsychological deficits, autotopagnosia and finger agnosia. The patient resumed creative activity by drawing and was able to use his slightly paralyzed hand. Other than before his illness he now acquired an altered emotional attitude towards his work. He started to sketch reclining female bodies with soft contours but did not seem to overcome a depressive anxiety when being artistically productive. In a later period he took up his preferred premorbid activity – sculpturing – and showed a preference for male bodies in quite a naturalistic manner. The concrete copying of bodies and also objects appeared to correspond to his actual capacities as he now had difficulties with abstract symbols. The artistic style of this academic sculptor had become more anxious and was characterized by a loss of symbols. In an often-quoted paper, Alajouanine [1948] presented observations in the fields of poetry, music and painting. Beside the description of the aphasia of Baudelaire and Ravel he reported a contemporary pictorial artist, Paul-Elie Gernez [Boller et al., 2005]. These three case studies led him to the conclusion that aphasia destroyed literary language in the writer, stopped sound expression in the musician, but left graphic realization untouched. The painter described by Alajouanine had Wernicke's aphasia, without motor disorders and was therefore able to continue painting with his dominant hand. For Alajouanine it seemed that 'the aphasic and the artist live together on two distinct planes'. The painter himself expressed this split as follows: 'There are in me two men, the one who paints, who is normal while he is painting and the other one... the fool who cannot manage words any more'. According to Alajouanine the painter's artistic activity remained at its customary high level and there were connoisseurs who maintained that the painter's work had actually gained a more intense and acute expression.

The patient of Gourevitch [1967], a retired professor of art, was rendered severely aphasic by a left-hemisphere stroke. He displayed expressive and motor disorders. However, he never finished communicating with his environment and compensated his language loss by a kind of communicative symbols, like hieroglyphs. Thus, he maintained an active correspondence. Nevertheless, this patient does not belong to the aphasic artists who were able to realize amazing creations without loss of quality even after their stroke. All the same, he demonstrated that drawing capacity is possible even after a high-grade aphasia and is able to compensate language to some extent. An art specialist could find a new kind of expression, like hieroglyphs. The case of a Bulgarian painter, ZB, i.e. Zlatio Boiyadjiev, described by Zaimov et al. [1969] also supports the finding that the ability to paint may not be affected by the loss of linguistic skills. ZB suffered a severe aphasia as well as paralysis of the right side of the body and retrained himself to paint with his left nondominant hand. However, his poststroke work showed an entirely new style. Whereas his prestroke art was characterized by a narrative style his later work displayed strange and fantastic dreamlike images. Although his style was entirely new, it was in no way inferior to his prestroke style. Contemporaries spoke of the birth of a new painter, fusion of reality and dream. The patient described by Reinvang [1987] was a 56-year-old right-handed male painter, OJH, who suffered a stroke resulting in a right-hemisphere infarction with initial left hemiparesis and a severe crossed aphasia. Reinvang's patient manifested a complete reversal of the pattern of deficit usually observed in a right hander. His ability to paint recovered completely. After the injury an art historian confirmed that there was no sign of pathology in his painting, but he showed some changes in his artistic style. He now preferred a technique with water colors, which appeals to spontaneity since the results are hard to control exactly. His style of painting had become naïve and concrete. Kaczmarek [1991] has presented a study of a prominent Polish painter, RL, who suffered a left-brain stroke resulting in right hemiparesis and aphasia. His drawing abilities were preserved on the performance level but he was not able to create the highly symbolic pictures he used to paint before the stroke. Premorbidly he preferred an abstract kind of art, whereas after his illness his artwork was quite different, there were now no more abstract, symbolic pictures, but concrete art. Thus RL produced above all landscapes and portraits of human beings. The patient GM, documented by Gardner et al. [1991], was a 62-year-old professional artist who developed a severe global aphasia after a large left-hemisphere stroke. GM began to paint and draw again a few months after his apoplexy, using his left hand. GM's work showed some alteration of style subsequent to the illness. Prior to the injury his creations were characterized by complexity of form and line, attention to depth, and interplay of shapes. GM's poststroke drawings exhibited less control of depth and layering of shapes. His artwork was now less sophisticated and he used amorphous forms in sharp contrast to the prestroke work.

Case Study: Art History

Carl Fredrik Reuterswärd, CFR, was born in Stockholm in 1934. His native tongue is Swedish and he attended Swedish schools until the age of 17. During this period he learned English and German, which he spoke fluently at school-leaving age. After graduating, CFR left for Paris and became scholar of Fernand Léger, which contributed to his international artistic success. CFR held exhibitions in the major art centers of the world. Thanks to the renowned surrealist artist, Meret Oppenheim, CFR moved to Switzerland in 1970. After living in a French-speaking area for about 20 years CFR mastered the French language both orally and in writing by the time of the onset of his illness. His everyday language, however, remained Swedish.

The most famous artistic production by CFR is certainly the sculpture *Non-Violence*, a kind of peace symbol in the shape of a 'knotted pistol', erected

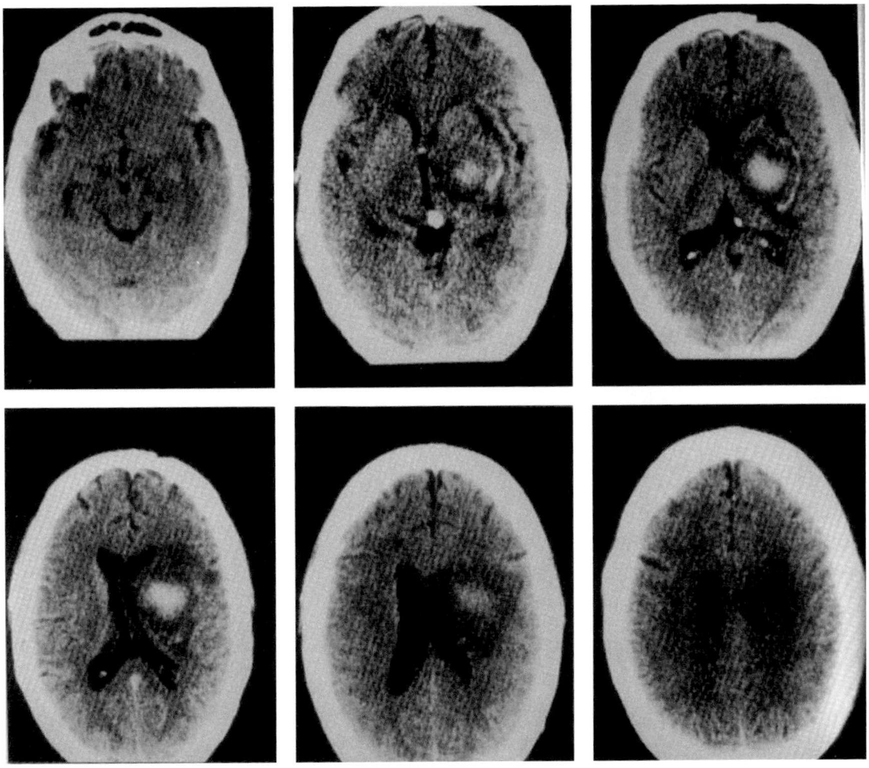

Fig. 1. CT scan: cerebral hemorrhage in the left capsular lenticular region.

in front of the UN building in New York. Furthermore his subtle portraits of famous personalities, representing impressive character studies are extremely fascinating. In 1962 CFR discovered the use of laser light for art purposes and also made holograms. In 1978 CFR invented a visual language, which explored the space inside and between letters and numbers. Besides drawing, painting and sculpture CFR was also an active literary: in 1988 he published his autobiography in Swedish.

History of Illness

CFR was a 55-year-old, right-handed man at the time of the onset of illness, when he suffered a cerebral hemorrhage. He presented a lesion in the left capsular lenticular region (fig. 1), which resulted in a right hemiplegia and sensory loss. He rapidly lost consciousness, which lasted for a few days.

Table 2. Neuropsychological assessment 6 months postonset

Apraxia	
Oral	–
Ideomotor	–
Ideational	–
Constructional	–
Neglect	–
Agnosia	
Visual	–
Associative visual	+
Spatial	–
Visual memory disorders	
Span	–
Learning	–
Recognition	–
Executive disorders	++
Nonverbal intellectual disorders	–

– = Absent; + = discrete; ++ = moderate; +++ = severe disorder.

Three weeks postonset, aphasia was apparent in all four languages spoken by the patient. The aphasia was global, with a special sparing for repetition of short words. Table 2 shows neuropsychological assessments 6 months postonset and revealed neither apraxia nor agnosia. CFR's state of health gradually recovered and 1 month postonset a thorough neuropsychological and neurolinguistic assessment was possible.

Language Assessment

CFR was first investigated in French, in which he displayed severe subcortical aphasia (table 3). His spontaneous speech was characterized by breaks in fluency, noticeable word finding problems, neologisms and jargon passages as well as code switches with Swedish components. The content was not informative. Repetition, auditory comprehension and reading were relatively well preserved, compared to the other modalities, realizing a kind of subcortical aphasia [Puel et al., 1986]. A Swedish assessment was made possible in addition to the French one and showed somewhat milder disturbance according to the 'primacy

Table 3. Language assessment

	French	Swedish
Intitial		
Spontaneous speech	+	+
Fluency	+	++
Repetition	++	++
Naming	0	++
Auditory comprehension	++	++
Token test	0	0
Reading aloud	++	+++
Comprehension	++	++
Writing	+	refused
1 year postonset		
Spontaneous speech	+++	++++
Fluency	++	++++
Repetition	++	+++
Naming	++	+++
Auditory comprehension	+++	+++
Token test	+++	++++
Reading aloud	++++	++++
Comprehension	++++	++++
Writing	++	+++

Performance: 0 = not possible; + = poor; ++ = moderate; +++ = good; ++++ = normal.

rule' by Ribot which states a better restitution of the first acquired language. In Swedish the patient revealed no language mixing and a simple conversation was possible since word finding was slightly better in this language. CFR totally refused the German language. The linguistic restitution was not the same in the different languages and since this area is not the main topic of the discussion, some aspects of the patient's language recovery are summarized. After an initial therapy of over 3 months in Swedish CFR's progress in this language was noticeable. Even if the competence level did not quite correspond to the premorbid high-developed state, CFR's results in a version of the Aachen Aphasia Test [Huber et al., 1983] adapted for Swedish were more or less within normal limits 1 year postonset. The French aphasia therapy which started after having finished the Swedish training also brought improvement: 1 year postonset French oral expression had improved remarkably and code switches had become rare, reading comprehension is now good, whereas writing difficulties are still present. An interesting detail can be observed in English: this deactivated language improved to a very high level without therapy. The German language, however, is still very disordered.

Artistic Creativity

What happened to the art of this artist with a paralyzed right hand after the injury? During a short period of a few weeks the patient refused to use his nondominant hand because he was still full of hope that his dominant right hand would recover. During a therapy session, the patient was stimulated and even persuaded to make his very first left-handed drawing as part of an exercise of body parts. This was the start of an extremely intense period of drawing. The recovery of artistic ability is – other than the restitution of language – CFR's own achievement, attained through exceptional willpower and a creative force, which initiated the use of the inexperienced left hand. At the end of the hospital stay, 6 months postonset, he had succeeded in drawing no more than about 3,000 sketches.

One year postonset, after intense exercise, the patient felt he mastered his movements enough to start regular artistic activity. This was to be drawing above all but also painting and sculpturing.

When asked about his feelings when drawing with his left hand, CFR said: 'Yes, much more agreeable…much more direct…much more spontaneous…much more…' and: 'It's the feeling that I have something in my hand and in my body…and the nit comes to my hand…and it is in my hand…on the paper…directly…it's marvellous…it's not a handicap…the left hand is the dreamer…the soul is localized in the left hand' [pers. comm., 1992]. These words attest CFR's firm belief that the new quality of his art originated from drawing and painting with his other hand. CFR uses the metaphor of Gulliver, arguing that the cerebral lesion constitute an extraordinary opportunity to completely change his perspective on art – or on the world, like Gulliver. Since then, CFR participated at different great international exhibitions with works realized with his left hand (Switzerland, Sweden, Denmark, Finland, France).

Art Critics

The appreciation of a change of style by a painter, during his artistic career or after a cerebral lesion, is without doubt a challenge. Art critics are specialized in analyzing artistic productions, but are not free from subjectivity. With this reservation, we choose to give some reports by art critics on CFR's productions.

Three and a half years postonset the authors visited CFR's studio together with Josef Helfenstein,[1] a specialist on Meret Oppenheim. According to Helfenstein [pers. comm., 1993], 'since the aphasia several modifications of style and perhaps also of content in the artwork of CFR are noticeable. These characteristics are partly due to the change of working hand. The changes, however, have not led to a loss of artistic quality in the work of CFR and are most obvious in his portraits. The drawing has changed fundamentally. As can be seen on the portrait of Léger (fig. 2), created before the injury, the lines are not interrupted and are conducted in an elegant way. We can compare this work with a portrait of Philip Sandblom (fig. 3), the art critic and author of *Creativity and Disease* [1991], made after the injury. Now the lines are separated, searching, awkward, but find their effect in a less styled manner. The apparent esthetic loss is replaced by a fresh vitality. The drawings are now expressive, the turn of the pen is more nervous, extremely sensitive, with a gain of psychic intensity.'

Sandblom [1991] described a 'renaissance of creativity' and emphasized a playful side of CFR, which the artist has been able to develop much more after the injury. This was demonstrated by the sketches of *Non-Violence* before and after the injury (fig. 4). 'Before the illness the lethal weapon had been presented with decisive heavy strokes; afterwards it looks more like an amusing toy pistol, never intended for killing' – said Sandblom.

Olle Granath[2] stated that CFR's art is very impressive because an enormous effort behind the work can be noticed. 'Before the stroke, CFR could easily draw and paint brilliantly, whereas now he has increased depth and concentration because he is forced to calm down, reflect and to give his utmost' [pers. comm., 1994].

All these commentaries appear to have one thing in common: the interrupted line has a symbolic character and seems in some way to reflect the biographical event of its creator. The artwork of CFR after his injury has provoked a change of style, which is unanimously judged as a gain in emotional intensity.

Discussion

Several scientists have studied the relationship between artistic creativity and cerebral lesion since the beginning of this century. There are few case reports on the effects of right-sided lesions. The relationship between aphasia

[1]Curator of the Klee Collection at the Museum of Art in Bern.
[2]Curator of the National Museum of Art in Stockholm.

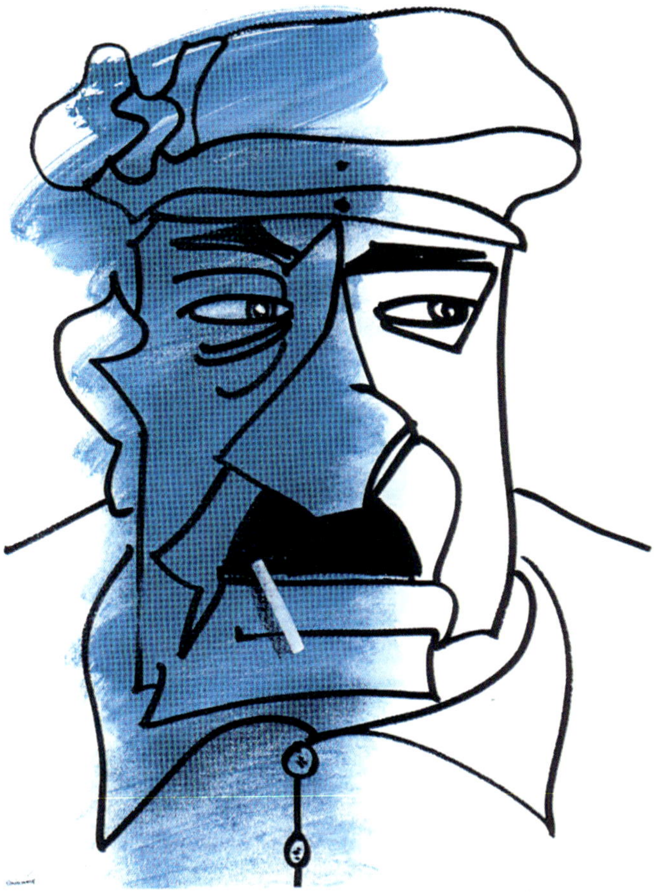

FERNAND LÉGER, 1955
Encre de Chine et gouache, 70 x 55 cm
Coll. Musée National, Stockholm

Fig. 2. Portrait of F. Léger, before the injury (with the right hand) (with the kind permission of the artist).

and artistic creativity will be discussed first, focusing on three questions: (1) is creative activity possible after aphasia?, (2) is a modification of style often observed?, and (3) if so, how to explain these phenomena? With the exception of Bay [1962] who hypothesized a drawing recovery according to language restitution, nearly all authors agree that graphic competence can exist at a high level despite a significant aphasia.

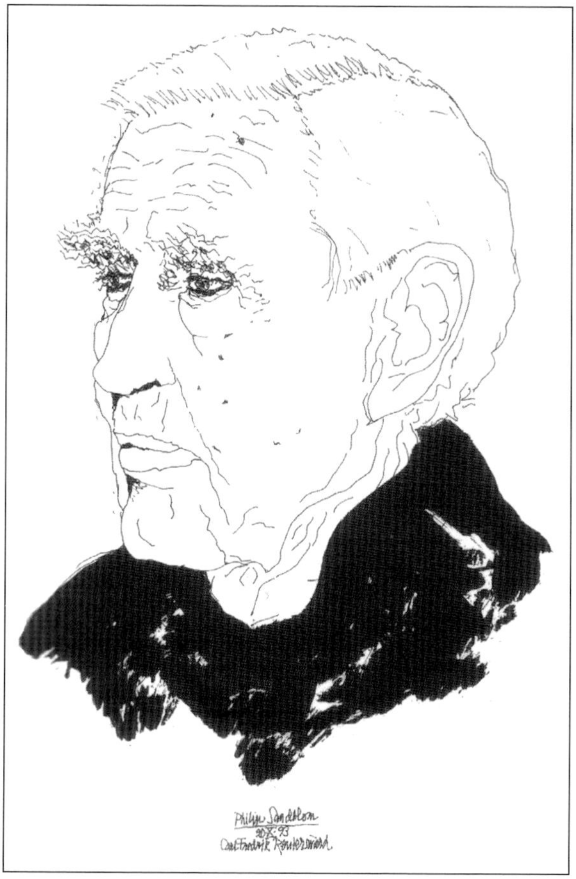

Fig. 3. Portrait of P. Sandblom, after the injury (with the left hand, 3 years postonset) (with the kind permission of the artist).

According to the literature, artistic creativity is possible in spite of a significant and permanent aphasia. Alajouanine [1948] deduced that graphic capacities in pictorial artists are preserved because of the different nature of their art production compared to writers and musicians. He stated that graphic capacities are not affected by aphasia since they work outside language; he thought that pictorial artists communicate their message to the viewer in a direct channel – without any symbolic medium. Gardner et al. [1977, 1991] confirmed the dissociation between graphic and linguistic capacities but rather looked for an explanation in the cerebral organization. In their noteworthy contribution to this topic, they supplied a critical review of the literature concerning

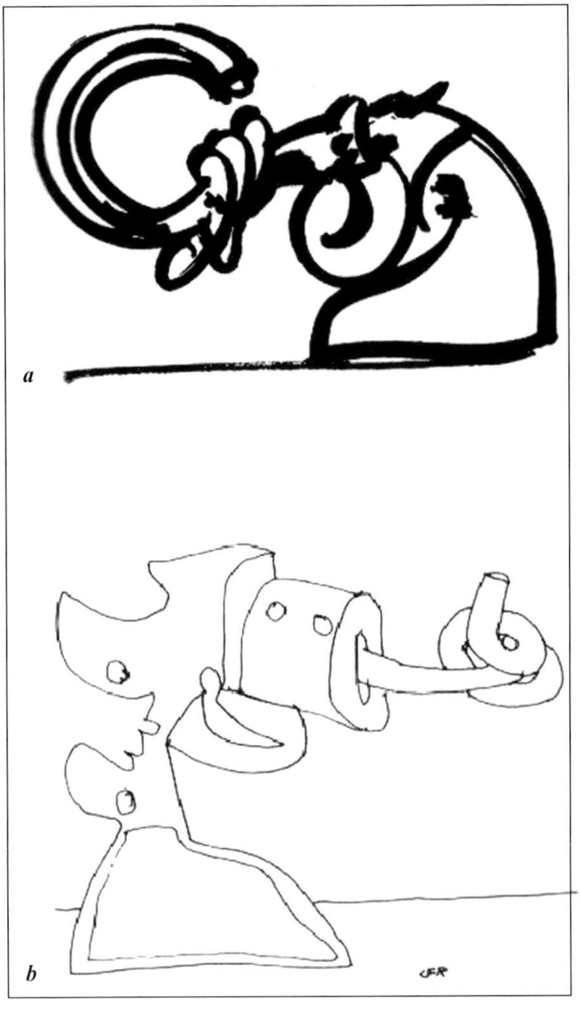

Fig. 4. Sketches of *Non-Violence* before (***a***) and after (***b***) the injury (with the kind permission of the artist).

cerebral organization and specialization. It seemed obvious that each cerebral hemisphere contributes different parts to the graphic process and it has been formulated that the left hemisphere proves particularly important for the details in a graphic production while the right hemisphere contributes to the general configuration of drawing [Kaplan, 1982]. This appears to be the case with unskilled individuals, whereas studies of painters with left-hemisphere damage have revealed that the left hemisphere of the skilled individual may play a less crucial graphic role. Whether the visual analysis of detail is preserved in the left-hemisphere-damaged artist because it is overlearned, or whether it is preserved because it is represented more widely in the brain is not known, since there exists no comparable group of normal and brain-intact artists. Gardner et al. concluded that the gifted visual artist is in general able to continue painting without loss of quality after left-hemisphere disease and severe aphasia.

A change of style subsequent to the stroke has been described in most of the case studies of skilled left-hemisphere-damaged painters. Changes of style are often characterized as leaning towards the more emotional, primitive, bizarre, dreamlike and so on. How to interpret this? One explanation according to Gardner and also to Landis [1988] would be the following: in non-brain-damaged individuals the dominant hemisphere – so defined according to language dominance – inhibits the nondominant hemisphere, which as a rule is the right half. As several studies have suggested, the right hemisphere is nevertheless dominant for visuospatial functions and emotional behavior. If it is less inhibited after a left-hemisphere injury it could be possible that emotion could be expressed in a more direct, spontaneous way, which mostly has been valued as a positive gain of expression. Another case of a painter, who suffered from frontotemporal dementia, showed once more 'that language is not required for, and may even inhibit, certain types of visual creativity' [Chang Mell et al., 2003]. However, according to a paper by Jung [1974] painters with right-hemisphere disease without symptoms of aphasia – like the two German expressionists, Corinth and Räderscheidt – also show style alterations when initial symptoms of neglect are overcome. Gardner et al. [1977, 1991] characterized these shifts as a more emotional, sensual and raw style of painting. Jung himself attributes these changes to psychological factors, reflecting the patient's general reaction to severe illness, whereas Gardner et al. rather find a neurological explanation and state that if the right hemisphere really is essential for emotional appropriateness, it seems conceivable that, as a result of their significant pathology, these patients will be affected by a different set of emotions after right-hemisphere brain damage. This observation nevertheless contradicts the observation of Vigouroux et al. [1990]: in their case of a right-hemisphere-lesioned painter with initial depression they observed a rich pictorial production with excellent spatial organization of the drawings. The style remained well recognizable and the favorite topics were unchanged. Change of style is also recognized by Annoni et al. [2005]: this change 'depends not only on the artist's personality, but also on the lesion site and the ability of the brain to reorganise'. As in their cases, the new painting style adopted by CFR may be attributed to mild changes in executive functions from one side to the change of hand to the other side. The initial hypothesis that change of hand – painting with the other hand – contributes to a modification of style is challenged by the cases of aphasic artists with left-hemisphere damage, who showed the same alterations without change of the working hand. Interestingly enough, according to Helfenstein, Klee who was right handed willingly used his left hand to paint and draw. This phenomenon is also specified by case 2 of Annoni et al. [2005]: 'the painter said that it was the use of the left hand that led him into this new artistic dimension and that figures executed with his left hand had more emotion strength'.

Changes of technique have often been described as a gain of artistic quality after aphasia. Whether these simpler, more direct works are preferred or not seems to be a rather subjective judgement, above all because the artwork of the different aphasic painters was not often evaluated by art specialists or with the same set of judgements.

Conclusion

With the report of CFR, a new case is added to the topic of art and aphasia, which fits very well into the pattern of the clinical literature. The relatively small number of case studies with major visual artists allows certain tentative generalizations. We suggest that although both cerebral hemispheres are important for graphic competence, the right hemisphere plays a dominant role for this ability, above all in skilled artists like CFR. The latter are able to continue their career with remarkable creativity in spite of aphasia and with the other hand. In all observations of left-hemisphere-damaged aphasic artists a change of style is described as having above all an increase in emotional intensity, which in the case of CFR was confirmed by several renowned art critics.

Acknowledgments

The authors thank Carl Fredrik Reuterswärd (CFR) for his kind permission to present his development of art and illness. They also thank Myriam Duc-Vuilleumier who did the therapy in French, and Dr. M. Gasser who died after having contributed to the scientific work on CFR.

References

Alajouanine T: Aphasia and artistic realization. Brain 1948;71:229–241.

Annoni J-M, Devuyst G, Carota A, Bruggimann L, Bogousslavsky J: Changes in artistic style after minor posterior stroke. J Neurol Neurosurg Psychiatry 2005;76:797–803.

Bay E: Aphasia and non-verbal disorders of language. Brain 1962;85:411–426.

Boller F, Sinforiani E, Mazzucchi A: Preserved painting abilities after a stroke. The case of Paul-Elie Gernez. Funct Neurol 2005;20:151–155.

Bonvincini G: Die Aphasie des Malers Vierge. Wien Med Wochenschr 1926;76:88–91.
Chang Mell J, Howard S, Miller BL: Art and the brain – the influence of frontotemporal dementia on an accomplished artist. Neurology 2003;60:1707–1710.
Chatterjee A: The neuropsychology of visual artistic production. Neuropsychologia 2004;42:1568–1583.
Engerth G, Urban H: Zur Kenntnis der gestörten künstlerischen Leistung bei sensorischer Aphasie. Z Ges Neurol Psychiatr 1933;145:753–787.
Gardner H: The pathology of art; in Gardner H (ed): The Shattered Mind. London, Routledge & Kegan, 1977.
Gardner H, Winner E, Rehak A: Artistry and aphasia; in Sarno MT (ed): Acquired Aphasia. San Diego, Academic Press, 1991, pp 373–404.
Gourevitch M: Un aphasique s'exprime par le dessin. L'Encéphale 1967;56:25–68.
Granath O: Personal communication, 1994.
Helfenstein J: Personal communication, 1993.
Huber W, Poeck K, Weiger D, Willmes K: Aachener Aphasie Test (AAT). Göttingen, Hogrefe, 1983.
Jung R: Neuropsychologie und Neurophysiologie des Kontur- und Formsehens in Zeichnung und Malerei; in Wieck HH (ed): Psychopathologie musischer Gestaltungen. Stuttgart, Schattauer Verlag, 1974, pp 29–88.
Kaczmarek BLJ: Aphasia in an artist: a disorder of symbolic processing. Aphasiology 1991;5:361–371.
Kaplan E: Process and achievement revisited; in Wapner S, Kaplan B (eds): Towards Holistic Developmental Psychology. Hillsdale, Erlbaum, 1982.
Landis T: Die Linke weiss nicht was die Rechte tut: Zur Interaktion der beiden Hirnhälften. Schweiz Med Wochenschr 1988;118:1779–1788.
Puel M, Cardebat D, Demonet J-F, Elghozi D, Cambier J, Guiraud-Chaumel B, Rascol A: Le rôle du thalamus dans les aphasies sous-corticales. Rev Neurol 1986;142:431–440.
Reinvang I: Crossed aphasia and apraxia in an artist. Aphasiology 1987;1:423–434.
Reuterswärd CF: Titta, jag är osynlig. Självbiografi. Baskerville, Gedins Förlag, 1988.
Reuterswärd CT: Personal communication, 1992.
Sandblom P: Creativity and Disease. London, Marion Boyars, 1991.
Vigouroux RA, Bonnefoi B, Khalil R: Réalisations picturales chez un artiste peintre présentant une héminégligence gauche. Rev Neurol 1990;146:665–670.
Zaimov K, Kitov D, Kolev N: Aphasie chez un peintre. Encéphale 1969;58:377–417.

Dr. Françoise Colombo-Thuillard
Department of Neuropsychology
Hôpital cantonal
CH–1708 Fribourg (Switzerland)
Tel. +41 26 426 7289, Fax +41 26 426 7297, E-Mail colombof@hopcantfr.ch

Bogousslavsky J, Hennerici MG (eds): Neurological Disorders in Famous Artists – Part 2.
Front Neurol Neurosci. Basel, Karger, 2007, vol 22, pp 184–192

Mozart in the Neurological Department – Who Has the Tic?

Thomas Kammer

Department of Psychiatry, University of Ulm, Ulm, Germany

Abstract

In Wolfgang Amadeus Mozart's medical history quite an impressive list of possible diseases has been collected. In the 1980s the diagnosis of Tourette's syndrome was added to the list. Evidence of vocal tics was derived from the scatological expressions found in the letters of Mozart. In addition there are a few contemporary reports on striking motor behavior suggesting the existence of motor tics. However, in a critical light the arguments for the diagnosis are quite weak. Most problematic is the concept that involuntary vocal utterances are transferred to the written form. One would expect to find similar written manifestations of vocal tics in the work of authors suffering from Tourette's syndrome. This is neither the case in the work of Samuel Johnson (1709–1784) nor in that of André Malraux (1901–1976). In conclusion, Tourette's syndrome is an inventive but implausible diagnosis in the medical history of Mozart.

Wolfgang Amadeus Mozart's 250th birthday brought us a surge of essays on almost every aspect of his short live. Given the fact that he is without doubt one of the greatest composers in human history this is not very surprising. His development from wunderkind to more or less reputed artist seems to be prototypical for the career of a genius. Many authors attempted to deduce the constituting factors of geniality from his biography but as Hildesheimer [1977] pointed out most of them failed. Mozart died at the early age of 35 which seems tragic considering what he might have written had he lived longer. The fact that Mozart worked on the famous *Requiem* in his last days seems even more mysterious. And the legend that his antagonist Antonio Salieri poisoned him contributed further to the Mozart mystery.

Unsurprisingly historians of medicine consistently wondered about Mozart's medical history. The focus of the scholarly discussions has not only been on the multitude of Mozart's illnesses during his lifetime but also on his final illness and death. The list of possible diseases leading to Mozart's death is quite impressive. It demonstrates the dilemma of any retrospective medical history. Historical medical reports are rarely thorough enough in their description of symptoms. Furthermore, the medicine of the past often misinterpreted side effects of treatments due to toxic doses of drugs or phlebotomy inducing severe anemia as a symptom. Many differences in hygiene and general nutrition have to be taken into account in historical medical cases. Finally, the range and the peculiarity of chronic diseases differ from century to century. In this essay I shall not touch on Mozart's early death but will focus on one aspect in his range of neurological disorders: Tourette's syndrome (TS).

Tourette's Syndrome

The neurologist Georges Gilles de la Tourette (1857–1904) was a coworker of Jean-Martin Charcot at Salpêtrière in Paris (fig. 1). Based on nine cases he described a 'maladie de tics' characterized by the combination of involuntary stereotyped movements and utterances – motor and vocal tics [Gilles de la Tourette, 1885]. TS usually manifests itself in early childhood and sometimes disappears with adulthood [for a review, see Jankovic, 2001; Leckman, 2002]. In more severe cases the tics persist throughout live. The severity of tics typically waxes and wanes, both throughout the day and during periods of weeks or months. According to actual criteria the diagnosis of TS requires multiple motor tics and at least one vocal tic persisting for at least 1 year. Tics are classified as simple or complex. Simple motor tics are brief rapid movements typically involving only one muscle group, e.g. face or shoulder. Complex motor tics can come as a coordinated sequence of movements that serves no purpose even though it seems to be purposeful. Simple vocal tics manifest as grunting, yelping or throat clearing. Complex vocal tics include syllables and phrases, as well as palilalia (the repetition of one's own words), echolalia (the repetition of other people's words) and coprolalia (utterance of obscene words). Although coprolalia is one of the best-known symptoms in TS it occurs in only about 10% of TS patients. TS cases with mild symptoms usually have a good prognosis. Important coexisting diagnoses often associated with TS are hyperkinetic disorders such as attention deficit hyperactivity disorder and other developmental problems in childhood as well as mood disorders and obsessive-compulsive disorders in adulthood.

The pathogenesis of TS is not yet clear. Genetic influences and damaging factors during gestation and birth have been suggested. A postinfectious autoimmune mechanism following rheumatic fever, like Sydenham's chorea,

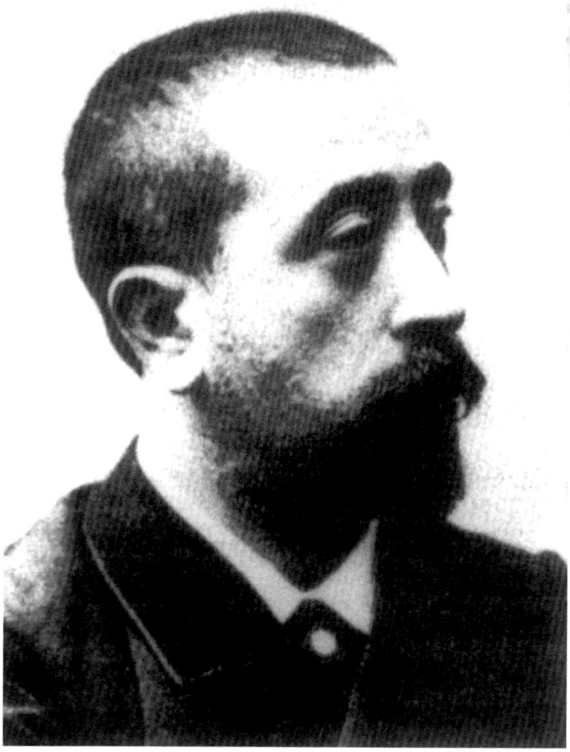

Fig. 1. Georges Albert Édouard Brutus Gilles de la Tourette (1857–1904), French neurologist. From Lees [1986]. Copyright Masson.

sharing target regions in the brain such as the basal ganglia and related cortical and thalamic sites might also contribute to the manifestation of TS.

The prevalence of TS in children aged 13–14 is estimated between 31 and 157 cases per 10,000 [Hornsey et al., 2001]. Considering this high prevalence the diagnosis of TS was surprisingly seldom in the past. Even after its first scientific description TS was rarely reported during the next 90 years. Tics were mainly explained in the framework of psychoanalysis and therefore were no longer considered as a separate disease. Most psychiatrists believed that patients with tics also suffered from unresolved psychological disturbances or psychosexual conflicts. Therefore, psychotherapeutic intervention based on psychoanalysis was the preferred method of treatment. This view only changed after first reports on successful TS treatment with haloperidol emerged [Caprini and Melotti, 1962; Shapiro and Shapiro, 1968]. Sacks' popular descriptions of TS cases [Sacks, 1985, 1995] led to increased public awareness. Nowadays

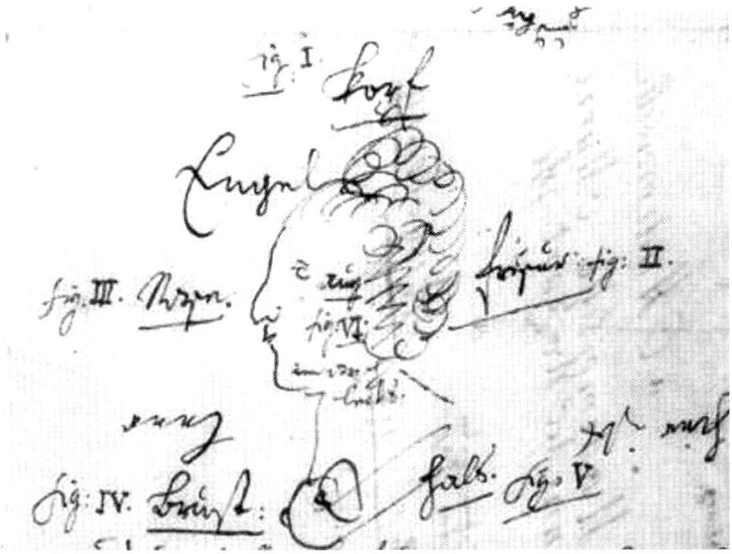

Fig. 2. Mozart's drawing of his cousin Maria Anna Tekla Mozart, nicknamed Bäsle, on his letter of May 10, 1779. Mozart dated the letter wrongly in order to get a rhyme: 'Salsbourg den 10ten May 1709ni, blass mir hint' aini. – gut ists, wohl bekomms' (blow into my rear, nothing could by finer, bon appétit) (by permission of The British Library, ZWEIG 64–67 Vol LXIV–LXVII).

support is available at many places to help patients and their families deal with the diverse medical and social aspects of the disease.

Mozart's Case

Today's readers feel challenged by quite a few passages of Mozart's letters as well as parts of his music. How could such an extraordinary artist express himself so vulgarly? How could a canon (K 231) be titled *Leck mich im Arsch* (lick my arse)? Out of shame musicology initially hushed up this aspect. This explains why text and title of the mentioned canon were changed when first published by Breitkopf: *Lasst uns froh sein* (let's be happy). Apart from the canons Mozart's impressive vulgarity shows most in his letters to his cousin Maria Anna Tekla Mozart, nicknamed Bäsle (fig. 2). Mozart wrote them between 1777 and 1781 (aged 21–25). They reveal an enthusiastic and light-hearted relationship or, possibly, a love affair. In his second letter Mozart wrote [translations by Spaethling, 2000]:

Mannheim, November 5, 1777

Deares cozz buzz!

I have received reprieved your highly esteemed writing biting, and I have noted doted thy my uncle garfuncle, my aunt slant, and you too, are all well mell. We, too thank god, are in good fettle kettle... You write further, indeed you let it all out, you expose yourself, you let yourself be heard, you give me notice, you declare yourself, you indicate to me, you bring me the news, you announce onto me, you state in broad daylight, you demand, you desire, you wish, you want, you like, you command that I, too, should could send you my Portrait. Eh bien, I shall mail fail it for sure. Oui, by the love of my skin, I shit on your nose, so it runs down your chin...

Mozart's widow Konstanze got the letters back after his death but did not publish them. In the very first edition of Mozart's letters the obscene parts had still been eliminated. Therefore, Mozart's admirers had to come to terms with the new insights into the genius's personality after the first unabridged edition was published. The vulgar expressions were not restricted to the Bäsle letters. They could also be found in several letters to his father, his mother, his sister as well as in letters to close friends.

Mozart to his father:

Augsburg, October 17, 1777

...A certain Pater Emilian, a conceited ass and simpleminded clerical wag, was there, full of sweetness. He wanted to flirt with Bäsle, but she instead had her fun with him... He sang a Canons... I was third in line to sing. But I sang a whole different text: 'P.E., o oh you prick, why don't you kiss my ass.' I sang it sotto voce to my Bäsle. We were laughing for half an hour.

A possible explanation for the well-documented vulgar utterances of Mozart could be the diagnosis of TS. This had been suggested for the first time at the World Congress of Psychiatry in Vienna in 1983 [Fog and Regeur, 1983]. Since then several scientists tried to diagnose the syndrome posthumously [Gunne, 1991; Simkin, 1992; Schaub, 1994; Fog, 1995]. They were promptly and harshly been criticized by others [Davies, 1993; Heyworth, 1993; Karhausen, 1993]. It is worthwhile to study the pros and cons in detail.

Simkin [1992] contributed a detailed analysis of all letters of Mozart with a statistical analysis of evidence of coprolalia, mostly scatological expressions and sexual insinuation. Simkin also counted the occurrences of palilalia, echolalia and comparable word plays. He found evidence of this in 63 out of 371 letters (17%) and interpreted it as a vocal tic in written form. Sorting the letters chronologically he identified several periods in the life of Mozart with an accumulation of coprolalia. These periods seem to correlate with putative phases of a particularly heavy emotional load in Mozart's life. Simkin took the passages of the letters as well as their striking periodicity as a proof for the existence of vocal tics and as a part of the diagnosis of TS. The motor tics required for a correct diagnosis of TS were derived from several statements of contemporaries. Mozart's restlessness was reported several times as finger playing, feet tapping, running around or even rollicking about. Sophie Haibel, Mozart's sister-in-law, mentioned [Haibel, 1965]:

> At a table he would often twist up a corner of a napkin and rub his upper lip with it, without appearing to know what he was doing, and he often made extraordinary grimaces with his mouth... Also, his hands and feet were always in motion, he was always playing with something, e.g. his hat, pockets, watch-fob, tables, chairs, as if they were a clavier.

Karoline Pichler, who took piano lessons with Mozart, mentioned in her memoirs [Pichler, 1965]:

> [After an improvisation on a melodie of Figaro]... he suddenly tired of it, jumped up, and, in the mad mood which so often came over him, he began to leap over tables and chairs, miaow like a cat, and turn somersaults like an unruly boy.

According to Simkin these and four other anecdotal citations fulfill the criteria of motor tics. Furthermore, the report of Pichler, mentioning the 'miaow', is the only one that might be taken as evidence of a vocal tic.

Discussion

The claim that Mozart suffered from TS was immediately and harshly criticized. Two main objections have been made: First, it is not proven whether written documents can account for the existence of a vocal tic. Second, the evidence of motor tics in Mozart's life is doubtful.

The scatological parts of Mozart's letters could be part of the conversation style typical for the region at that time. Indeed, southern Bavaria and the Salzburg region are known for quite a crude language style. From contemporary sources we can also conclude that roughness in spoken language was not even restricted to a certain region [Aterman, 1994]. The language of Luther in the 16th century is a nice example, and even Goethe allows his Götz von Berlichingen to reply to the Bishop of Bamberg: 'He can lick my ass!'. Furthermore, it could be argued that Mozart deliberately used rough language to demonstrate his disrespect of the nobility.

Although the conversation style was different in the 18th century the scatological parts in Mozart's letters have been considered to be a sign of a very special relationship between Mozart and his parents as well as his sister.

Ortheil [1982] suggests that the Bäsle letters should be read in their chronological relation to the letters Mozart wrote to his father. At the age of 21, Mozart was for the first time travelling without his father, seeking an independent position in Munich, Mannheim and Paris. He did not have the expected success and from Salzburg Mozart's father tried to help his son go to the right places. In his frequent correspondence the father felt that his son had started to emancipate himself from his rigid regime and he diligently admonished his son. In his letters Wolfgang tried to follow his father's suggestions without losing his new liberty. According to Ortheil the Bäsle letters are an outlet for this complex father-son constellation. The whole pressure caused by the father's exhortations

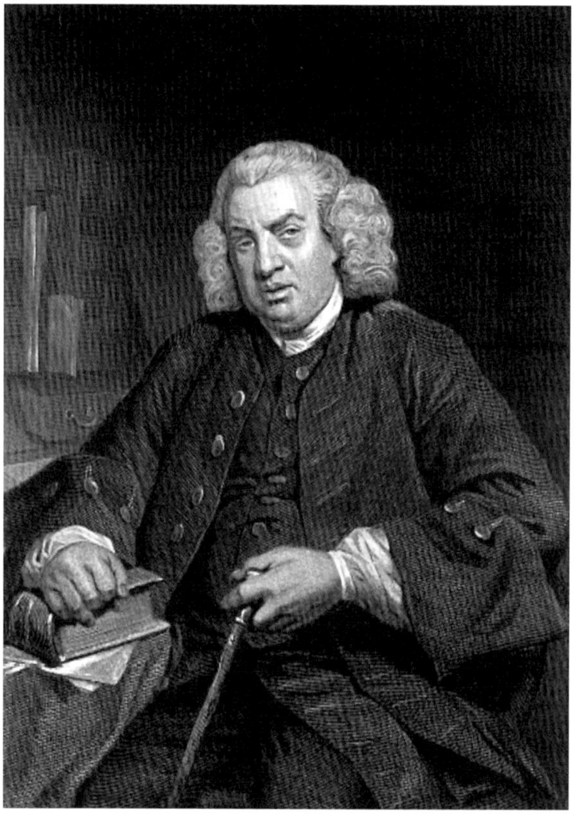

Fig. 3. Dr. Samuel Johnson (1709–1784), English writer and lexicographer, suffering from TS. From Duyckinick [1873].

in combination with the disappointing development of his career was transferred by Mozart into the radical messages to Bäsle.

Mozart's letters demonstrate undoubtedly an unusual delight to play on words. Mieder [2003] presents a detailed analysis of Mozart's use and alteration of proverbs. He demonstrates Mozart's inventive use of language to express such different things as his love for Konstanze or his disreputable dismissal from the Salzburg Court. He often took the role of the tomfool annotating facts with clownish phrases. From this point of view the examples of echolalia and palilalia have to be interpreted differently. Reading the letters aloud even makes the musicality of the phrases obvious.

The written documents that seem strange at first glance can be taken as an inventive and imaginative verbalism against the backdrop of the specific language culture of the time.

Can written documents be a proof of vocal tics of the author? In the history of literature, two prominent authors are known to have suffered from TS: Samuel Johnson (1709–1784, fig. 3) and André Malraux (1901–1976). Both wrote a voluminous opus with a large spectrum of different genres. But in none of their writings are there signs of involuntary passages. In contrast, Johnson stands for his witticism which is frequently quoted. In 1933 André Malraux received the Prix Concourt, the most prestigious prize in French literature, for his novel *La condition humaine*. The claim that involuntary utterances influence the content of written documents seems quite questionable from this point of view.

What about the reports suggesting that Mozart suffered from motor tics? In my view they are the most important part of the diagnosis. However, even these documents leave some questions unanswered. Why is there no mentioning of tics in Mozart's childhood? Although adult onset of TS has been described [Marneros, 1983; Chouinard and Ford, 2000] first manifestation in childhood is much more common. Leopold Mozart probably would have mentioned some of his son's motor tics or other motor problems had there been any. Also the reports of Mozart's motor tics seem insignificant in comparison with the documented evidence of tics of Samuel Johnson.

Conclusion

Although the idea seems to be compelling the evidence is too small to claim that Mozart suffered from TS. A definite statement about the retrospective diagnosis is impossible due to the lack of sufficient sources. The concept has its own charm, in particular if one follows the distinction of Sacks [1992] between the stereotypical form and the phantasmagorical form of TS. He emphasizes the possibility of a patient mastering his TS and directing it into an orderly flow with extraordinary creative features. Yet it is important not to confuse a disorder with an extraordinary creativity. The long debate on a link between creativity and mental illness has not been resolved yet [e.g. Waddell, 1998]. However, the equation has a very romantic touch, but it fails to explain ingenuity. There is no need to listen to the marvellous music of Mozart with a switched on 'syndrome filter' in mind.

References

Aterman K: Did Mozart have Tourette's syndrome – some comments on Mozart's language. Perspect Biol Med 1994;37:247–258.

Caprini G, Melotti V: Un grave sindrome ticcosa guarita con haloperidol. Riv Sper Freniatr Med Leg Alien Ment 1962;86:191–196.

Chouinard S, Ford B: Adult onset tic disorders. J Neurol Neurosurg Psychiatry 2000;68:738–743.
Davies PJ: Mozart's scatological disorder. Br Med J 1993;306:521–522.
Duyckinick EA: Portrait Gallery of Eminent Men and Women in Europe and America. New York, Johnson, Wilson & Comp., 1873.
Fog R: Mozart's bizarre verbal behavior: a case of Tourette syndrome? Maledicta 1995;11:59–62.
Fog R, Regeur L: Did W.A. Mozart suffer from Tourette's syndrome? World Congress of Psychiatry, Vienna, 1983.
Gilles de la Tourette G: Étude sur une affection nerveuse caractérisée par l'incoordination motrice accompagnée d'écholalie et de coprolalie. Arch Neurol (Paris) 1885;9:19–42, 158–200.
Gunne LM: Hade Mozart Tourettes syndrom? Läkartidningen 1991;88:4325–4326.
Haibel S: Memoirs, 1828; in Deutsch OE: Mozart, a documentary biography. Stanford, Stanford University Press, 1965:537.
Heyworth MF: Mozart's scatological disorder. BMJ 1993;306:522.
Hildesheimer W: Mozart. Frankfurt am Main, Suhrkamp, 1977.
Hornsey H, Banerjee S, Zeitlin H, Robertson M: The prevalence of Tourette syndrome in 13–14-year-olds in mainstream schools. J Child Psychol Psychiatry 2001;42:1035–1040.
Jankovic J: Tourette's syndrome. N Engl J Med 2001;345:1184–1192.
Karhausen LR: Mozart's scatological disorder. BMJ 1993;306:522.
Leckman JF: Tourette's syndrome. Lancet 2002;360:1577–1586.
Lees A: Georges Gilles de la Tourette: the man and his times. Rev Neurol (Paris) 1986;142:808–816.
Marneros A: Adult onset of Tourette's syndrome: a case report. Am J Psychiatry 1983;140:924–925.
Mieder W: 'Now-I-sit-like-a-rabbit-in-the-pepper': proverbial language in the letters of Wolfgang Amadeus Mozart. J Folk Res 2003;40:33–70.
Ortheil HJ: Mozart im Innern seiner Sprachen. Frankfurt am Main, Fischer, 1982.
Pichler K: Memoirs (1843–44); in Deutsch OE: Mozart, a documentary biography. Stanford, Stanford University Press, 1965:556.
Sacks O: Tourette's syndrome and creativity. BMJ 1992;305:1515–1516.
Sacks OW: The Man Who Mistook His Wife for a Hat and Other Clinical Tales. New York, Summit Books, 1985.
Sacks OW: An Anthropologist on Mars: Seven Paradoxical Tales. New York, Knopf, 1995.
Schaub S: Mozart und das Tourette-Syndrom. Acta Mozartiana 1994;41:15–20.
Shapiro AK, Shapiro E: Treatment of Gilles de la Tourette's syndrome with haloperidol. Br J Psychiatry 1968;114:345–350.
Simkin B: Mozart scatological disorder. Br Med J 1992;305:1563–1567.
Spaethling R: Mozart's Letters, Mozart's Life. London, Faber & Faber, 2000.
Waddell C: Creativity and mental illness: is there a link? Can J Psychiatry 1998;43:166–172.

Dr. Thomas Kammer
Department of Psychiatry, University of Ulm
Leimgrubenweg 12
DE–89075 Ulm (Germany)
Tel. +49 731 500 61544, Fax +49 731 500 61542, E-Mail thomas.kammer@uni-ulm.de

Bogousslavsky J, Hennerici MG (eds): Neurological Disorders in Famous Artists – Part 2.
Front Neurol Neurosci. Basel, Karger, 2007, vol 22, pp 193–205

Hans von Bülow: Creativity and Neurological Disease in a Famous Pianist and Conductor

Johannes C. Wöhrle[a,b], *Frithjof Haas*[c]

[a]Department of Neurology, Katholisches Klinikum, Koblenz, [b]Department of Neurology, University of Heidelberg, Universitätsklinikum Mannheim, Mannheim, and [c]University of Music and Badisches Staatstheater Karlsruhe, Karlsruhe, Germany

Abstract

Hans von Bülow (1830–1894) was a conductor and pianist of worldwide reputation and founder of many stylistic interpretations of classic and romantic symphonies. The close friendship with Richard Wagner, but not the enthusiastic admiration of his dramatic musical opus, ended abruptly when Hans von Bülow became aware of the betrayal of his wife Cosima and Richard Wagner. Hans von Bülow reported symptoms and signs of neurological disease in many letters that were kept and edited by his second wife Marie. For decades he suffered from chronic neuralgiforme headaches, which were caused by a tumor of the cervical radicular nerves. At the age of 45 years, he suddenly developed a motorsensory deficit in the right arm and hand and a contralateral facial deficit, suggestive of brainstem infarction. He recovered and celebrated even greater successes as a musician, although phases of major depression also interfered with his professional life. In the last, phase of his life, he experienced the consequences of generalized atherosclerosis and cerebral microangiopathy. It was a second cerebrovascular accident of the brainstem that caused his death, only 10 months after his last concert performance. Although his death occurred in Egypt, an autopsy was performed by Professor Ludwig Edinger and the results will be presented.

Hans von Bülow: Musician and Person

Hans von Bülow (1830–1894) was a man of worldwide reputation for his extraordinary achievements both as classical pianist and conductor of concerts and operas (table 1). His master and teacher Franz Liszt regarded him his legitimate successor. He was chosen by Richard Wagner as his closest collaborator,

Table 1. Biography of Hans von Bülow [Haas, 2002]

January 8, 1830	Born in Dresden
	Piano education started at 8 years of age
1848–1850	Studies in Leipzig and Berlin (philology, history, literature, law)
1850/1851	Conductor under the directorate of Richard Wagner in Zürich and St. Gallen
1851–1853	Student of Franz Liszt in Weimar, subsequently concert tour as pianist
1855	Piano teacher at Stern's Conservatory in Berlin
August 18, 1857	Marriage to Cosima Liszt in the St. Hedwig's Church, Berlin
1865	Private pianist to the Bavarian King Ludwig II in Munich, Cosima von Bülow worked as secretary for Richard Wagner
April 10, 1865	Birth of Isolde, the first child of the liaison between Cosima and Richard Wagner
June 10, 1865	Bülow conducted the premier performance of *Tristan und Isolde*, and on June 21, 1868 of *Die Meistersinger von Nürnberg* in Munich
1866/1867	Bülow escaped from Munich and worked as a piano teacher in Basel
May 1, 1867	Returned to Munich, working as first royal conductor and director of the Royal School of Music
1869–1871	Residency in Florence; divorce from Cosima on July 18, 1870
1873–1875	Concert tours as pianist and conductor throughout Germany, Russia and England
April 1875	Cerebral stroke in England, recovery on the Isle of Wight
October 1875	Start of a concert tour as pianist with 139 performances in the USA
May 1876	Premature end of the tour because of physical and psychological breakdown
1876/1877	Stay in Hannover, rehabilitation in Bex/Vaud, Bad Kreuznach, Baden-Baden
1877–1879	Opera and concert conductor in Hannover
1880–1885	Director and conductor of the Royal Orchestra of Meiningen
July 19, 1882	Second marriage to the actress Marie Schanzer
November 1, 1886	Director of the new subscription concert series in Hamburg
October 1, 1887	Chief conductor of the Berlin Philharmonic Orchestra
June 1891	Because of major depression and severe neuralgia rehabilitation in Schöneck, on the Lake of Lucerne
December 1892	Treatment in a hospital in Pankow for nervous disease
March/April 1893	Conducting his last concerts in Hamburg and Berlin, then phase of severe terminal illness
February 12, 1894	Died in Cairo, Egypt, at the age of 64 years

and he conducted the first performances of *Tristan und Isolde* (June 10, 1865) and *Die Meistersinger von Nürnberg* (June 21, 1868). During his appointments as chief conductor in Munich, Hannover, Meiningen and Berlin and on the occasions of worldwide tours as guest conductor, he established ways and rules for orchestral discipline and stilistic interpretations of classic and romantic symphonies which are still valid today. He became the idol of all subsequent conductors. His instructive editions of the piano pieces of Johann Sebastian Bach, Ludwig van Beethoven and Frédéric Chopin gave testimony to the virtuosity and spirit of the performing concert pianist (figs. 1, 2) [Haas, 2002].

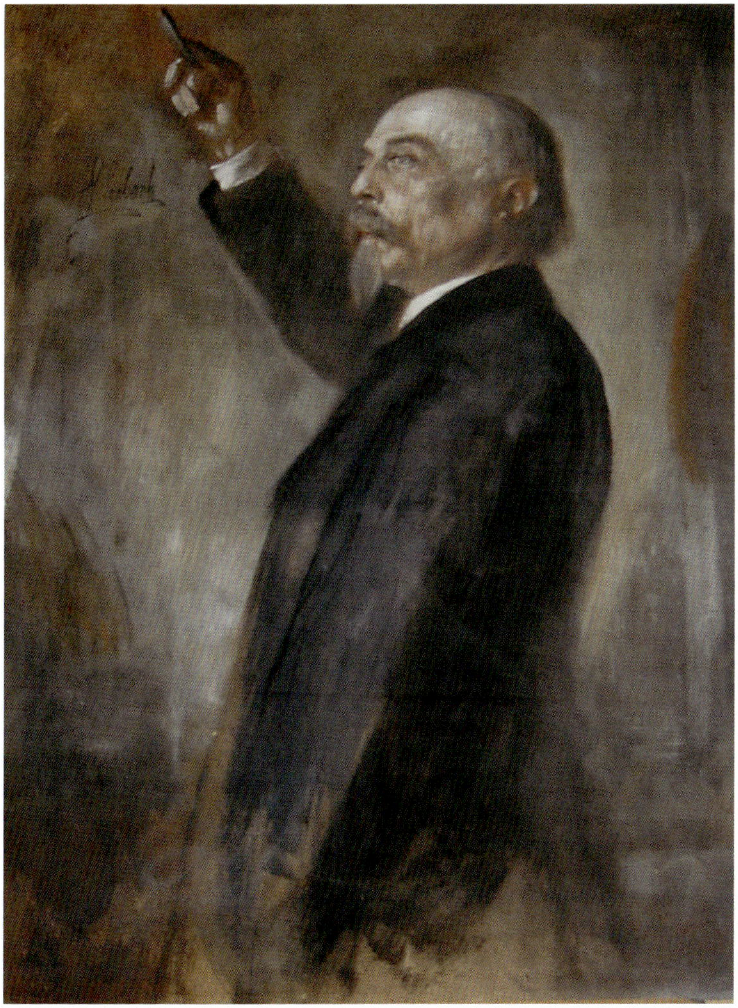

Fig. 1. Hans von Bülow – the conductor. Painting in oil by Franz von Lenbach, Bavarian State Opera [from Haas, 2002, with permission].

Hans von Bülow had a seemingly limitless capacity to memorize the finest details. He knew his entire repertoire for orchestra and piano by heart. On the podium, he never used music. The foundation for his universal education in literature and music and his brilliant spirit was laid at home by his family. His father wrote novels and he was a translator of Roman languages. His mother, an acquaintance of Liszt, had received an education in music. She spoke French with her son. At the age of 4 years, Hans von Bülow had to learn poems and

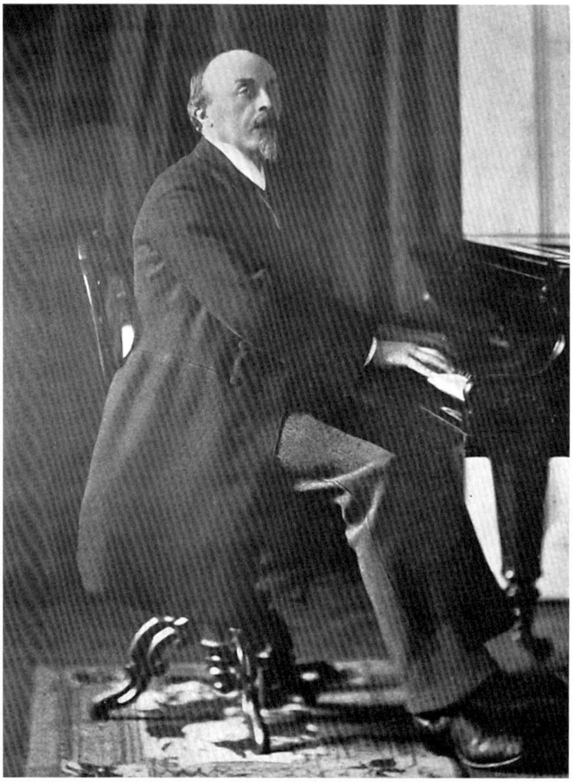

Fig. 2. Hans von Bülow – the pianist. Photograph, approximately 1885 [from Haas, 2002, with permission].

fables in order to recite them to his parents on weekends. It was here that the pattern of his later life – a life involving largely musical and intellectual activity – was set. Leisure and recreation were options that only became available when disease or complete exhaustion made them a necessity. When on concert tours, he always took along a large number of books, which he read during the night and later passed on to friends. He seems to have always found the time to keep up to date with the latest literature which he discussed in his correspondence with friends. He spoke and corresponded in perfect French, Italian and English.

The composers Franz Liszt and Richard Wagner entered the life of Hans von Bülow early, and they greatly influenced him as a musician. It was only in his later years that he came into contact with Johannes Brahms, whose works he propagated with great passion. However, Hans von Bülow admired Richard Wagner most of all, although he broke off all personal contacts and correspondence with him after Wagner's liaison with Cosima. Bülow adored his wife Cosima,

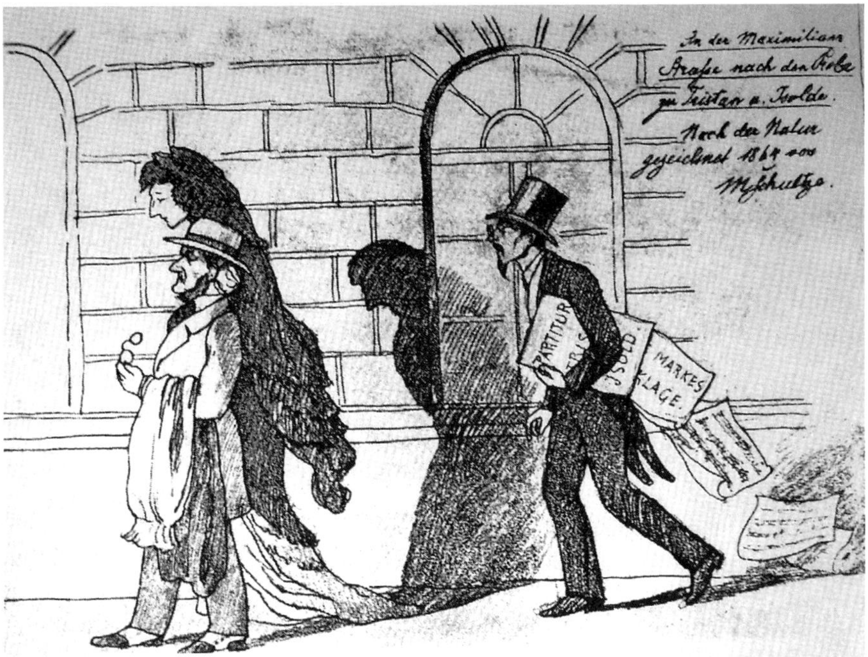
In der Maximilian
Straße nach der Probe
zu Tristan u. Isolde.
Nach der Natur
gezeichnet 1864 von
M. Schultze.
PARTITUR
ISOLD
MARKES KLAGE.

Fig. 3. Richard Wagner and Cosima with Hans von Bülow following behind after the revision of *Tristan und Isolde*, on Maximilian's Street in Munich (1864). Caricature by M. Schultze [from Haas, 2002, with permission]. Note that Cosima – at that time still Bülow's wife and Wagner's secretary – walks side by side with Richard Wagner, while the dwarfed Hans von Bülow can hardly keep up their pace.

Franz Liszt's daughter, like no other woman, and his adoration continued even after she divorced him in order to marry Richard Wagner. Once Hans von Bülow realized that Cosima and Wagner betrayed him, he wanted to duel with Wagner, but eventually recognized that this would bring no solution. He consented that only with Cosima at his side could this great composer fulfill the great dramatic opus *Der Ring des Nibelungen*. He agreed that his two daughters Blandine and Daniela would grow up together with the other children of Wagner in their household at Wahnfried in Bayreuth. At the same time, he was agonized by the deep wound of having failed as husband to live up to the demands of Cosima (fig. 3). One gets the impression that in his later life he wanted to compensate for this failure by extraordinary artistic achievements, irrespective of the frailty of his body and mind.

Hans von Bülow's work as conductor and pianist was accompanied by a permanent struggle against many illnesses. He reported one of them to his mother and friends as 'névralgie', 'Kopfneuralgie', or 'Kopfgrippe' (neuralgia, cranial neuralgia, or cranial cold). Only extreme self-discipline allowed him to give his regular performances as conductor and pianist. The immeasurable energy with which he fulfilled his duties was fuelled by the great catastrophe of his life – his separation from Cosima and the betrayal by Wagner. Although at first after this incident Bülow had a psychological and physical breakdown, eventually he was driven to more and more extraordinary artistic activities: in all major German cities he gave recitals of the last 5 piano sonatas by Ludwig van Beethoven, which in those days were regarded as incomprehensible. He went on a European tour with the Royal Orchestra of Meiningen, whose 45 musicians had been so well trained over years that this small orchestra celebrated more frequent and greater successes in the European metropolitan centers of music than the philharmonic orchestras of Berlin or Vienna with almost twice the number of musicians. In addition, he was the first to perform the piano concertos of Beethoven and Brahms without conductor but with himself leading the orchestra from the concert piano as 'conducting pianist'.

After an extremely strenuous concert tour throughout Russia and England in 1875, Hans von Bülow – at the age of 45 years – had a stroke with paralysis of his right arm. He wrote to his mother: 'The result of meticulous investigations is: site of trouble in the brain – disrupture of a small vessel – an apoplectiform insult, so to speak' [von Bülow, 1900–1908a]. After some recuperation in Tirol, he traveled to the Isle of Wight. Here, in tranquil isolation, he trained his impaired arm and hand at the piano for many hours per day. This severe disease that troubled him for the rest of his life was associated with the great catastrophe that he had experienced with Cosima and Richard Wagner. To participate in the opening of the first Bayreuth Festival in 1876 would have been the fulfillment of Bülow's career as a musician, having been the closest friend of Wagner for many years. However, because of his desire and need to stay as far away from Bayreuth as possible, he contracted to perform as a pianist at an incredibly large series of concerts that required a 150 performances and were held in every major US city during the 1875/1876 season even though he had recently suffered stroke. After concert number 139 he had a physical and psychological breakdown, which forced him to refrain from any musical activity for many months. His clinical state was described by his friend Hans von Bronsart, director of the theater in Hannover, who took care of Bülow after his return from America: 'I have seen Bülow in states, which would indicate near death to lay people' [von Bronsart, 1900–1908]. But Bülow again recovered within 1 year, and was able to accept a position as conductor and director of the Hannover Opera and Concert House. Subsequently, the positions as director of the Royal Orchestra of Meiningen and chief conductor of the Berlin Philharmonic Orchestra led him to the peak of his brilliant career and laid the foundation for his reputation as the ideal modern conductor.

During the last 7 years of his musical vocation he simultaneously held the positions of director and conductor of the concert series in both Hamburg and Berlin, and for two winter seasons in addition in Bremen. Despite relapsing attacks of agonizing neuralgia, these years were most important for his achievements. He was an unusual and fascinating conductor, which was reflected by an enthusiastic audience and confirmed by newspaper commentaries:

> One must have witnessed, how Mr. von Bülow conducts each instrument in the orchestra more by a twist of his heart or a glimpse of his eye, as if the orchestra were a mere extension of his own personality, and how he thus demonstrates the mystical depth of the piece of art [Krause, 1892].

The fervent responses to his late performances reinforced Bülow to persevere until his mental and physical powers eventually failed. The 10 months following his last concert in Berlin were filled with agony, only supported by the hope to find relief and recovery during a stay in Egypt, where he died just 3 days after his arrival at the age of 64 years.

Diseases of Hans von Bülow

Neuralgia

In his letters Bülow gave many accounts of terrible states of headaches that were characterized by him as neuralgia, cranial neuralgia ('Kopfneuralgie'), or 'névralgie'. He described these pains as 'stabbing, as if one was to become mad'. These pains occurred in attacks lasting for days to weeks and they were so disabling that Bülow stopped working apart from giving some piano lessons. He tried several treatments like arsenic and electricity. He reasoned that his past was responsible for these headaches combined with his ambitious return to work once the headaches had subsided [von Bülow, 1900–1908b]. The episodes of occipital neuralgia accompanied von Bülow throughout his life, and the cause was accounted for by Ludwig Edinger, Professor of Anatomy and Pathology in Frankfurt am Main, who had the opportunity to examine his brain postmortem. Edinger reported a large tumor that had involved and compressed the two uppermost cervical roots of one side. He suggested that this tumor would have been present since adolescence – perhaps due to an affection of the meninges, but he explicitly stated that there were no 'specific' changes due to tuberculosis or syphilis in this tissue [Edinger, 1900–1908]. Occipital neuralgia has been described due to a solitary fibrous tumor – a mesenchymal tumor staining positive for CD34 antigen – amongst other local compressive, vascular or inflammatory causes [Gaetani et al., 2004], but the true nature of the tumor of Hans von Bülow remains unknown.

First Stroke

After an extremely strenuous concert tour throughout Russia and England, in April 1875, Hans von Bülow – at the age of 45 years – had a stroke with paresis and sensory deficit of his right upper extremity. He reported to his mother on May 29, 1875: 'To write causes me a terrible effort – also my hand feels icy cold...' and a few days later he told her the result of Professor v. Buhl's examination: 'The result of meticulous investigations is: site of trouble in the brain – disrupture of a small vessel – an apoplectiform insult, so to speak. This explains the strange likeness of the state of my right side of the body with the left side of the face, i.e. no hint of typical or untypical gout' [von Bülow, 1900–1908a]. In September 1875, Hans von Bülow gives another account of his health after having moved from his resort on the Isle of Wight to America:

> My state is still very unsatisfactory and tantalizing because of the permanent uncertainty, the swing between hope and desperation... Often dizziness – and my head and memory still feel wrong, however the fingers are improved, despite their frequent coldness and stiffness – what a wonder! After 120 hours of exercises! Perhaps the crossing has a charitably revolutionary effect on my totally ruined nerves [von Bülow, 1900–1908c].

These symptoms point to an infarction in the left pontomedullary region of the brainstem, leading to crossed symptomatology with contralateral right-sided paresis and sensory dysfunction of the right arm and hand and sensory and possibly motor dysfunction of the ipsilateral left face. Also the dizziness he complained about would be most compatible with an infarction in this region. Von Bülow worked very hard to regain the function of his right hand but also his ability to concentrate and memorize, and in autumn 1875, he presented the first world performance of a piano concerto by Tchaikovsky hitherto unknown to him.

Episodes of Depression

Hans von Bülow had barely recovered from his stroke in April 1875, when he fell ill again during his extremely strenuous American concert tour in May 1876 after having performed 139 concerts in 7 months. The symptoms of this illness were announced by von Bülow in his letter to his mother from Cleveland:

> ...the sequelae of my stroke 13 months ago manifest in a similar way – instead of disappearing! My mind is weak, my 'famous' memory impaired by continuous dizziness, and during the day, I need to practice the most familiar concert programs before the public performance at night, in order not to produce a fiasco [von Bülow, 1900–1908d].

Four weeks later, he wrote to his mother from New York that his fatigue was so 'radical' that he had to stop and flee to New York in order to seek medical attention for his state that was described as 'nervous prostration' [von Bülow, 1900–1908e]. Thereafter, Hans von Bülow was unable to perform any artwork. He wrote to Louise von Welz: 'You cannot imagine the total disruption of my nervous capacities. I can only sit outside, I am barely able to walk, to talk, to read, to think,...' [von Bülow, 1900–1908f]. At the same time, in July 1876, the first Bayreuth Festival was to be opened, the event of a lifetime Hans von Bülow would have liked to attend and participate in as conductor. However, he had to stay away because of the tragic loss of his wife Cosima and of his friend and admired genius Richard Wagner; reflecting on this, he concluded in his letter to Louise von Welz: 'My mental state of exhaustion has become even worse, I am a mere animal shadow of my former self...' [von Bülow, 1900–1908g]. His mental state was so depressed that his doctors feared he had to be transferred to a mental asylum, had there not been his friend Hans von Bronsart who offered him care and company at his home in Hannover. From the symptoms and signs major depression would have been the modern diagnosis for this episode of incapacity to work that lasted for more than 500 days. Hans von Bülow went into a similar episode of severe depression, when he received the news of Richard Wagner's death in 1883. Stunned by this message, he uttered that with the 'Feuergeist' Wagner also his spirit had died, and that his body was a mere fragment from now on. The message came to him as such a severe shock that his mind was paralyzed, he fell into a deep depression, and he was subsequently unable to work as a pianist or conductor for 6 months.

Terminal Phase of Illness

The last year of Hans von Bülow's life was determined by various sufferings and multiple medical treatments. One major complaint was his 'Kopfgicht' and Hans von Bülow increasingly took to strong medications such as antipyrine, codeine, caffeine, cocaine, morphine, and bromide to overcome his headaches and insomnia. Apparently, he often used these drugs as self-medication, but they were also prescribed by the treating physicians, even during his stay from December 1892 to March 1893 in Pankow in the clinic of Dr. R. Gnauck, who was a specialist for nervous diseases and who practiced hypnotism [Vetter, 1994]. However, medical success was not achieved, and Hans von Bülow went to Berlin to receive therapy by the ear, nose, and throat (ENT) surgeon Dr. Wilhelm Fliess, who was a friend of Sigmund Freud and a protagonist of the new theory of nasal reflex neurosis. This theory claimed a causal relationship between the nasal turbinates and the genitals in women and men. As treatment, it suggested galvanic and chemical cauterizations of the nasal mucosa and even osteotomy of the nasal bone in order to cure headaches but also distant ailments of the genitourinary system, gastrointestinal tract, the lungs and heart [Vetter, 1994; Young, 2002]. Fliess operated on Bülow's nose, and he performed cauterizations in several sessions that Hans von Bülow reported to his wife as 'infernalement douloureuse' and leading to subsequent episodes of severe nasal bleedings [von Bülow, 1900–1908h]. After Marie von Bülow had made it known that she profoundly disagreed and was unhappy with this therapy, Fliess suggested a change of climate. Thus, Hans von Bülow traveled to St. Blasien in the Black Forest, where he was going to receive Brown-Séquard injections. These were injections of testicular extracts of dogs and guinea pigs that according to a report of a self-experiment of the distinguished French neurologist and physiologist Charles E. Brown-Séquard in 1889 had dramatic rejuvenating effects. However, even to the present day, androgen treatment in healthy middle-aged or elderly men has not convincingly shown positive effects on their well-being; furthermore, the extract according to the method of Brown-Séquard has recently been shown to have biologically inefficient levels of androgens [Cussons et al., 2002]. By intuition, Marie von Bülow seemed to have suspected that the injections were ineffective, since at her request they were replaced by placebo injections of distilled water [von Bülow, 1900–1908i]. But the painful occipital neuralgias persisted and Hans von Bülow moved to Aschaffenburg, where hypnosis, iodine and quinidine for the provisional diagnosis of malaria were administered. Eventually, the ophthalmologist Professor Michel from Würzburg was consulted and he made the diagnosis of Bright's disease of the kidneys. Bright's disease was a term used synonymously for 'glomerulonephritis' which at that time stood for any kind of kidney disease although it was already known through early work of the great French neurologist Jean-Martin Charcot, who died in 1893, that small kidneys were pathoanatomically associated with diseases of chronic duration and large kidneys with acute renal failure [Fogazzi, 1998]. Obviously, Professor Michel had found the characteristic retinal lesions of malignant arterial hypertension that were referred to as 'inflammatory' lesions of the retina. Later on, Hans von Bülow developed severe leg edema presumably due to albuminuria [von Bülow, 1900–1908i]. Already 2 years earlier, Hans von Bülow had reported repeated attacks of difficulties in breathing, suggestive of congestive heart failure, and continuous memory deficits suggestive of subcortical vascular encephalopathy, both being caused by arterial hypertension [von Bülow, 1900–1908j]. Although he had overcome pneumonia, Hans von Bülow's condition worsened in November 1893. He had heard of miraculous cures in Egypt and with his last strength he undertook his final journey to Cairo where he died 3 days after his arrival, on February 12, 1894. An autopsy was performed by Dr. P. Kaufmann, of which only a brief note in the appendix of Marie von Bülow's editions of Hans von Bülow's letters has been preserved. Kaufmann gave the final diagnosis: 'Chronic hemorrhagic nephritis with renal shrinkage, cardiac hypertrophy, bronchitis, bulbar paralysis? (to be examined microscopically)' [von Bülow, 1900–1908k]. The conserved brain was transported separately from Egypt to Frankfurt, where the neuropathologist and Professor of Anatomy

Dr. Ludwig Edinger performed the autopsy of the brain. He described severe atherosclerosis of all arteries, including arteries of middle caliber. He could not find the hemorrhage of the medulla oblongata that was described by Dr. Kaufmann, and he concluded that its site must have been on the cut surface where the brain was disconnected from the medulla for conservation. The bleeding must have been fresh and most likely was the immediate cause of death as no secondary changes were present in the tissue preparations. Tissue preparations of the cortex gave no clues to brain disease. Edinger assumed:

> ... that the extreme wall thickening of all cerebral and medullary arteries had certainly caused the states of exhaustion of the nervous system in the later years due to an abnormal blood supply.... The severely progressed sclerosis and calcification of the arteries frequently occur in professionals of mental occupations at this age and they easily progress amongst other processes to the kidneys [Edinger, 1900–1908].

He said that together with the tumor of the first two cervical roots of one side: 'the results of his investigations explained at least some of the symptoms Hans von Bülow suffered during his life while other phenomena of more psychologic interest remained unanswered' [Edinger, 1900–1908]. Today a new field of behavioral medicine has developed founding the basis for causal relationships between psychosocial stress factors and organic disease of the cardiovascular system. Chronic states of major depression are associated with an increased risk of cardiovascular disease or death, arterial hypertension and arteriosclerosis [Rozanski et al., 2005]. Even acute emotional stress can result in acute cardiac disease similar to a myocardial infarction mediated by sympathetic mechanisms [Wittstein et al., 2005]. This direction of causality is contrasted by frequent observations of depressive episodes after cerebral infarctions [Kronenberg et al., 2006]. Hans von Bülow himself always favored the idea that his tragic connection to Cosima and Richard Wagner was the source of the frailty of his health. At least, this situation was an ongoing factor of psychosocial stress in both his private and professional life. Apart from organic risk factors for stroke, factors of lifestyle may also have contributed to his cerebrovascular diseases such as the lack of physical exercise, smoking, nutrition at least during extensive traveling and perhaps even excessive work. Possibly, Professor Edinger alluded to these factors when he stated that: 'sclerosis and calcification of the arteries frequently occur in professionals of mental occupations at this age' [Edinger, 1900–1908].

Concluding Remarks

In modern terms, Hans von Bülow's diagnoses were occipital neuralgia due to a unilateral tumor (mesenchymal?) of the upper two cranial nerves; arterial hypertension with widespread atherosclerosis, subcortical vascular encephalopathy and recurrent brainstem strokes (final stroke/hemorrhage of medulla oblongata confirmed at autopsy); hypertensive kidney disease with chronic renal failure, and relapsing episodes of major depression and substance abuse. All his diseases resulted in prolonged or chronic states of impairment, and interactions between lifestyle and disease were most likely. Due to his most enduring character and enormous amount of self-discipline in conjunction with his brilliant education in arts and music from an early age, Hans von Bülow led an extremely productive and successful life as a conductor and pianist in the world of music of the 19th century in Europe and overseas. Modern medicine could certainly have provided more exact diagnoses during his lifetime and better treatment for Hans von Bülow, but it remains open to debate whether the interactions between the sufferings as a human being and the pursuit of perfect harmony in the art of music were prerequisites for his outstanding musical achievements.

References

Cussons AJ, Bhagat CI, Fletcher SJ, Walsh JP: Brown-Séquard revisited: a lesson from history on the placebo effect of androgen treatment. Med J Aust 2002;177:678–679.

Edinger L: Autopsy report of Hans von Bülow's brain; in von Bülow M (ed): Hans von Bülow Briefe. Leipzig, Breitkopf & Härtel, 1900–1908, vol 7, pp 490–492.

Fogazzi GB: Bright's disease and albuminuria as seen by the famous neurologist Jean-Martin Charcot. Nephrol Dial Transplant 1998;13:2407–2408.

Gaetani P, Di Ieva A, Di Rocco MG, Aimar E, Debernardi A, Tancioni F, Rodriguez y Baena R: Arnold's neuralgia caused by solitary fibrous tumor. Case report. J Neurosurg Sci 2004;48:49–53.

Haas F: Hans von Bülow – Leben und Wirken. Wilhelmshaven, Noetzel, 2002.

Krause T: Der Reichsbote, March 1892, No 76, suppl 2.

Kronenberg G, Katchanov J, Endres M: Poststroke-Depression – Klinik, Epidemiologie, Therapie, pathophysiologische Konzepte. Nervenarzt 2006;77:1176–1185.

Rozanski A, Blumenthal JA, Davidson KW, Saab PG, Kubzansky L: The epidemiology, pathophysiology, and management of psychosocial risk factors in cardiac practice – the emerging field of behavioral cardiology. J Am Coll Cardiol 2005;45:637–651

Vetter I: Hans von Bülows Irrfahrt durch die Medizin. Mit Briefen und anderen unveröffentlichten Zeugnissen aus seinem letzten Lebensjahr. Südthüringer Forschungen 28, Beiträge zum Kolloquium: Hans von Bülow – Leben, Wirken und Vermächtnis. Schweinfurt, Weppert, 1994, pp 100–118.

von Bronsart H: Letter to Hans von Bülow's brother-in-law Jan 1877; in Marie von Bülow (ed): Hans von Bülow Briefe. Leipzig, Breitkopf & Härtel, 1900–1908, vol 5, p 394.

von Bülow H: Letter to his mother 29.05.1875; in von Bülow M (ed): Hans von Bülow Briefe. Leipzig, Breitkopf & Härtel, 1900–1908a, vol 5, pp 268–269.

von Bülow H: Letters to Eugen Spitzweg, 23.10.1870 to 21.05.1871; in von Bülow M (ed): Hans von Bülow Briefe. Leipzig, Breitkopf & Härtel, 1900–1908b, vol 4, pp 434–483.

von Bülow H: Letter to Mr. and Mrs. v. Welz, Isle of Wight, 06.09.1875; in von Bülow M (ed): Hans von Bülow Briefe. Leipzig, Breitkopf & Härtel, 1900–1908c, vol 5, p 273.

von Bülow H: Letter to his mother, Cleveland, 27.04.1876; in von Bülow M (ed): Hans von Bülow Briefe. Leipzig, Breitkopf & Härtel, 1900–1908d, vol 5, p 362.

von Bülow H: Letter to his mother, 22.05.1876; in von Bülow M (ed): Hans von Bülow Briefe. Leipzig, Breitkopf & Härtel, 1900–1908e, vol 5, p 373.

von Bülow H: Letter to Mrs. v. Welz, Godesberg, 01.07.1876; in von Bülow M (ed): Hans von Bülow Briefe. Leipzig, Breitkopf & Härtel, 1900–1908f, vol 5, p 381.
von Bülow H: Letter to Mrs. v. Welz, Godesberg, 01.08.1876; in von Bülow M (ed): Hans von Bülow Briefe. Leipzig, Breitkopf & Härtel, 1900–1908g, vol 5, p 385.
von Bülow H: Letter to his wife, Berlin, 29.04.1893; in von Bülow M (ed): Hans von Bülow Briefe. Leipzig, Breitkopf & Härtel, 1900–1908h, vol 7, p 434.
von Bülow M: Letters to Toni Petersen; in von Bülow M (ed): Hans von Bülow Briefe. Leipzig, Breitkopf & Härtel, 1900–1908i, vol 7, pp 442–459.
von Bülow H: Letter to his wife, Schöneck, 20.07.1891; in von Bülow M (ed): Hans von Bülow Briefe. Leipzig, Breitkopf & Härtel, 1900–1908j, vol 7, p 340.
von Bülow M (ed): Hans von Bülow Briefe. Leipzig, Breitkopf & Härtel, 1900–1908k, vol 7, p 490.
Wittstein IS, Thiemann DR, Lima JAC, Baughman KL, Schulman SP, Gerstenblith G, Wu KC, Rade JJ, Bivalacqua TJ, Champion HC: Neurohumoral features of myocardial stunning due to sudden emotional stress. N Engl J Med 2005;352:539–548.
Young AR: Freud's friend Fliess. J Laryngol Otol 2002;116:992–995.

Prof. Dr. med. Johannes C. Wöhrle
Department of Neurology, Katholisches Klinikum, Marienhof/St. Josef gGmbH
Kardinal Krementz-Strasse 1-5
DE–56073 Koblenz (Germany)
Tel. +49 261 496 6445, Fax +49 261 496 6280, E-Mail j.woehrle@kk-koblenz.de

Bogousslavsky J, Hennerici MG (eds): Neurological Disorders in Famous Artists – Part 2.
Front Neurol Neurosci. Basel, Karger, 2007, vol 22, pp 206–222

Synaesthesia, the Arts and Creativity: A Neurological Connection

Catherine M. Mulvenna

Institute of Cognitive Neuroscience, University College London, London, UK

Abstract

For over 100 years the link between synaesthesia and the arts has attracted controversy. This has been spurred by the production of auditory, literary and visual art by famous individuals who report experiences synonymous with the neurological condition. Impressive protagonists in this discussion include Arthur Rimbaud, Charles Baudelaire, Vasily Kandinsky, Vladimir Nabokov, Alexander Scriabin, Olivier Messiaen and David Hockney. Interdisciplinary debates have concerned whether synaesthesia can actively contribute to an artist's ability, whether it is a driving force or a mere idiosyncratic quirk and whether, fundamentally, it is a distinct idiopathic condition or an unusual metaphorical description of normal perception. Recent psychological and neuroscientific evidence offers a new level to the debate. Coherent patterns of a neural basis of synaesthesia have been confirmed with high spatial resolution brain imaging techniques and the link with the arts is transpiring to be more than superficial or coincidental. Moreover, the neural distinction of the synaesthete brain may prove to be a window into a neural basis of creative cognition, and therefore conducive to the expression of creativity in various media.

Synaesthesia in the Arts

A question of much interest in these days is that of color hearing... repeatedly discussed in the daily press, literary and scientific reviews, medical theses... poetry, in romance and even in the theatre.

Alfred Binet, 1893

If you think you may experience synaesthesia or for more information go to www.icn.ucl.ac.uk/cmulvenna

For more information on the artists please go to www.rowan-hull.co.uk/ and www.soundingart.com/

'Colors are very important to me because I have a gift – it's not my fault, it's just how I am – whenever I hear music or even if I read music, I see colors.' He claimed peculiarities like 'the lower range of C-sharp was "copper with gold highlights", D flat was "orange with stripes of pale yellow, red and gold"'. [Duffy, 2001; Cytowic, 2002]

French composer *Olivier Messiaen*

'There are pale blue spots on the yellow glare. Only my eyes saw the pale blue spots. They did my eyes good. Why didn't anyone else?' [Kandinsky, 1981]

Russian painter *Vasily Kandinsky*

'Sounds are clothed in colors and colors in music.' [Baudelaire, 1971]

French symbolist poet *Charles Baudelaire*

'"B" has the tone called burnt sienna by painters… dull green, combined somehow with violet is the best I can do for "W".' [Nalokov, 1947]

Russian novelist *Vladimir Nabokov*

'The letter G is black with glints of yellow in it. I can't figure out why the yellow glints are there; it's just the way G looks.' [Duffy, 2001]

American writer *Patricia Lynne Duffy* (living classified synaesthete)

'I listened to *Dieu Parmi Nous* (God amongst us) and I thought it was wonderful... I could see dark blue's/orange and numerous complementary colours playing against each other.' [pers. commun.]

Mark Rowan-Hull (living classified synaesthete)

'The vibraphone… makes a round shape, each note is like a little gold ball falling. That's what the sound is, it couldn't be anything else.' [from Cytonic, 1993]

(living classified music-colour synaesthete)

'When I see equations, I see the letters in colours – I don't know why. As I'm talking, I see… light-tan j's, slightly violet-blueish n's and dark brown x's flying around. And I wonder what the hell it must look like to students.' [Feynman, 1988]

American Nobel Prize-winning physicist *Richard Feynman*

Fig. 1. Highly creative individuals over 100 years have been describing cross-sensory experiences highly indicative of synaesthesia.

Synaesthesia is certainly not a new phenomenon and has enjoyed uncommon topicality in both the sciences and the arts. The link to the latter is often fuelled by the seemingly peculiar comments made by highly creative individuals like those in figure 1. Much to the bewilderment of many of their contemporaries, these individuals all describe experiences highly indicative of music-colour and grapheme[1]-colour synaesthesia: when internally generated

[1]Letters and/or digits.

colours are experienced in consistent, automatic reaction to hearing music or verbalisations, or seeing graphemes.

In addition to anecdotal reports, we can observe synaesthesia playing a considerable active role in the history of visual art. Notably, between 1909 and 1914 Kandinsky produced a large group of abstractions on the theme of visual music. It is argued that he instigated the complex and revolutionary doctrine of abstraction based on synaesthesia. Examples of other painters labelling their works with reference to musical form were plentiful in this period (e.g. *Blue and Green Music* 1921, Georgia O'Keeffe; *Andante* 1908, Konstantinas Ciurlionis) and synaesthesia became a staple of Romantic and Symbolist schools of thought. Synaesthetic experiences began to be labelled the result of a heightened state of aesthetic awareness. Kandinsky maintained they were even indicative of a heightened state of spirituality. Thus, for a period, it was artistically and spiritually fashionable to experience synaesthesia and to not only represent it through ones work (be it painting, composing or poetry) but aim to generate a similar cross-sensory state in audiences [Van Campen, 1997]. In this context the term 'synaesthesia' became diluted to include cross-sensory experiences that were common to everyone and far from perceptually unusual. Instances of these include generalized matching of light colours to high notes and vice versa [for more examples see Marks, 1978], which is not considered what we now term 'developmental synaesthesia'. Therefore, while the individuals highlighted in figure 1 are an impressive group spanning 100 years of the arts and sciences, some inevitable questions present themselves: did they all have synaesthesia per se or were they describing typical cross-sensory fusion, or metaphor? Furthermore, even if they did, is the subsequent link between synaesthesia and the arts merely a coincidental bias in the media attending to these apparently eccentric comments of artists? (fig. 2).

In the following sections we shall outline the profile of synaesthesia drawn from psychological observation, recent neuro-imaging evidence of its neurological basis, and parallels with neural states known to be conducive to high creativity, acknowledging a new landmark in this century-long discussion. Additionally, synaesthesia was understood to be extremely rare but has recently been shown to occur in a remarkable 4% of the population [see Simner et al., in press]. We cannot formally test historical figures who may have had synaesthesia, but their reports can be reassessed in light of current evidence. The presence of synaesthesia continues in the contemporary arts. Furthermore, the propensity for different types of creativity between the synaesthete and non-synaesthete populations can now be investigated empirically.

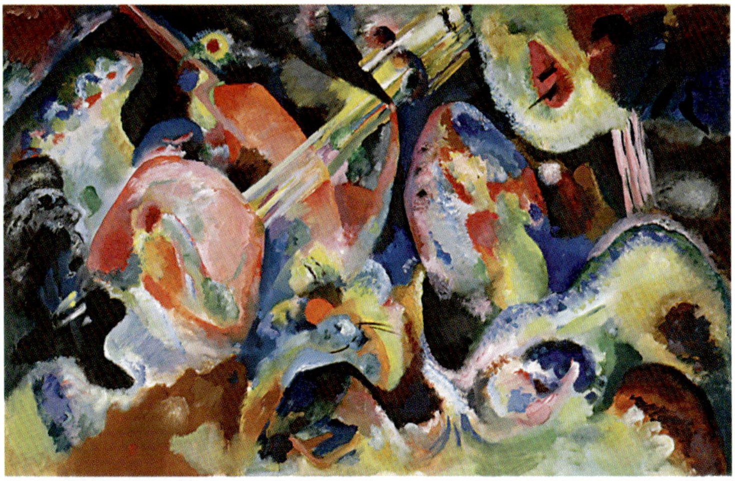

Fig. 2. Russian painter Vasily Kandinsky's *Flood Improvisation*, 1913, oil on canvas, Städtische Galerie im Lenbachhaus, Munich, Germany (with kind permission). Between 1909 and 1914 Kandinsky produced a large group of abstractions on the theme of visual music. It is argued that he instigated the complex and revolutionary doctrine of abstraction based on synaesthesia.

The Profile of a Synaesthete

One of these accounts sounds more wild and lunatic than the next[2].

Sir Francis Galton, 1883

The occurrence of developmental synaesthesia[3] will be indicated by several key factors. A healthy individual will report that particular stimuli (e.g. alphabetic letters or musical pitches) naturally but inexplicably trigger specific secondary sensations such as the experience of a colour or a taste in their mouths. Considerable attention has been drawn to music-colour synaesthesia, but the phenomenon can actually involve a crossing of experiences between or within the senses of vision, sound, touch, smell and taste. From the possible

[2]In Duffy [2001].

[3]Developmental synaesthesia, coined by Baron-Cohen et al. [1996], is the term given to naturally occurring synaesthesia that is present from birth and has the profile discussed here. It is distinguished from what others might call acute episodes of synaesthesia such as drug-induced or meditation-induced states of sensory fusion.

Song
A man sits in
A narrow ring,
A narrow ring
Of thinness.
He has no ear.
And doesn't have his eyeballs.
He cannot find
What's left behind
Of red sounds of the sun ball.
Whatever falls
Stands up again.
And what was dumb,
It sings a song.
Until the man,
Who has no ear,
And doesn't have his eyeballs,
Will start to find
Signs left behind
Of red sounds of the sun ball.

Fig. 3. A poem by Vasily Kandinsky in a collection entitled *Sounds* [Kandinsky, 1981, p. 110] (reprinted with kind permission from Elsevier). A cross-sensory poem offering the novel perspective of the confusion and frustration with which non-synaesthetes can be viewed. Note that Kandinsky believes determination and enlightenment can grant the 'eyeballs' of synaesthesia with time. This is a view not held by neuroscientists today, but it depicts the common feeling that the synaesthetic sensation feels both natural and obvious to the individual who experiences them, so natural it is hard to imagine how others do not experience them.

combinations of double sensations emerges distinct subtypes such as lexical-chromatic synaesthesia [the sight or sound of words will induce a sensation of colour, e.g. Baron-Cohen et al., 1987], lexical-gustatory synaesthesia [the sight or sound of words will induce a sensation of taste in the mouth, e.g. Ward and Simner, 2003] or pitch-chromatical synaesthesia (particular frequencies of sound will induce a sensation of colour). The extent to which synaesthesia is experienced in each individual can range from one strand of one subtype (e.g. the sight or sound of days of the week will induce colour sensations, but not other words) or be poly-synaesthetic with multiple subtypes [Mulvenna et al., 2004; Simner et al., in press].

The synaesthetic colour occurs automatically like a reflex [see Rich and Mattingley, 2002], illustrated by Messiaen's defensive claim of 'it's not my fault, it's just how I am'. It also occurs involuntarily in that the individual cannot consciously choose the second sensation – it can often be a colour or taste that they dislike. The synaesthetic colours are also characteristically specific for each individual. For instance, the sound of the name Rachel can induce 'black with red surrounding it' [Mulvenna, 2003] or a sequence of pitches can induce 'gold, yellow and white moving upwards and at an angle to the right, like a rippling stream' [Mulvenna and Walsh, 2005] (fig. 3). Likewise in figure 1, the colour descriptions from reputed synaesthetes in the arts are not general but highly particular, e.g. 'pale blue spots on the yellow glare', 'dull green, combined somehow with violet', 'copper with gold highlights'. This attention to

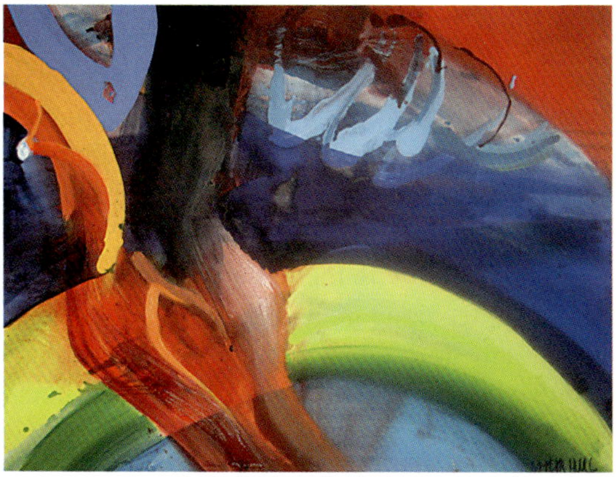

'I have always been aware that music and visual art are one and the same for me... I will listen to a piece of music over and over again... be aware of different colours and different shapes and when they come in. Then paint what I see.'

a

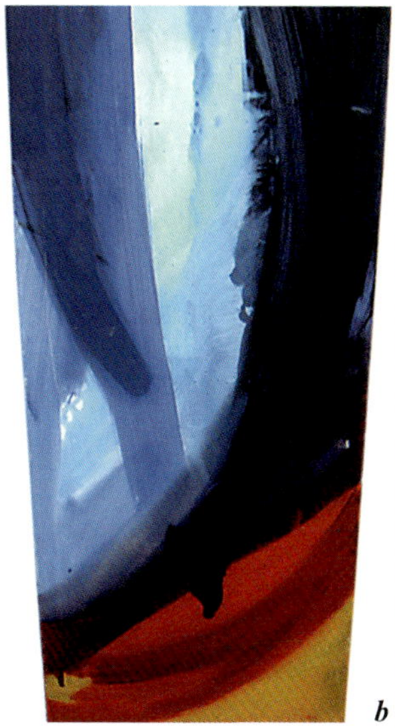

b

Fig. 4. ***a*** *Aloof, Aloft*, 2006, oil on canvas, 183 × 153 cm, collection of St. Hugh's College Oxford. ***b*** *Turangalîla ii*, 2005, oil on canvas, 183 × 46 cm, collection of the artist (reprinted with kind permission from the artist). Mark Rowan-Hull is a professional artist based in London. He automatically and consistently experiences moving coloured forms in response to musical auditory stimuli (tone-colour/form synaesthesia). Like most synaesthetes, there are parameters to his 'trigger' stimuli: He does not have visual experiences in response to general environmental sounds (generalized sound-triggered synaesthesia) or to the sound of the spoken word (phoneme-triggered synaesthesia), but namely for musical sequences.

detail is typical of synaesthetic experiences reported from Galton [1883] to Baron-Cohen et al. [1993], who demonstrated that even a colour matrix of over 250 colours could not sufficiently cover the specificity and variety of synaesthetes' colour descriptions.

Sense pairs can (and typically do) differ between synaesthetes, but within each synaesthete the exact sense pairs will remain consistent from early childhood and they will strongly resist suggestions to the contrary, typified in the synaesthetic comment above: 'That's what [colour] the sound is, it couldn't be anything else.' For instance, if Olivier Messiaen was a true synaesthete, the sound of D flat would never change from orange and yellow to green or blue. If an entire musical piece induces a complex series of specific moving colours and shapes, this will be reproduced unchanged every time the synaesthete hears that piece played with the same instruments. Modern artists with synaesthesia, such as Rowan-Hull and Mackay (see fig. 4), report listening to a piece over and over when painting it, in order to replicate on a physical canvas that they retrieve from their mental canvas.

Synaesthetes are not known to seek a 'cure' or report their experiences to a physician. They are an everyday, seemingly natural and often pleasant occurrence. In contrast to other neurological states, synaesthetic colours, for example, do not occur in acute episodes (epilepsy, migraine, Charles Bonnet syndrome, dementia with Lewy bodies), they do not appear to the synaesthete to have consciousness or try to communicate with them, do not appear to have been placed there by any external agent (schizophrenia-related hallucinations), are not psychedelic in appearance or appear to interact with external surroundings (drug-induced states), nor are they accompanied by any obvious detriments except in very rare extreme cases.

Since 1987 the first-pass behavioural method of formally classifying synaesthesia has focused on the consistency of sense pairs over time [Baron-Cohen et al., 1987]. When individuals are presented with 100 items (such as notes, letters or words) and report a second sensation that 'goes best' with it, synaesthetes' responses will be ~90% consistent over time (even when the second test is a not expected and is 1 year later) and non-synaesthetes will be ~30% consistent (even when a test of consistency is expected and tests are as little as 2 weeks apart). The perceptual strength of the synaesthetic colours withstands robust measures, such as applications of the Stroop test [see Rich and Mattingley, 2002].

A Neurological Movement in Synaesthesia Research

The neuroscientific evidence regarding synaesthesia both validates the behavioural reports and triggers a range of debates about the basis and consciousness of internally generated perceptions. Neuro-imaging techniques can be employed *during* the synaesthetic experience, including the high spatial resolution of functional magnetic resonance imaging (fMRI). The resultant data indicate that synaesthesia obeys the same rules as other conscious experiences in that it relies on neural activity in appropriate sensory cortical areas [Grossenbacher and Lovelace, 2001]. In other words, the synaesthetic brain behaves to a certain extent as if it were normally experiencing a vision of colour when the synaesthete reports it. This is comparable to evidence from more classically recognized conditions that involve visual hallucinations. For example, patients with Charles Bonnet syndrome experience sporadic involuntary episodes of complex visual hallucinations that also correlate with activity in the visual cortex [Ffytche et al., 1998].

Neural correlates of different subtypes of synaesthesia focusing on colour have been investigated, and consistencies have emerged involving activation of

V4, an area in the fusiform gyrus that is normally activated when an individual perceives colour [Zeki et al., 1991]. For phoneme-colour synaesthesia (the sound of words induce colours), V4 is active when synaesthetes' eyes are closed while listening to vocal words [Nunn et al., 2002]. No such activation is observed when the synaesthetes are listening to auditory stimuli that do not induce colour sensations (in this instance, auditory tones), nor in control participants. Furthermore, this activation withstands comparison to non-synaesthetes who are specifically trained to mentally associate colours with verbal words during fMRI [Nunn et al., 2002]. Such data differentiate the synaesthetic experience from forced colourful mental imagery. While the behaviour of associating sense pairs could be learned by the non-synaesthete, the neural sensory co-activation was not[4]. This indicates that, far from being fanciful with their vocabulary or visual imagination, synaesthetes have a distinctly and neurally driven, different experience to non-synaesthetes.

This activation of colour-sensitive areas during 'live' synaesthetic colour experiences has been replicated in different subtypes of the phenomenon and with different techniques. It occurs in synaesthetes who report colours for letters [e.g. Sperling et al., 2006; Weiss et al., 2005] and activation in the left dorsal visual stream (including Brodmann's areas 19, 7, 39 and 40) in synaesthetes who report colours for digits or numerical concepts [Elias et al., 2003], and subthreshold V4 with positron emission tomography for verbal words contrasted with auditory tones [Paulesu et al., 1995].

However, there is certainly complex additional activation during the synaesthetic experience that creates different possibilities concerning how the second (synaesthetic) sensation is internally generated. For example, secondary visual areas such as V4 are normally only activated after primary visual areas in the striate cortex, suggesting that the internally generated colours may follow different pathways than externally perceived colours. One possibility is a direct connection between the area corresponding to the trigger sensation (i.e. the letter or pitch that caused the synaesthesia) and the colour-sensitive area V4 (see fig. 5). The connection is either not used for this function in non-synaesthetes [Grossenbacher and Lovelace, 2001] or anatomically not present in non-synaesthetes [Ramachandran and Hubbard, 2001][5], or involves areas of normal

[4]More recently it has been shown that an auditory stimulus can elicit a response in visual cortex after classical conditioning. However, no explicit contrasting with synaesthetic co-activation was attempted, leaving it unclear whether this provides conflicting evidence for the comparability of synaesthesia with mental imagery [see Tanabe et al., 2005].

[5]The connections could be entirely absent or simply occur in less abundance in non-synaesthetes.

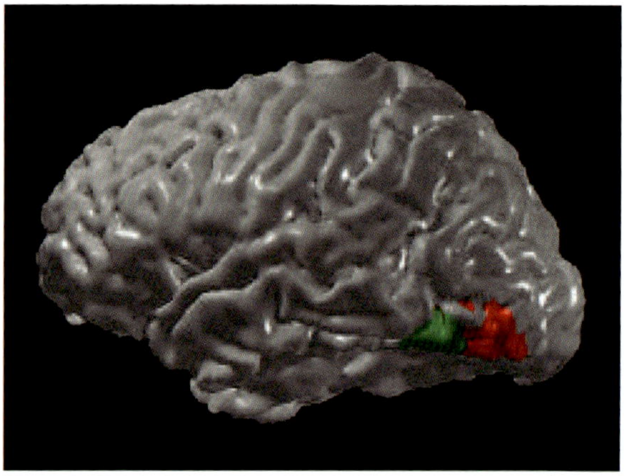

Fig. 5. Sensory cross-activation in the synaesthete brain. This schematic depicts the colour-sensitive area V4 (red) and the grapheme-sensitive area (green) adjacent to each other in the fusiform gyrus. These areas are thought to be cross-activated in grapheme-colour synaesthetes [Ramachandran and Hubbard, 2001] (reprinted with kind permission from Imprint Academic).

visual binding such as the intraparietal sulcus [Esterman et al., 2006; Mulvenna and Walsh, 2006]. This is one of the significant questions about synaesthesia that has recently made it a desirable model for investigating plasticity and variability of sensory integration in the normal brain. It inevitably leads to the issue of how these seeming 'extra connections' come to exist (fig. 6).

From behavioural tests on infants and more invasive techniques with neonatal hamsters and kittens, it is argued that all human infants up to around 4 months old naturally experience sensory input in an undifferentiated way: hyperdense interconnections temporarily exist between sensory systems in the brain before normal pruning processes enable them to be more distinct and specialized [Maurer, 1993]. Adult synaesthesia could therefore be the product of this sensory modularity never reaching typical maturity, through delayed apoptosis or a partial failure of the pruning process that naturally eliminates the neural connections or inhibits their usage [Baron-Cohen et al., 1993]. Synaesthesia is perhaps not the consequence of extra, 'synaesthetic' connections in the cortex, but rather an intriguing yet harmless perceptual marker of an early difference in sensory pruning and plasticity. This also suggests that, to a neurological extent, we were all synaesthetes in at least the first few months of life.

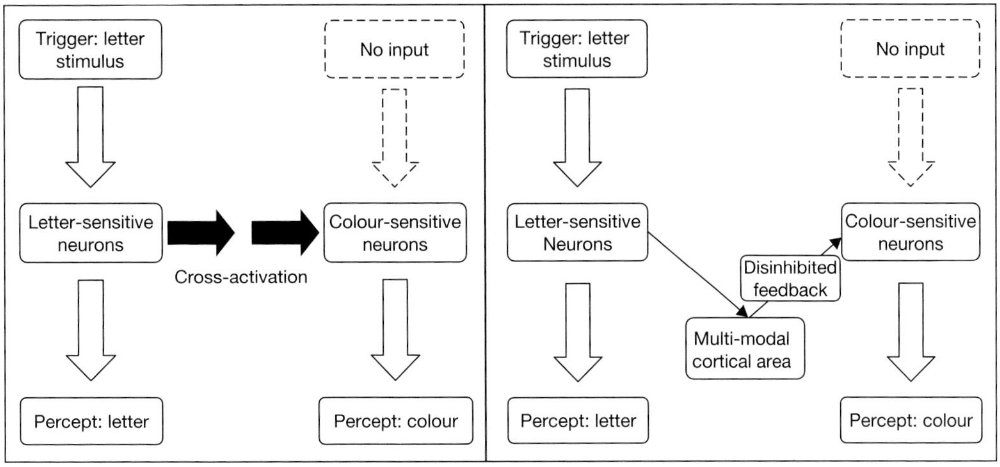

Fig. 6. How is the synaesthetic sensation internally activated? Synaesthesia involves co-activation of an externally generated sensation and an internally generated sensation. The exact connection between the cortical areas corresponding with the double activation is not known. Theories include (1) a *structural* difference of excess direct connections between neurons sensitive to the trigger stimulus and neurons sensitive to the secondary percept, and (2) a *functional* difference of abnormal communication to and from multimodal areas [from Mulvenna and Walsh, 2006] (reprinted with kind permission from Elsevier).

A Relationship between Synaesthesia and Creativity

Since Binet [1893] and Sokolov [1901] originally suggested that synaesthetes possessed a lively visual imagination and were more often than not artistic, investigations into this relationship have been ongoing. There is one obvious bias that lends itself to synaesthetes succeeding in creative pursuits: the continual inspiration provided by the automatic visual experiences that only they are privy to. Within the subtype of auditory-visual synaesthetes, famous examples such as Kandinsky, Hockney, Rowan-Hull and Mackay (see figs. 2, 4, 7) represent synaesthetes who are driven to portray their atypical visual experiences through visual art; they physically depict what they internally 'see'. In contrast, Messiaen (fig. 1) represents auditory-visual synaesthetes who are driven to compose music dictated by the aesthetics of the visual experiences the notes produce; they compose pieces by the colours and shades of the notes.

As discussed in the chapter by Pollak et al., pp. 75–88, this behaviour is not limited to synaesthesia. Individuals who develop dementia with Lewy bodies late in adulthood begin to experience highly complex visual and auditory hallucinations, sometimes accompanied with a drive to communicate them through artistic output such as visual art or poetry [e.g. Miller, 1998]. Indeed, this behavior is

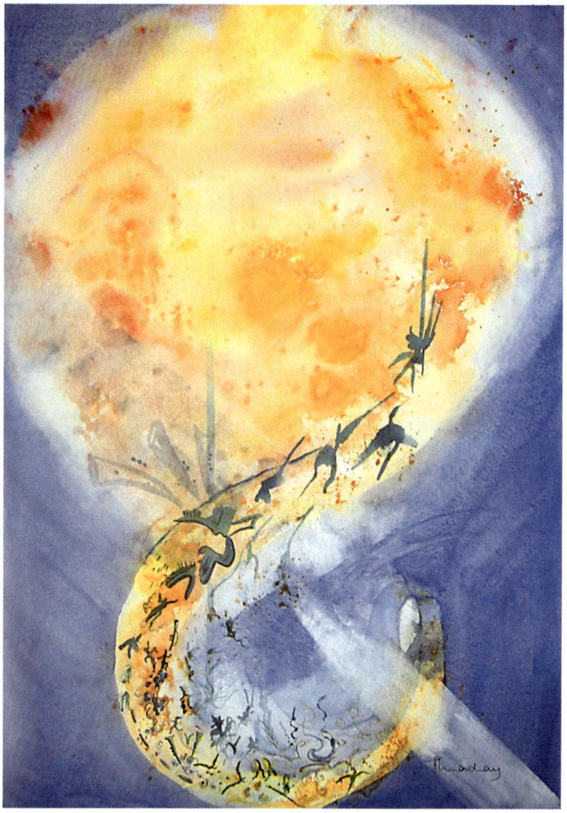

Fig. 7. Sound of the flute by synaesthetic artist Jane Mackay, 1993, watercolour on paper, 59 × 42 cm, held in private collection in Cambridge, painted from visual experiences responding to *Spring Symphony op. 44* by Benjamin Britten (reprinted with kind permission from the artist). It is suggested that what separates synaesthetic artists like Rowan-Hull and Mackay from other synaesthetes is that they possess the combination of specific mechanisms necessary for successful *creative ouput* in addition to the higher propensity for *creative cognition* that synaesthetes as a population benefit from [e.g. Mulvenna and Walsh, 2007]. A former medical practitioner and Artist in Residence with Cambridge University Musical Society, Mackay is now a professional artist whose work has attracted considerable media attention and is best known for her *Britten Series* paintings, over two hundred of which are distributed in collections worldwide. She reports her 'synaesthetic' images are a constant source of creative inspiration and, together with her love and knowledge of the classical repertoire, fundamental to her life as an artist.

actively encouraged for disorders such as schizophrenia, 'allowing exploration of the patient's inner world in a non-threatening way' [Ruddy and Milnes, 2005].

Therefore, a higher prevalence of synaesthetes among successful artists, poets and novelists [Dailey et al., 1997; Domino, 1989] may not be surprising:

they are frequently exposed to additional sensory inspiration yet do not suffer the detriments associated with the other neurological states discussed. The phenomenon could be used as a method of isolating and exploring mechanisms involved in the creative process.

Synaesthesia and Creative Cognition

A definitive criterion for creativity is a matter of ongoing debate that reaches far beyond the territory of synaesthesia. One fundamental division is between *creative cognition* [Finke et al., 1992; Smith et al., 1995] and *creative output* [e.g. Amabile, 1983, 1996]. *Creative cognition* involves the production of concepts through problem solving and idea generation, can be referred to as abstract/divergent thinking, and can undergo reliable empirical measurement. It can be successfully applied to a wide variety of lifestyles (e.g. from small business owners, to chefs, to plumbers, to charity fundraisers, to research scientists, to budgeting homemakers) and therefore does not rely on artistic pursuit. *Creative output*, on the other hand, focuses on the attempt to communicate such concepts through a medium in the arts. It relies on a culmination of specific mechanisms, including production-relevant skills (the motor skills to paint, the auditory skills for memory and differentiation between sounds etc), domain-relevant knowledge, and the intrinsic motivation to communicate through the secondary medium such as poetry, composition or painting. While anecdotal reports and examples of successful synaesthetes in the arts suggest that the synaesthete population has a higher incidence of *creative output*, empirical evidence suggests that the population difference lies instead in *creative cognition* abilities.

Synaesthetes as a group (n = 61) score significantly higher on reliable tests of divergent thinking compared to non-synaesthetes [Domino, 1989]. It has also been shown that individuals from the typical population (non-synaesthetes), who score higher in cognitive creativity tests involving conceptual association, also score higher in physiognomic tests consistently matching auditory tones and auditory vowels to colours [Dailey et al., 1997].

One argument for synaesthetes' higher creative thinking scores focuses on their awareness of belonging to a specialist group. However, studies have tested individuals who previously did not know they had synaesthesia, and still did not know during creative thinking tests.[6] For example, a large student population

[6]Often individuals with synaesthesia will believe the rest of the world has experiences just like they do. Among those who do realize this is not the case, very few are aware it is a recognized neurological phenomenon.

(n = 445) was randomly screened for synaesthesia and blindly tested on measures of divergent thinking and mental flexibility[7] *before* being classified as a synaesthetes. The scores on the tests were then compared to a group of non-synaesthetes from the same population who were matched for age, university attended, subject studied, year group, nationality, and remained naive to their synaesthetic/non-synaesthetic status. The study demonstrated that synaesthetes have a higher ability in divergent thinking than non-synaesthetes in the absence of knowledge of synaesthesia, and in the absence of creative output[8] [Mulvenna, 2003; Mulvenna et al., 2004].

The question poses itself: why would synaesthetes have this propensity for creative thought? Possible explanations range form social to cognitive to neural. Firstly, the awareness of having perceptual experiences atypical to the norm over a lifetime could predispose individuals with synaesthesia to conceptually divergent alternatives in the long term. However, this theory is compromised somewhat by the last piece of evidence involving synaesthetes with no previous awareness of the phenomenon.

A second possibility is that the cognitive processes underlying synaesthesia share faculties with the classic cognitive processes underlying creative thought. For instance, 'the ability to change things – to produce or even just to allow transformations – is central to the creative process' [Barron and Harrington, 1981]. Since as early as 1906 the capacity of thinking by analogy has been one of the fundamental examples of transformation. This juxtaposition of two concepts to encourage greater understanding of one (or both) can be directly paralleled to the spontaneous, neurally driven acceptance that the letter P is also 'dark green' or the sound of a particular musical note is also 'like gold balls dropping from the sky'. This ability to pair across senses could either predispose synaesthetes to the classic creative thinking processes of transformation and pattern formation or vice versa; such a process present in them could have driven the generation of synaesthetic experiences in early childhood. From current evidence the direction cannot be ascertained. However, such a transformational process is an automatic feature of the synaesthetic process and also underlies pursuits of high creative output (compositions, poetry or paintings) and creative cognition (urban planning, business innovation or mathematics).

[7]The Torrance Test of Creative Thinking measures six classic aspects of creative cognition for fluency, flexibility and originality during idea generation and problem solving.

[8]They were all students of literature or psychology.

The Neurology of Creative Thought and Synaesthesia

The third strand of explanations draws evidence from neuroscience, offering parallels between the neural co-activation/'modularity leakage' in the synaesthete's brain and the neurobiological basis of creative thought. For example, we have observed how synaesthetes have additional neural activation during the synaesthetic experience over and above activation involved in typical mental imagery. This may occur only during the synaesthetic experience, or may be one outward marker of a greater pattern of cross-modal activation across the cortex. For instance, the angular gyrus shows greater activation in synaesthetes [e.g. Weiss et al., 2005; Nunn et al., 2002], and consistent with its strategic location at the crossroads between the temporal, parietal and occipital lobes, is understood to serve in the function of cross-modal association. Indeed, a lesion in this area leads to an individual presenting with literal mindedness [Gardner, 1975] pointing to problems in metaphorical thought [Ramachandran and Hubbard, 2001].

Moreover, the synaesthetic co-activation in different sensory modes creates a de-focus of attention from just the trigger sensation to another sensation. Broadened cortical activation is also correlated with an increase in ideation productivity and, importantly, a decrease in 'fixation' that stunts creative thought in the typical population [Howard-Jones and Murray, 2003]. Electroencephalographic (EEG) evidence demonstrates an increase of anatomically distributed coherence of EEG oscillations during creative thought [e.g. Jausovec and Jausovec, 2000]. Potentially, this could explain how synaesthetes, who experience an excess co-activation in different areas of the cortex continually in everyday life, can have a propensity for high creative thinking abilities.

Further to broaden cortical activation, the synaesthete's brain is employing one network architecture in the brain to express another. To be exact, when a sound-colour synaesthete such as Kandinsky or Rowan-Hull (see figs. 2, 4, 7) processes the properties of acoustic stimulus, they will activate the typical networks involving acoustic processing. This will be observed in imaging techniques like fMRI, in the auditory cortex. However, they also employ, and to some extent 'borrow', part of the network architecture of visual processes, to treat colours as a property of the sound. This is demonstrated by activation in the colour-sensitive area V4 (and for some other sound synaesthetes, the visual areas associated with movement, V5, V3A) [Mulvenna et al., in preparation]. This is significant to the understanding of synaesthesia and creative cognition because the ability to use one network architecture to represent another is hypothesized to enable escape of constraints in the original network and lead to novel associations, solutions and subsequent innovative pattern formations [see Heilman and Nadeau, 2003].

To draw on a famous demonstration, Nobel Prize-winning physicist Richard Feynman created abstract visual representations of his theories which he then transformed into mathematical terms. The visual representations and their alternative architecture of networks supplied the basis of creative innovation by allowing the manipulative freedom to escape traditional mathematical formulae [Heilman and Nadeau, 2003]. Coincidently, Feynman was a digit-colour synaesthete. Therefore, in a separate but perhaps not unrelated way, he had a neural predisposition to employ properties of visual networks when processing digits (i.e. co-activation of grapheme and colour-sensitive areas in the fusiform gyrus). He was not directly *using* his synaesthesia when transforming complex visual representations into innovative mathematics, but the fact of his synaesthesia may be an outward marker of a neural capability to move between network architectures like this.

Conclusions

Synaesthesia is now undoubtedly recognized as a neurological phenomenon and a valuable method of investigating cross-sensory integration. The contemporary art world enjoys the ongoing presence of synaesthetic art produced by individuals who, unlike Kandinsky and Messiaen, can be reliably tested for developmental synaesthesia. Investigations are yet to conclude whether the phenomenon plays an active role in the drive or abilities necessary for successful *creative output*, or whether the apparent high incidence of synaesthetic artists is an illusory result of media bias. However, repeated investigations have found the synaesthetic population to have higher abilities in *creative cognition*. The cross-disciplinary approach of psychology and neuroscience offers parallels between the basis of synaesthesia and the neural correlates and cognitive processes involved in creative thinking. It gives new insight into the relationship between synaesthesia and creativity, and introduces a fresh debate of whether such cognitive strengths are related to the level of normal cross-modal activity in all individuals.

Acknowledgements

Sincere thanks to Mark Rowan-Hull, Jane Mackay, Professor Chris Frith, Patricia Lynne Duffy, Dr. Colleen McKenna, Professor Vincent Walsh, Dr. Edward Hubbard, Dr. Mike Dixon, Dr. Mark Lythgoe, and the synaesthete participants who made all of the research discussed possible.

References

Amabile TM: The Social Psychology of Creativity. New York, Springer, 1983.

Amabile TM: Creativity in Context. Boulder, Westview Press, 1996.

Baron-Cohen S, Harrison J, Goldstein LH, Wyke M: Coloured speech perception: is synaesthesia what happens when modularity breaks down? Perception 1993;22:419–426.

Baron-Cohen S, Wyke M, Binnie C: Hearing words and seeing colours: an experimental investigation of a case of synaesthesia. Perception 1987;16:761–767.

Baron-Cohen S: Is there a normal phase of synaesthesia in development? Psyche 1996;2:2.

Barron F, Harrington D: Creativity, intelligence and personality. Annu Rev Psychol 1981;32:439–476.

Baudelaire C: Artificial Paradise. New York, Herder & Herder, 1971.

Binet A: The problem of color hearing. The Chautaquan 1893;16:1447 (translated and reprinted from Revue des Deux Mondes).

Cytowic R: The Man Who Tasted Shapes. New York, Putnam, 1993.

Cytowic R: Synaesthesia: A Union of the Senses, ed 2. Cambridge, MIT Press, 2002.

Dailey A, Martindale C, Borkum J: Creativity, synesthesia, and physiognomic perception. Creativity Res J 1997;10:1–8.

Domino G: Synaesthesia and creativity in fine arts students: an empirical look. Creativity Res J 1989;2:17–29.

Duffy PL: Blue Cats and Chartreuse Kittens: How Synesthetes Color Their Worlds. New York, Henry Holt, 2001.

Elias LJ, Saucier DM, Hardie C, Sarty GE: Dissociating semantic and perceptual components of synaesthesia: behavioural and functional neuroanatomical investigations. Brain Res Cogn Brain Res 2003;2:232–237.

Esterman M, Verstynen T, Ivry RB, Robertson LC: Coming unbound: disrupting automatic integration of synaesthetic color and graphemes by TMS of right parietal lobe. J Cogn Neurosci 2006;18: 1570–1576.

Feynman R: What Do You Care What Other People Think? Further Adventures of a Curious Character. New York, Norton, 1988.

Ffytche DH, Howard RJ, Brammer MJ, David A, Woodruff P, Williams S: The anatomy of conscious vision: an fMRI study of visual hallucinations. Nat Neurosci 1998;1:738–742.

Finke RA, Ward TB, Smith SM: Creative Cognition. Theory, Research and Applications. Cambridge, Bradford/MIT Press, 1992.

Galton F: Inquiries into Human Faculty and Its Development. London, Dent, 1883.

Gardner H: The Shattered Mind: the Person after Brain Damage. New York, Knopf, 1975.

Grossenbacher PG, Lovelace CT: Mechanisms of synesthesia: cognitive and physiological constraints. Trends Cogn Sci 2001;5:36–41.

Heilman KM, Nadeau SE: Creative innovation: possible brain mechanisms. Neurocase 2003;9:369–379.

Howard-Jones PA, Murray S: Ideational productivity, focus of attention, and context. Creativity Res J 2003;15:153–166.

Jausovec N, Jausovec K: EEG activity during the performance of complex mental problems. Int J Psychophysiol 2000;36:73–88.

Kandinsky V (translation Napier ER): Spring 2; in Sounds. New Haven, Yale University Press, 1981.

Marks LE: The Unity of the Senses. New York, Academic Press, 1978.

Maurer D: Neonatal synesthesia: implications for the processing of speech and faces; in de Boysson-Bardies B, de Schonen S, Jusczyk P, McNeilage P, Morton J (eds): Developmental Neurocognition: Speech and Face Processing in the First Year of Life. Dordrecht, Kluwer Academic Publishers, 1993.

Miller BL, Cummings JL, Mishkin F, Boone K, Prince F, Ponton M, Cotman C: Emergence of artistic talent in frontotemporal dementia. Neurology 1998;51:978–982.

Mulvenna CM: The Relationship between Synaesthesia and Creativity; BA Dissertation, University of Glasgow, 2003.

Mulvenna CM, Hubbard EM, Ramachandran VS, Pollick F: Synaesthesia and creativity. J Cogn Neurosci Suppl 2004;16:188.

Mulvenna CM, Walsh V: Synaesthesia. Curr Biol 2005;15:R399–R400.
Mulvenna CM, Walsh V: Synaesthesia: supernormal integration? Trends Cogn Sci 2006;10:350–352.
Mulvenna CM, Walsh V: Synaesthesia and Cognitive Creativity. American Synesthesia Association Annual Meeting. University of South Florida, St Petersburg, 2007.
Mulvenna CM, Stewart L, Ward J, Griffiths T: Functional magnetic resonance imaging of auditory-kinetic colour synaesthesia. In preparation.
Nabokov V: Speak Memory. New York, Random House, 1947.
Nunn JA, Gregory LJ, Brammer M, Williams SCR, Parslow DM, Morgan MJ, et al: Functional magnetic resonance imaging of synesthesia: activation of V4/V8 by spoken words. Nat Neurosci 2002;5: 371–375.
Paulesu E, Harrison J, Baron-Cohen S, Watson J, Goldstein L, Heather J, Frackowiak J, Frith C: The physiology of coloured hearing: a PET activation study of colour-word synesthesia. Brain 1995;118:661–676.
Ramachandran VS, Hubbard EM: Synaesthesia – a window into perception, thought and language. J Conscious Stud 2001;8:3–34.
Rich AN, Mattingley JB: Anomalous perception in synaesthesia: a cognitive neuroscience perspective. Nat Rev Neurosci 2002;3:43–52.
Ruddy R, Milnes D: Art therapy for schizophrenia or schizophrenia-like illnesses (Cochrane Review). Cochrane Database Syst Rev 2005;4:CD003728. DOI:10.1002/14651858.CD003728.
Simner J, Mulvenna C, Sagiv N, Tsakanikos E, Whitherby SA, Fraser C, Scott K, Ward J: On segregation of the senses: when modularity breaks down. Perception, in press.
Smith SM, Ward TB, Finke RA: The Creative Cognition Approach. Cambridge, MIT Press, 1995, pp 327–335.
Sokolov P: L'individuation colorée. Rev Philos 1901;51:36–46.
Sperling JM, Prvulovic D, Linden DEJ, Singer W, Stirn A: Neural correlates of colour-graphemic synaesthesia: a fMRI study. Cortex 2006;42:295–303.
Tanabe HC, Honda M, Sadato N: Functionally segregated neural substrates for arbitrary audiovisual paired-association learning. J Neurosci 2005;25:6409–6418.
Van Campen C: Synesthesia and artistic experimentation. Psyche 1997;3:1–7.
Ward J, Simner J: Lexical-gustatory synaesthesia: linguistic and conceptual factors. Cognition 2003;89: 237–261.
Weiss PH, Zilles K, Fink GR: When visual perception causes feeling: enhanced cross-modal processing in grapheme-color synesthesia. Neuroimage 2005;28:859–868.
Zeki S, Watson JGD, Lueck CJ, Friston KJ, Kennard C, Frackowiak RSJ: A direct demonstration of functional specialization in human visual cortex. J Neurosci 1991;11:641–649.

Catherine M. Mulvenna
Neuropsychologist
Institute of Cognitive Neuroscience, University College London
17 Queen Square
London WC1N 3AR (UK)
Tel. +44 20 7679 1128, Fax +44 20 7813 2835, E-Mail c.mulvenna@ucl.ac.uk

Bogousslavsky J, Hennerici MG (eds): Neurological Disorders in Famous Artists – Part 2.
Front Neurol Neurosci. Basel, Karger, 2007, vol 22, pp 223–235

The Hallucinating Art of Heinrich Füssli

Christian Baumann[a], *Franziska Lentzsch*[b], *Marianne Regard*[a], *Claudio Bassetti*[a]

[a]Department of Neurology, Universitätsspital Zürich and
[b]Kunsthaus Zürich, Zürich, Switzerland

Abstract

Der Nachtmahr (*The Nightmare*) was painted 1781 by the Swiss-born artist Heinrich Füssli (1741–1825). Neurologists, sleep medicine specialists and sleep researchers are familiar with this popular work, which became a symbol for the phenomenon of sleep paralysis. Notably, Füssli created this work decades before the first scientific description of the syndrome. Therefore, the following chapter aims to reflect the painting against the background of Füssli's biography, neuropsychological interpretations, and of pathophysiological and neurobiological considerations on sleep paralysis.

Der Nachtmahr (*The Nightmare*), painted in 1781 by the Swiss-born artist Heinrich Füssli (in England, he was called Henry Fuseli), is a hallucinating – dramatic, weird, insinuating, confusing – painting that cannot be forgotten easily (fig. 1). The artist portrays a woman with pale and shimmering skin, lying on her back on a divan, her head and arms hanging over the edge. The lady suffers from the burden of an incubus sitting on her chest, smirking maliciously at the viewer. A horse with ghostly eyes pushes his head through the ponderous curtains behind her, smothering the boudoir scene in a spooky atmosphere. Füssli obviously succeeded in depicting all the hallmarks of sleep paralysis with hypnagogic hallucinations. This painting, in its combination of dream and sexual drive, eroticism and demonic aspects, shocked the public when it was presented for the first time at the annual exhibition at the Royal Academy in London (1782). On the other hand, this scandal made Füssli famous, also because of the subsequent wide diffusion of replications of the painting. From this very moment on, Füssli was known worldwide as an eccentric artist. Until today *Der Nachtmahr* is one of the most interpreted paintings in the history of art. Later

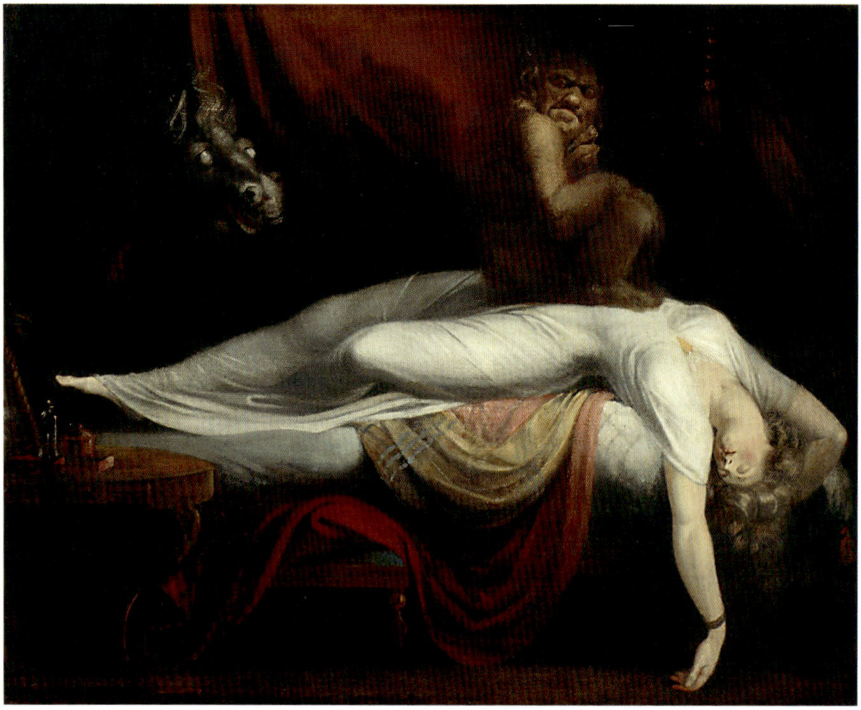

Fig. 1. *Der Nachtmahr (The Nightmare)* (1781), oil on canvas, 101 × 127 cm. Founders Society Purchase with funds from Mr. and Mrs. Bert L. Smokler and Mr. and Mrs. Lawrence A. Fleischman. Photograph copyright 2005, The Detroit Institute of Arts (with kind permission).

on, the work became a symbol for the sleep-wake disorder narcolepsy. Who was the artist creating such a thrilling painting, and – to the best of our knowledge – who was the first to depict sleep paralysis? Did he suffer from sleep paralysis, or from narcolepsy? If not, where did his inspiration come from? The aim of this work is to examine the art and character of Füssli in the light of the current understanding of sleep paralysis and narcolepsy.

Biography

Heinrich Füssli was born in Zürich in 1741 [Knowles, 1831; Lentzsch et al., 2005; Schiff, 1973]. Many generations of his family were active in various artistic sectors. Füssli's talent, his interest in and his passion for the arts was noticed very early – nonetheless his parents forbade him to become a painter.

His elder brother Rudolf followed in his father's footsteps – he was a well-known painter of portraits, and wrote famous books on art. For Heinrich, on the other hand, an intellectual education, and the very popular studies of theology were arranged. During his studies, Füssli became familiar with the circle of men of letters around Johann Jacob Bodmer, who greatly inspired German intellectual society, and formed Füssli's personality and spirit. In 1761, Füssli's first sermon as a pastor – about the vice of curiosity – constituted the end of his theological career. His ingenuous and impetuous character and his thinking of being able to cure the world's ills prompted him – together with his friends Johann Caspar Lavater and Felix Hess – to write a pamphlet denouncing a corrupt provincial governor, who was subsequently drummed out of town. But this had repercussions for him: Füssli and his friends were forced to leave Switzerland. They stayed a couple of months in Germany, where they interacted with intellectuals such as Johann Joachim Spalding and Johann Georg Sulzer. During this stimulating period, Füssli became convinced that emigrating entirely would be more advantageous to his further development and intellectual growth than going back to Zürich.

In 1764, Füssli, protégé of Andrew Mitchell, the English ambassador in Berlin at that time, traveled to London with influential recommendations. Andrew Mitchell introduced him to numerous persons of great significance for his future career. Thus, he was soon known as a somebody conversing ingenuously and eloquently with an extravagant style and remarkable poise (fig. 2).

In London, he spent 6 unsteady years as a man of letters, critic and translator with moderate success, but he also continued to draw and carry out commissions as an illustrator. The metropolis offered him a new world. The London theater scene influenced him, especially the actor and director of the Drury Lane Theatre, David Garrick, who revolutionized the art of acting by breaking with the traditional, classical and rigid style, by introducing and adopting a style regarded as realistic and natural. This style – full of emotions, facial expressions and gestures – clearly influenced Füssli's drawings. Encouraged by Joshua Reynolds, the President of the Royal Academy, and financially supported by his friend, the banker Thomas Coutts, he left London in 1770 and traveled to Rome for further artistic education. In Michelangelo, he found an example and also the justification for his artistic concept which was based on heroic and exaggerated expressions. In 1779, returned to London via Zürich. In London, finally, his mannerism in life and in art became widely accepted: his expressive and exaggerated figures, sometimes extremely fashionable and with extravagant coiffures, the daring poses which are supposed to turn into the grotesque, the subjectively interpreted emotional scenes which strived after originality, ignoring iconographic traditions, the conspicuous compositions without embellishment, erotic scenes – all these factors suddenly turned out to

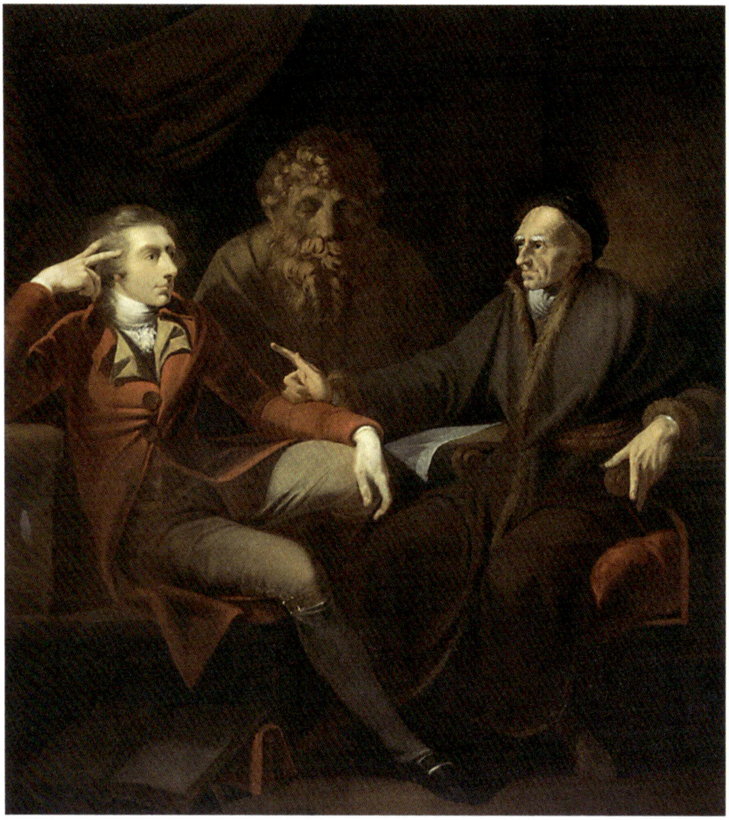

Fig. 2. Bodmer and Füssli with a bust of Homer (1778–1780), oil on canvas, 163 × 150 cm. Kunsthaus Zürich (with kind permission).

make his art sensational. Even though he was a foreigner, he was soon a well-known and popular illustrator of Shakespeare's scenes.

In 1790, Füssli became a full member of the Royal Academy. In 1801, he was elected a professor, and in 1804, he even became Keeper of this famous institution. As he was very liberal, and as he accepted many ideas and inspirations, Füssli was a popular professor among his students – not least because of his intellect and thorough knowledge in different areas. For Füssli, this position meant primarily a secure livelihood, allowing him to put his ideas into practice even if he had no special commission for them.

As much as Zürich and the years in Rome were important for Füssli's understanding and perception of art, London was crucial for his career. This city which was economically and socially advanced was also inspiring for artists. There was no court dictating the arts, and no tradition to obstruct creativity. At this time, and until the late 18th century, English artists were focussed on portraying and landscape painting. Füssli's close relations to the intellectual society of London, and his knowledge of world literature – he knew in details the works of Homer and Dante, he read meticulously the *Nibelungenlied*, the works of Shakespeare, Milton, as well as of contemporary English writers – helped him to realize his very personal ideas in his paintings. The overcrowded annual exhibitions at the Royal Academy advanced his obsessive genius, his urge to attract attention, and to stand out of mediocrity [Riding, 2006]. *Der Nachtmahr* was the first successful work to achieve these aims. Later, Füssli painted other versions of *Der Nachtmahr*, which proves his serious interest in this topic.

With his works, however, Füssli failed to conquer the English art market. But the development of his individual style led to a brilliant academic career up to the second highest position at the Royal Academy, and guaranteed him a lasting presence in the English art world. Füssli was a healthy person until he died at the age of 84 in 1825. He was buried with much pomp in London's St. Paul's Cathedral.

Heinrich Füssli and Der Nachtmahr from a Neurological Perspective

Neurologists, sleep medicine specialists and sleep researchers are familiar with Füssli's most famous painting, which became a symbol for the phenomenon of sleep paralysis [Schneck, 1969]. Various aspects of medicine have long been represented in art, frequently prior to scientific descriptions. Similarly, Füssli outlined parts of the narcoleptic syndrome in his most famous painting (1781) decades before the first scientific descriptions of sleep paralysis [Binns, 1842] and narcolepsy [Westphal, 1877; Gélineau, 1880].

Füssli labeled his painting *Der Nachtmahr* (*The Nightmare*). In the English tradition, 'mare' stands for a demon as well as for the female horse. Therefore, and as the horse is an old symbol of sexuality, the painting often has been interpreted to allegorize demonic sexual connotations. Also, the incubus has been interpreted to have intercourse with his female victim. In ancient northern German popular belief, however, the Nachtmahr was a sinister night ghost that sits on the chest of sleeping men and causes anxiety. The suffix 'mare' in nightmare is possibly derived from 'maren', which means 'to crush'. Thus the nightmare would be the night crusher. This would suggest that the term nightmare might have been originally coined to describe sleep paralysis with hypnagogic or hypnopompic hallucinations rather than bad dreams during sleep.

Füssli's painting obviously shows significant elements of sleep paralysis and hypnagogic hallucinations, including paralysis, hallucination, sleep, and breathing disturbances. All these elements have been described meticulously [Cheyne, 2001, 2002; Cheyne et al., 1999]. At the center of the painting there is a limp (paralyzed) supine and evidently helpless woman half asleep, with a demonic goblin sitting heavily on her chest, thus interfering with her respiration, and a horse in the background of the painting peering out from behind a dark curtain, indicating a visual hallucination. The painting clearly depicts the sensations of weight and constriction contributing to the feeling of suffocation and anxiety. An impressive artistic description of sleep paralysis with hypnopompic hallucinations is found in Guy de Maupassant's *Le Horla* [de Maupassant, 1886; Schneck, 1994]:

> … I sleep, for a while, two or three hours – then a dream, no, a nightmare seizes me in its grip, I know full well that I am lying down and that I am asleep … I sense it and I know it … and I am also aware that somebody is coming up to me, looking at me, running his fingers over me, climbing on my bed, kneeling on my chest, taking me by the throat and squeezing … with all its might, trying to strangle me. I struggle, but I am tied down by that dreadful feeling of helplessness which paralyzes us in our dreams. I want to cry out, but I can not. I want to move – I can't do it. I try, making terrible, strenuous efforts, gasping for breath, to turn on my side, to throw off this creature who is crushing me – but I can not! Then, suddenly, I wake up … I am alone.

In clinical terms, sleep paralysis can be defined as a period of inability to perform voluntary movements at the onset of sleep or on awakening, while the sufferer can recall every detail of the surroundings. Vivid hallucinoid experiences often accompany sleep paralysis. Patients frequently report feeling a 'presence' that is often described as malevolent, threatening, or evil.

Ohayon et al. [1999] found a prevalence of 6–7% for sleep paralysis (sample size: n = 494). Other studies found even higher prevalence rates [Fukuda et al., 2000; Cheyne et al., 1999]. Chronic sleep deprivation (today referred to as behaviorally induced insufficiency sleep syndrome) is associated with sporadic (isolated) sleep paralysis. Sleep paralysis may be genetic in some cases (familial form) or associated with psychiatric disorders. Several studies found an association of sleep paralysis with mental disorders such as bipolar and anxiety disorders [Ohayon et al., 1999; Otto et al., 2006]. Rosenthal [1939] described an association between schizophrenia and sleep paralysis. Finally, sleep paralysis occurs as one of the symptoms of narcolepsy, which also comprises excessive daytime sleepiness (typically leading to involuntary naps and sleep attacks), cataplexy (sudden bilateral loss of muscle tone, provoked by strong emotions such as laughter or anger) and hypnagogic/hypnopompic hallucinations [Bassetti and Aldrich, 1996]. The latter are defined as visual, auditory, proprioceptive, and tactile hallucinations, as well as out-of-body experiences, which occur at sleep onset (hypnagogic) or on waking up (hypnopompic), and last for a few seconds to minutes. Also in narcolepsy, sleep paralysis and hallucinations often appear concurrently. Only a minority of narcoleptic patients develop the full tetrad, whereas isolated symptoms of the tetrad may also occur in healthy nonnarcoleptic individuals.

The pathophysiology of sleep paralysis is still not exactly known. Historically, sleep paralysis has been linked to rapid eye movement (REM) sleep states, because they both share elements such as muscle atonia and dreaming [Hishikawa and Kaneko, 1965]. Sleep paralysis is often associated with vivid, terrifying multimodal, and sometimes elaborate nightmare hallucinations [Cheyne, 2005]. It can, however, not be put on par with REM sleep intrusions into wakefulness. REM in association with nightmares differs from dream-related REM in that there is no loss of waking consciousness, and no or only little blocking of exteroceptive stimulation [Hishikawa, 1976]. In a recent study, Girard and Cheyne [2006] hypothesized whether sleep paralysis may sometimes reflect the maintenance of REM sleep consciousness when waking, and whether associated hallucinations may be a continuation of dream experiences into waking life. Thus, sleep paralysis may also result from failure to maintain sleep during REM sleep periods. The disintegration of different sensory systems is another theory for the pathophysiology of sleep paralysis. A failure of integrating proprioceptive, tactile and visual information has been hypothesized to underlie out-of-body experiences and autoscopy, which are also common phenomena of sleep paralysis with hallucinations [Blanke et al., 2004; Cheyne, 2005].

Similarly, the underlying neurobiological processes are not yet known: Cheyne et al. [1999] postulated an involvement of brain stem- and thalamus-induced activation of amygdala and anterior cingulate underlying hallucinations, and paralysis of the major antigravity muscles underlying feelings of suffocation, as the thoracic contribution to breathing is lower during REM sleep, and hypotonia can result in increased airflow resistance. In the same study, they postulated that central features of this neurobiological model of sleep paralysis are consistent with studies on schizophrenia-associated hallucinations [Silbersweig et al., 1995].

It is not known where Füssli's inspiration for this masterwork came from. Did he himself suffer from sleep paralysis or narcolepsy or rather somebody he knew? According to studies of experts in art history, almost all of Füssli's paintings could be traced back to historical or literary sources, but not *Der Nachtmahr*, which he painted several times at different periods. As he often depicted scenes from William Shakespeare's plays, he might have taken his inspiration from Mercutio's Queen Mab speech in *Romeo and Juliet* (probably 1591) [Shakespeare, 1967]:

Drums in his ear, at which he starts and wakes,
And being thus frighted, swears a prayer or two,
And sleeps again. This is the very Mab,
That plaits the manes of horses in the night,
And bakes the elf-locks in foul sluttish hairs,
Which once untangled much misfortune bodies.
This is the hag, when maids lie on their backs,
That presses them, and learns them first to bear,
Making them women of good carriage.

Nonetheless, because of the facts that (1) Füssli's painting goes much more into (clinically correct) details of sleep paralysis than previous descriptions of writers, and that (2) his repeated occupation with this topic may be interpreted as an outstanding personal interest, we believe that inspirations other than Shakespeare must be considered.

In various biographies and numerous letters [Muschg, 1942; Weinglass, 1982; Bircher and Guthke, 1973; Mason, 1944; Lentzsch et al., 2005], there is no evidence that Füssli might have suffered from sleep paralysis, hypnagogic/hypnopompic hallucinations or narcolepsy. He never alluded to sleepiness at daytime or to increased sleep need. On the contrary, Füssli seemed to work day and night without resting or sleeping. He describes his almost addictive attitude towards writing, which is associated with a lack of need for sleep, for instance, in a letter to his friend Lavater (November 13, 1763): 'It is midnight – I should go to bed – but sleep is not mandatory for me because of you. I do not feel my body – how many pages haven't I filled with sweet palaver, which is the true sign of affectionate friendship' [Muschg, 1942]. Furthermore, in his biography and letters, we found just as little evidence for sleep paralysis or narcolepsy in Füssli's friends or relatives.

A Neuropsychological Interpretation

The graphic collection of Heinrich Füssli in the Kunsthaus Zürich is testimony of the productive artist already as a young boy. His drawings at the age of 10 and older show a strong attraction to themes and figures from ancient mythology and a high interest in famous literary works. In one of his drawings, an artist sitting in front of big body parts is 'in despair over the grandeur of Antique remains'. A huge foot and, more interestingly, a right hand can be seen (fig. 3). Who could ever draw a right hand if not with his left while observing his right hand? This and the hatching in many of his drawings (see for example fig. 4) descending from the left to the right [Lanthony, 1995] suggest that Füssli may have used his left hand to draw. Left-handedness, if not so-called familial, is often associated with a number of neurological signs and symptoms related to

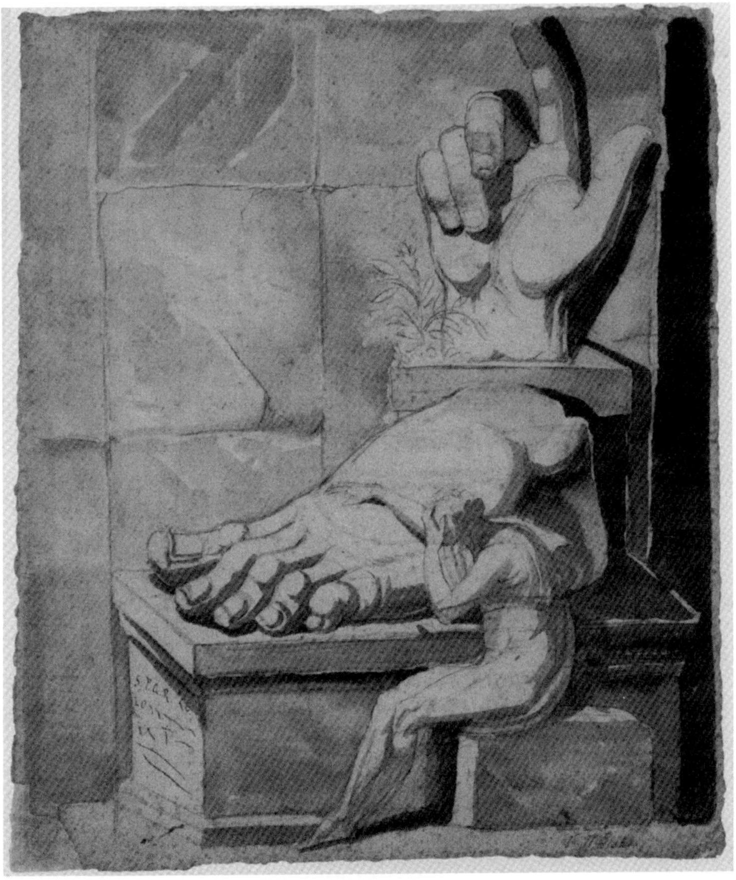

Fig. 3. The artist in despair over the grandeur of Antique remains (1778–1780), red chalk and brown wash, 42 × 36 cm. Kunsthaus Zürich (with kind permission).

cerebral dysfunctions. These are acquired early in life, at birth or during pregnancy, and typically, disturb or delay the development of left-hemispheric functions [Geschwind and Galaburda, 1985]. Following this line of thought, Füssli's handwriting (most likely the product of his right hand) and other verbal skills may not be as impressive as his visual artistic skills as a painter. Left-handed men have been shown not only to have symptoms of a weak immune system, a heightened risk of developing addictions and other neuropsychiatric signs, but frequently dyslexic problems including poor orthography. His writings written in 'Kurrentschrift' (italic fonts, see for example fig. 5) contained errors and many corrections [see comments by Muschg 1942, p. 42; by Bircher and Guthke, 1973, pp. 105, 119] and he was not a gifted poet. Assuming that

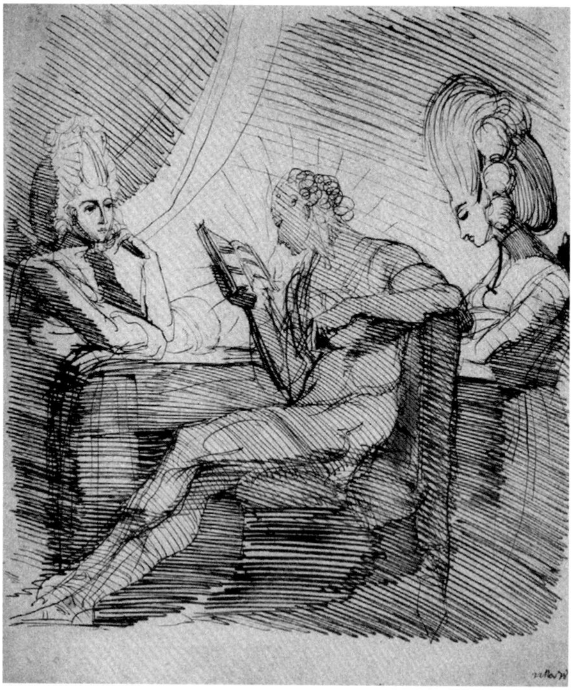

Fig. 4. Füssli reading to the Hess sisters (1778), pen, 36.4 × 30.9 cm. Kunsthaus Zürich (with kind permission).

Füssli was not a 'regular' right-hander, he should be gifted in nonverbal skills such as the visual arts or mathematics and may, besides writing problems, have other handicaps or oddities be it in the motor, cognitive or behavioral domain. In his letters to Lavater for example, one finds aspects of a somewhat diminished control of impulses. He lacked respect of authorities and was not shy to criticize others while pointing out his own superiority [Muschg, 1942]. He seems to have been rather small in stature, always on the go, in his own words, restless. His contemporaries perceived him as eccentric. He was careful in the way he dressed and was obviously powdering his hair. Besides becoming a famous painter, many of his works have a daring erotic content. His letters reflect that Füssli was a socialite and befriended a number of, sometimes controversial, men of his time. Women are hardly mentioned and seem to have played a minor role in his life. He married only at age 47. Because his works present women as macabre or dominating men, it has been concluded that he was a misogonist. About a bisexual woman friend, who approached him and his wife, Füssli said: 'I hate clever women, they are only troublesome.' Men, on the other hand, were often painted nude and muscular. Johann Caspar Lavater wrote

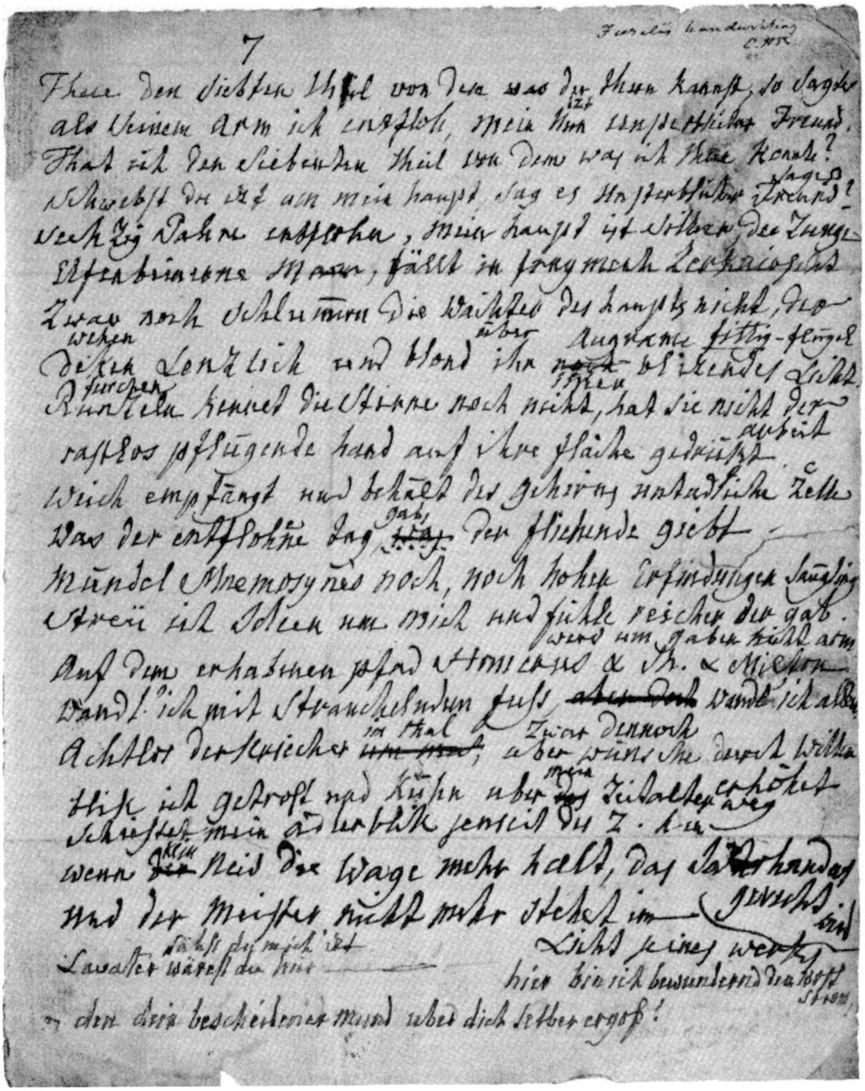

Fig. 5. Autograph of Füssli: Poem No. 40 [Bircher and Guthke, 1973].

of Füssli: 'Specters, demons and madmen's phantoms, exterminating angels; murders and acts of violence – such are his favorite subjects; yet, I repeat, no one loves with more tenderness' [Mason, 1951]. He may have been gay, at least in mind, another sign associated with a higher incidence of left-handedness [Maidment, 2001; Lalumiere et al., 2000]. Although he grew up in a family of artists and was surrounded by inspiring contemporaries, some of Füssli's behavioral manifestations suggest 'impulsive nonconformity' [Nettle, 2006], today better known as part of a hyperactivity syndrome or schizotypy related to minimal brain dysfunction, of unknown origin. In line with this notion is his obsessive interest in entomology. On a trip to the Binn Valley in southern Switzerland to study minerals and insects and accompanied by his wife Sophia Rawlins and his friend, the British painter William Blake, as he once wrote in a letter to Blake, he was experiencing mysterious bizarre sounds of unknown dancing creatures. It may well be that such experiences coming from strong imagination, hallucinatory proneness and magical ideation inspired his paintings. It is likely that his schizotypical thinking and perception of the world was enhanced by his lack of sleep and the drugs he used but this is subject of further studies.

In conclusion, the source of Füssli's inspiration for his famous painting *Der Nachtmahr* and his work in general remains elusive. There are three arguments in favor of the hypothesis that Füssli himself might have suffered from sleep paralysis with hallucinations. First, his depiction of sleep paralysis and its associated features was very appropriate in clinical terms. To the best of our knowledge, there was no comparably correct description in the world literature, which was the inspiration for most of his paintings. Second, his devotion to this topic clearly exceeds his interest in other themes, for he created several versions of *Der Nachtmahr*. Third, epidemiologic considerations, his chronic sleep deprivation, and his personality with schizotypical traits corroborate the hypothesis that Füssli himself might have had first-(left) hand information on sleep paralysis.

References

Bassetti CL, Aldrich MS: Narcolepsy. Neurol Clin 1996;14:545–571.

Binns E: The Anatomy of Sleep; or the Art of Procuring a Sound and Refreshing Slumber at Will. London, Churchill, 1842.

Bircher M, Guthke KS: Johann Heinrich Füssli. Sämtliche Gedichte. Zürich, Orell Füssli, 1973.

Blanke O, Landis T, Spinelli L, Seeck M: Out-of-body experience and autoscopy of neurological origin. Brain 2004;127:243–258.

Cheyne JA: The ominous numinous. Sensed presence and other hallucinations. J Consciousness Stud 2001;8:1–18.

Cheyne J: Situation factors affecting sleep paralysis and associated hallucinations: position and timing effects. J Sleep Res 2002;11:169–177.

Cheyne JA: Sleep paralysis episode frequency and number, types, and structure of associated hallucinations. J Sleep Res 2005;14:319–324.

Cheyne JA, Newby-Clark IR, Rueffer SD: Relations among hypnagogic and hypnopompic experiences associated with sleep paralysis. J Sleep Res 1999;8:313–318.

Cheyne JA, Rueffer SD, Newby-Clark IR: Hypnagogic and hypnopompic hallucinations during sleep paralysis: neurological and cultural construction of the night-mare. Consciousness Cogn 1999;8: 319–337.

de Maupassant G: Le Horla. Paris, Editions Gallimard, 1886.

Fukuda K, Ogilvie RD, Takeuchi T: Recognition of sleep paralysis among normal adults in Canada and in Japan. Psychiatry Clin Neurosci 2000;54:292–293.
Gélineau JBE: De la narcolepsie. Lancette Française (Gazette des Hôpitaux Civils et Militaires) 1880;53:626–628.
Geschwind N, Galaburda AM: Cerebral lateralization. Biological mechanisms, associations, and pathology. II. A hypothesis and a program for research. Arch Neurol 1985;42:521–552.
Girard TA, Cheyne JA: Timing of spontaneous sleep-paralysis episodes. J Sleep Res 2006;15:222–229.
Hishikawa Y: Sleep paralysis; in Guilleminault C, Dement WC, Passouant P (eds): Narcolepsy. New York, Spectrum, 1976, pp. 97–124.
Hishikawa Y, Kaneko Z: Electroencephalographic study on narcolepsy. Electroencephalogr Clin Neurophysiol 1965;18:249–259.
Knowles J: The life and writings of Henry Fuseli, Esq. M.A.R.A., vol 1: The Life of Henry Fuseli. London, 1831.
Lalumiere ML, Blanchard R, Zucker KJ: Sexual orientation and handedness in men and women: a meta-analysis. Psychol Bull 2000;126:575–592.
Lanthony P: Left-handed painters. Rev Neurol 1995;151:165–170.
Lentzsch F, Becker C, Klemm C, Myrone M, von Waldkirch B: Fuseli – The Wild Swiss. Zürich, Scheidegger & Spiess, 2005.
Maidment I: Fuseli, Henry; in Aldrich R, Wotherspoon G (eds): Who's Who in Gay and Lesbian History from Antiquity to World War II. London, Routledge, 2001, pp 172–173.
Mason EC: Heinrich Füssli. Aphorismen über die Kunst. Basel, Schwabe, 1944.
Mason EC: The Mind of Henry Fuseli. London, Routledge & Kegan Paul, 1951. www.kirjasto.sci.fi/fuseli.htm.
Muschg W: Heinrich Füssli. Briefe. Basel, Schwabe, 1942.
Nettle D: Schizotypy and mental health amongst poets, visual artists, and mathematicians. J Res Pers 2006;40:876–890. online www.sciencedirect.com.
Ohayon MM, Zulley J, Guilleminault C, Smirne S: Prevalence and pathologic associations of sleep paralysis in the general population. Neurology 1999;52:1194–1200.
Otto MW, Simon NM, Powers M, Hinton D, Zalta AK, Pollack MH: Rates of isolated sleep paralysis in outpatients with anxiety disorders. J Anxiety Disord 2006;20:687–693.
Riding A: Spirits, gothic fantasies and sex, please, we are British. The New York Times, Feb 27, 2006.
Rosenthal C: Ueber das Auftreten von halluzinatorisch-kataplektischem Angstsyndrom, Wachanfällen und ähnlichen Störungen bei Schizophrenen. Monatsschr Psychiatr Neurol 1939;102:11–38.
Schiff G: Johann Heinrich Füssli 1741–1825, 2 Volumes. Zürich, Oeuvrekataloge Schweizer Künstler, 1973.
Schneck JM: Henry Fuseli, nightmare, and sleep paralysis. JAMA 1969;207:725–726.
Schneck JM: Guy de Maupassant's 'The Horla' and sleep paralysis. J Clin Psychiatry 1994;55:544.
Shakespeare W: Romeo and Juliet. London, Penguin Classics, 1967.
Silbersweig DA, Stern E, Frith C, Cahill C, Holmes A, Grootoonk S, Seaward J, McKenna P, Chua SE, Schnorr L, et al: A functional neuroanatomy of hallucinations in schizophrenia. Nature 1995;378: 176–179.
Weinglass DH: The Collected English Letters of Henry Fuseli. Millwood, Kraus International, 1982.
Westphal C: Eigenthümliche mit Einschlafen verbundene Anfälle. Arch Psychiatr 1877;7:631–635.

Prof. Claudio L. Bassetti
Department of Neurology
University Hospital
Frauenklinikstrasse 26
CH-8091 Zürich (Switzerland)
Tel.: +41 44 255 5503, Fax +41 44 255 4649, E-Mail claudio.bassetti@usz.ch

Author Index

Assal, G. 44, 169
auf der Horst, C. 105

Bassetti, C. 223
Baumann, C. 223
Bäzner, H. 1, 30
Blanke, O. 14
Bogousslavsky, J. 44, 89, 121

Colombo-Thuillard, F. 169

Dieguez, S. 44, 121

Espinel, C.H. 150

Haas, F. 193
Hennerici, M.G. 1, 30

Kammer, T. 184

Lentzsch, F. 223
Lythgoe, M.F. 75

Mulvenna, C.M. 75, 206

Pollak, T.A. 75

Regard, M. 223

Wöhrle, J.C. 193

Subject Index

Aichinger-Kassek, Wolfgang, art after right-hemisphere stroke 6, 7
A la recherche du temps perdu 101, 102
Aloof, Aloft 211
Alzheimer's disease, *see* de Kooning, Willem; Dementia
Anamnesis, Heine 107
Anosodiaphoria, definition 69
Anosognosia
  Baudelaire 142
  definition 69
  Visconti and Fellini studies 53, 54, 67–69
Aphasia
  Baudelaire
    art effects 145–147
    Broca's versus global aphasia 136, 137
    catastrophic reactions 141, 142, 145
    evaluation 133–136
    expletive use 137–141
  literature review of painters 170–172
  Reuterswärd
    creativity effects 176, 178–180
    evaluation 174–176
  self-portrait effects 22, 23, 28
Artistic drive, de novo artistic output after brain injury 82–86
ArtScience, *see* Thinking Methods
Asomatognosia, definition 69

Baudelaire, Charles
  aphasia
    art effects 145–147
    Broca's versus global aphasia 136, 137
    catastrophic reactions 141, 142, 145
    evaluation 133–136
    expletive use 137–141
  biography 122–124
  medical history
    nervous disorders 127–129
    stroke 129–132, 143–145
    synaesthesia 147
    syphilis 126, 127
    visceral and gastrointestinal disorders 127
  overview of works 124, 125
  rehabilitation efforts 142, 143
Berlin unter den Linden 42
Birth of Venus 41
The Black Mask 41
Bright's disease, *see* Glomerulonephritis
Brown, Reynold, art after right-hemisphere stroke 8, 9, 12

Carmencita 41
Chambers, Danae, Alzheimer's disease effects on self-portraits 25
Combray 103
Composition 1955 155
Corinth, Lovis
  biography 31, 32
  hemineglect 31
  illness history 32–36
  self-portraits 19–22, 36–38
  true art discovery 43
Creating in the Midst of Dementia syndrome 163–166

Creative cognition
synaesthesia 217, 218, 220
versus creative output 217
Creativity
de novo artistic output after brain injury 82–86
synaesthesia relationship 215–217

de Kooning, Willem
Alzheimer's disease effects
daily function 159, 160
masterpieces 151–153
painting technique 160
self-portraits 24
specificity of response 164, 165
care 159
Creating in the Midst of Dementia syndrome 163–166
symptoms 159
Thinking Methods analysis
cognitive analysis
episodic memory 162, 163
procedural memory 162
semantic memory 163
short-term memory 161, 162
specificity of diagnosis 164
creation mechanisms 164, 165
gathering of information
colors 158
lines 157
surfaces 157, 158
overview 151, 156
recognizing the observed 158, 159
Dementia, *see also* de Kooning, Willem; Frontotemporal dementia
abstract art creation 151
Creating in the Midst of Dementia syndrome 163–166
de novo artistic output 75–77, 79, 80
self-portrait effects 23–27
Depression, von Bülow 200, 201, 203
Dix, Otto
biography 4
paintings after right-hemisphere stroke 4–6
La Dolce Vita 56
Dürer, Albrecht, self-portraits 16, 17

Exhumed 23, 24

Fellini, Federico
biography 54–58
medical history 58, 59, 61, 63–65
neorealism 45
right-hemisphere stroke
effects 7, 8, 59–64
humor effects 64, 65, 72
neglect syndrome features 61, 63, 65–67
personality effects 69–72
Visconti comparison 44, 45
Les Fleurs du Mal 123
Flood Improvisation 209
Frauenraub 41
Frontotemporal dementia (FTD), de novo artistic output 75–77, 79, 80
Füssli, Heinrich
biography 224–227
Der Nachtmahr, interpretation 223, 224, 227, 229, 234
sleep paralysis 227, 228

Glomerulonephritis, von Bülow 202
Greenshield, Tom, art after right-hemisphere stroke 9, 10
Gruppo di famiglia in un interno 51, 53, 54

Hallucinations, *see* Füssli, Heinrich; Sleep paralysis
Heine, Heinrich
anamnesis 107
medical history reconstruction 105, 106
opium abuse and cause of death 116–119
physicians and applied therapies 107–110
syphilis
evidence 112, 113
treatments 113, 115, 116
tabes dorsalis 110
Hemiconcern, definition 69
Hemineglect
awareness and processing 66, 67
Fellini 61, 63, 65–67
painting effects after right-hemisphere stroke 8–10, 12

self-portraiture effects 19, 21, 22
Hemispheric model, de novo artistic output after brain injury 81, 82
The Hygiene of the Neurasthenic 102
Hypergraphia, de novo artistic output after brain injury 80, 81

In despair over the grandeur of Antique remains 230, 231
The Innocent 52–54
The Interior before the Mirror 41

Kandinsky, Vasily, synaesthesia 208, 210
Knecht Franz 41

Ladri di Biciclette 46
Le temps retrouvé 102
Lusignoli, Gugliemo, art after right-hemisphere stroke 11

Mackay, Jane, synaesthesia 211, 216
Las Meninas 17
Misoplegia, definition 69
Mozart, Wolfgang Amadeus
cause of death 185
Tourette's syndrome evidence 188–191
vulgarity 187, 188

Der Nachtmahr 223, 224, 227, 229, 234
Neorealism 45
Neuralgia, von Bülow 199
Non-Violence 172

On the Balcony in Bordighera 42
Opium abuse, Heine 116–119

Parkinson's disease, de novo artistic output 81
Personification, definition 69
Pieta 42
Poetry, de novo artistic output after brain injury 80, 81
Portrait of the Painter Bernt Grönvold 41
Prosopagnosia, right-hemisphere stroke 2
Proust, Marcel
medical history 89–91, 94–97
neurology and medicine in works 101–103
physician interactions 91, 92, 94, 97–101

Quo Vadis 23, 24

Räderscheidt, Anton
biography 2
paintings after right-hemisphere stroke 2–4, 22
prosopagnosia 2
Rembrandt, self-portraits 17
Requiem 23, 184
Reuterswärd, Carl Fredrik
aphasia
creativity effects 176, 178–180
evaluation 174–176
art critic response after stroke 176, 177
biography 172, 173
medical history 173, 174
style change after stroke 176, 177, 181, 182
Roma, Città Aperta 45
Romanzero 109, 110, 112
Rowan-Hull, Mark, synaesthesia 211

Samson Blinded 42
Schiele, Egon, self-portraits 17, 18
Schwitters, Kurt, art after right-hemisphere stroke 11
Seated Woman 154
Self-portraits
Aichinger-Kassek 7
aphasia effects 22, 23, 28
Corinth 19–22, 36–38
dementia effects 23–28
Dix 5
embodiment and disembodiment 16–19
Hume's philosophy of self 14, 15
neglect effects 19, 21, 22
neurocognitive theory of self 15, 16
neuropsychological mechanisms 19, 28
Räderscheidt 22
Sleep paralysis
definition 228
Füssli 227, 228
left-handedness 230, 231
neuropsychological interpretation 230–234
pathophysiology 229
prevalence 228
writings 231, 233

Somatoparaphrenia, definition 69
Sound of the Flute 216
Still Life with Flowers, Skull, and Oak Leaves 41
Stroke
de novo artistic output 75, 76
left-hemisphere stroke
Baudelaire 129–132, 143–145
Reuterswärd and art effects 174–182
von Bülow 200
psychological versus physical consequences in style 38–42
right-hemisphere stroke effects on art
Aichinger-Kassek 6, 7
Brown 8, 9, 12
Corinth, *see* Corinth, Lovis
Dix 4–6
Fellini, *see* Fellini, Federico
Greenshield 9, 10
hemineglect 8–10, 12, 19, 21, 22
Lusignoli 11
Räderscheidt 2–4
Schwitters 11
unilateral body schema disorders 69
unnamed artists 10, 11
Visconti, *see* Visconti, Luchino
Susanna and the Elders 41
Synaesthesia
Baudelaire 147
classification 209, 210, 212
cortical connections 214
creative cognition 217, 218, 220
creativity relationship 215–217
definition 147
electroencephalography and neurology 219, 220
examples in creative individuals 207, 208
functional imaging studies 212–214
profile 209–212
Syphilis
Baudelaire 126, 127
Heine, evidence 112, 113
history of study 106
treatments in 19th century 113, 115, 116

Tabes dorsalis, Heine 110
Thiel, Johannes, paintings after right-hemisphere stroke 6
Thinking Methods, ArtScience analysis
de Kooning art analysis
cognitive analysis
episodic memory 162, 163
procedural memory 162
semantic memory 163
short-term memory 161, 162
specificity of diagnosis 164
creation mechanisms 164, 165
gathering of information
colors 158
lines 157
surfaces 157, 158
recognizing the observed 158, 159
overview 151, 156
Thomas with a Hat in His Hands 41
Tourette's syndrome (TS)
diagnosis 185
epidemiology 186
history of study 185
Mozart, evidence 188–191
pathogenesis 185, 186
treatment 186, 187
Turangalîla ii 211

Untitled XIII 152
Utermohlen, William, Alzheimer's disease effects on self-portraits 25, 26

Velazquez, self-portraits 17, 18
Visconti, Luchino
biography 46–49
Fellini comparison 44, 45
medical history 49–53
neorealism 45
right-hemisphere stroke
films after stroke 51, 52
personality effects 69–72
von Bülow, Hans
autopsy 202, 203
biography 193–199
medical history
depression 200, 201, 203
glomerulonephritis 202
neuralgia 199
overview 203, 204
stroke 200
treatments 201, 202